AF334015

Pharmacotherapy
of Asthma

LUNG BIOLOGY IN HEALTH AND DISEASE

Executive Editor

Claude Lenfant
Former Director, National Heart, Lung, and Blood Institute
National Institutes of Health
Bethesda, Maryland

The opinions expressed in these volumes do not necessarily represent the views of the National Institutes of Health.

Pharmacotherapy of Asthma

Edited by

James T. Li
Mayo Clinic College of Medicine
Rochester, Minnesota, U.S.A.

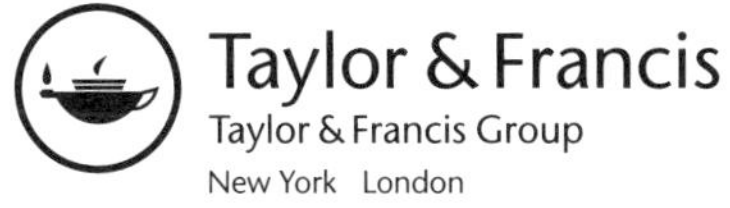

Taylor & Francis
Taylor & Francis Group
New York   London

Published in 2006 by
Taylor & Francis Group
270 Madison Avenue
New York, NY 10016

© 2006 by Taylor & Francis Group, LLC

No claim to original U.S. Government works
Printed in the United States of America on acid-free paper
10 9 8 7 6 5 4 3 2 1

International Standard Book Number-10: 0-8493-3710-0 (Hardcover)
International Standard Book Number-13: 978-0-8493-3710-9 (Hardcover)

Library of Congress Cataloging-in-Publication Data

Catalog record is available from the Library of Congress

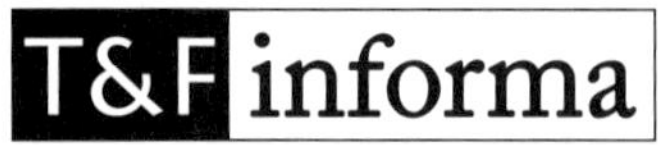

Taylor & Francis Group
is the Academic Division of T&F Informa plc.

**Visit the Taylor & Francis Web site at
http://www.taylorandfrancis.com**

Introduction

Over many decades, the treatment of asthma has evolved and improved considerably, largely because of the availability of several classes of medications. This was recently reviewed and analyzed in an excellent publication by Chu and Drazen (1).

The current concept of asthma treatment is to achieve control of symptoms, rather than reacting to changes in the severity of the disease. This approach, which may lead to a "steady state" of the disease, is dependent on knowing what works, and what does not, in a specific patient. The identification of the best therapy also depends on the realization that "asthma (is) liable to great variety in different individuals." This view (and actually a matter of fact) was first advanced in the late 1800s by Henry Hyde Salter (2), a physician in Charing Cross Hospital in London, and the first to describe the role of environment in the etiology and the course of asthma.

Physicians who treat asthma patients today have in hand a variety of classes of medications with different mechanisms of action. The knowledge and understanding of these medications is fundamental to ensure the most optimal treatment for a given patient.

This new volume of the series of monographs Lung Biology in Health and Disease, edited by Dr. James T. Li, gives the reader a thorough review of all the classes of available medications and how and when they will benefit the patients most. Thus, the physician will be aided in making a decision about the specific medication to prescribe.

Much has happened over the centuries that physicians have been interested in asthma, but surely we are on the eve of even better and more significant progress. Indeed, asthma may be the condition that will be the first to benefit from genomic research and the concept of so-called personalized medicine (3). The notion that tests (hopefully easy and inexpensive ones) can be designed to provide information to a physician on whether or not a given medication will work in a specific patient will be an important and fundamental step forward. However, for this to happen the knowledge of the mechanism of action of the medications must be known; this is what this volume provides the readers.

As the executive editor of this series, I am grateful to Dr. Li and the expert group of contributors who have assembled for the opportunity to present this monograph to the readership.

Claude Lenfant, MD
Gaithersburg, Maryland, U.S.A.

References

1. Chu EK, Drazen JM. Asthma: One hundred years of treatment and onward. Am J Resp Crit Care Med 2005; 171:1202–1205.
2. Salter HH. On Asthma: Its Pathology and Treatment. New York: William Wood and Co, 1882.
3. Israel E, Chinchilli VM, Ford JG, Boushey HA, Cherniack R, Craig TJ, Deykin A, Fagan JK, Fahy JV, Fish J, et al. Use of regularly scheduled albuterol treatment in asthma: genotype-stratified, randomised, placebo-controlled cross-over trial. Lancet 2004; 364:1505–1512.

Preface

Asthma continues to be a significant cause of morbidity and mortality. According to Centers for Disease Control's surveillance statistics for asthma, there are approximately 27 million persons with asthma in the United States, 11 million of which experience an asthma attack in any given year. There are 14 million school days missed every year because of poorly controlled asthma, and another 14 million workdays missed by adult workers with asthma. Annually, asthma accounts for 10 million office visits, over 400,000 hospitalizations, and over 4500 deaths.

Fortunately, medications can be highly effective in reducing the burden of asthma for many people. Clinical studies show that proper treatment of asthma with appropriate medications can reduce deaths, hospitalizations, and symptoms. As new drugs for asthma are developed, the complexity of determining the proper drug treatment for individual patients with asthma increases. The recommended practice of using multiple drugs in the treatment of asthma adds to the complexity.

Providing health care for patients with asthma is not easy. No two persons with asthma are alike. Practice guidelines for the treatment of asthma are helpful resources, but treatment programs must be individualized. New, effective medications and biologic agents for asthma are now available.

Clinicians must have the knowledge and skills to instruct patients on how to use asthma drugs effectively and safely.

Prompt and proper treatment of acute asthma can be life-saving. The drug treatment of asthma in the emergency department, hospital, and intensive care unit may be very different from the outpatient treatment of chronic asthma. Health care professionals caring for severely ill patients with asthma should have a complete understanding of the variety of inpatient asthma therapies available.

This book is intended to provide comprehensive, practical, and clinically useful information on the drug treatment of asthma for clinicians who care for persons with asthma. Medical students, residents-in-training, primary care physicians, specialty physicians, asthma educators, respiratory care providers, nurses, and physicians who care for asthma patients should find the information and recommendations in this book helpful.

The opening chapter reviews the place of pharmacotherapy in the overall management of asthma. The recommendations in published practice guidelines are an excellent starting point. The importance of asthma education and adherence to treatment plans is included in this chapter.

Chapters 2 through 11 cover all the currently available drugs used in the treatment of asthma. All drug-specific chapters include a review of pharmacology, mechanisms of action, efficacy, safety, special concerns and situations, and recommendations. Readers can use the information in these chapters to help guide decisions about asthma therapy. One chapter in this section reviews the use of immunosuppressive agents for severe asthma. Another covers the indications and risks of inhaled corticosteroids. There is a comprehensive chapter on the most appropriate use of leukotriene modifiers. The final chapter in this section reviews allergen immunotherapy for asthma in a rigorous, evidence-based manner.

Chapter 12 reviews the intricacies of outpatient pharmacotherapy of asthma, including combination therapies. The final chapter is a detailed review of drug treatment of asthma in the emergency department, hospital floor, and intensive care unit.

The editor and contributors hope that this book offers clear, comprehensive, and clinically useful information and guidance for the drug treatment of asthma. Individualization of treatment and appropriate selection of asthma therapy should result in a decreased burden of asthma for our patients.

James T. Li

Contributors

Richard Beasley   Medical Research Institute of New Zealand, Wellington, New Zealand, and University of Southampton, Southampton, U.K.

David I. Bernstein   Division of Allergy-Immunology, University of Cincinnati College of Medicine, Cincinnati, Ohio, U.S.A.

Guy G. Brusselle   Department of Respiratory Diseases, Ghent University Hospital, Ghent, Belgium

Roland Buhl   Pulmonary Department, Mainz University Hospital, Mainz, Germany

Mark S. Dykewicz   Division of Allergy and Immunology, Department of Internal Medicine, Saint Louis University School of Medicine, St. Louis, Missouri, U.S.A.

Anthony J. Frew   University of Southampton School of Medicine, Southampton General Hospital, Southampton, U.K.

Ruth H. Green   Department of Respiratory Medicine and Thoracic Surgery, Institute for Lung Health, Glenfield Hospital, Leicester, U.K.

Nicholas J. Gross   Loyola University Stritch School of Medicine, VA Hospital, Hines, Illinois, U.S.A.

Jesse Hall   Section of Pulmonary and Critical Care Medicine, University of Chicago Hospitals, Chicago, Illinois, U.S.A.

Shaun Holt   P3 Research, Wellington, New Zealand

S. G. O. Johansson   Department of Medicine, Unit of Clinical Immunology and Allergy, Karolinska University Hospital, Stockholm, Sweden

Kevin J. Kelly   Department of Pediatrics, Children's Mercy Hospital, University of Missouri Kansas City, Kansas City, Missouri, U.S.A.

J. P. Kress   Section of Pulmonary and Critical Care Medicine, University of Chicago Hospitals, Chicago, Illinois, U.S.A.

Margaret Lowery   Department of Pediatrics (Allergy/Immunology), Medical College of Wisconsin, Milwaukee, Wisconsin, U.S.A.

Matthew Masoli   Medical Research Institute of New Zealand, Wellington, New Zealand

Romain A. Pauwels   Department of Respiratory Diseases, Ghent University Hospital, Ghent, Belgium

Philippa Shirtcliffe   Medical Research Institute of New Zealand, Wellington, New Zealand

Dave Singh   North West Lung Research Centre, South Manchester University Hospitals Trust, Manchester, U.K.

Ajeet G. Vinayak   Section of Pulmonary and Critical Care Medicine, University of Chicago Hospitals, Chicago, Illinois, U.S.A.

Andrew J. Wardlaw   Department of Respiratory Medicine and Thoracic Surgery, Institute for Lung Health, Glenfield Hospital, Leicester, U.K.

Mark Weatherall   Wellington School of Medicine and Health Sciences, Wellington, New Zealand

Michael E. Wechsler Pulmonary and Critical Care Division, Department of Medicine, Brigham and Women's Hospital and Harvard Medical School, Boston, Massachusetts, U.S.A.

Miles Weinberger Department of Pediatrics, Allergy and Pulmonary Division, University of Iowa College of Medicine, Iowa City, Iowa, U.S.A.

Ashley Woodcock North West Lung Research Centre, South Manchester University Hospitals Trust, Manchester, U.K.

Contents

1

Pharmacotherapy According to Published Guidelines

DAVID I. BERNSTEIN

Division of Allergy-Immunology, University of Cincinnati College of Medicine
Cincinnati, Ohio, U.S.A.

I. Introduction

In the past 30 years, physicians have been introduced to a myriad of new
pharmacologic agents that have gained Food and Drug Administration
(FDA) approval for treatment of persistent asthma. Many of these agents
have arisen from advances in basic and translational research that have
elucidated pathogenetic mechanisms of human asthma and airway inflammation. At the same time, epidemiologic research conducted in longitudinal
childhood studies and adult populations have provided valuable insights
into the natural history of human asthma and defined phenotypic and environmental determinants of disease morbidity. Despite impressive advances
in our knowledge, asthma is a major health care problem and, in the past
two decades, incidences have steadily risen worldwide along with costs
related to drugs and medical care. Data showing rising incidence rates,
costs, hospitalizations, and asthma-related deaths on a worldwide basis
have provided strong impetus for development and dissemination of asthma
treatment guidelines. At the same time, investigators worldwide continue to

search for underlying causes of rising asthma incidence rates, hoping that new information may lead to effective primary preventive strategies.

The National Heart, Lung, and Blood Institute (NHLBI) asthma treatment guidelines were first published in 1991 under the auspices of the National Asthma Education and Prevention Program (NAEPP). The treatment guidelines, entitled *Guidelines for Diagnosis and Management of Asthma*, summarized the recommendations of the first NAEPP expert panel (1). The stated objective of the first report was to provide general recommendations for diagnosing and managing asthma based on best available data and scientific evidence. The first edition was subsequently revised and expanded in 1997 (2). In 2002, the NAEPP expert panel released an "Update on Selected Topics" (3), which addressed the use of combination therapy in children, patient monitoring of symptoms and peak expiratory flow rates (PEFR), and symptom-based written action plans.

In 1993, the NHLBI convened a workshop in collaboration with the World Health Organization (WHO) which was attended by an international panel of experts and entitled *Global Strategy for Asthma Management and Prevention.* At that time, the Global Initiative for Asthma (GINA) was started to broadly disseminate new information pertaining to asthma to physicians, public health officials, and lay groups. The first report of this workshop appeared in 1995 and was subsequently updated in 2002 (4). Treatment guidelines contained in both of these documents are evidence based and designed for patients according to similar disease severity classifications. As general goals of management, the latest GINA guidelines stress the importance of normalizing lung function, instituting anti-inflammatory drugs, and initiating patient education and self-management programs. These guidelines propose a management plan with interrelated parts, which include education, assessment and monitoring of asthma severity, avoidance of risk factors, establishing medication plans for long-term control, and designing individual strategies for managing exacerbations (Table 1). The 2002 GINA guidelines go further than the NHLBI document in presenting extensive reviews of the pathophysiology, mechanisms and epidemiology of asthma (5). Specifically, asthma definitions, airway pathology,

Table 1 Global Initiative for Asthma (GINA) Six Part Asthma Management Plan

---

1. Educate patients to develop a partnership in asthma management
2. Assess and monitor asthma severity with both symptom reports and, as much as possible, measurements of lung function
3. Avoid exposure to risk factors
4. Establish individual medication plans for long-term management in children and adults
5. Establish individual plans for managing exacerbations
6. Provide regular follow-up care

---

asthma mortality, risk factors, genetic susceptibility, environmental causes, and triggers of asthma are discussed extensively. These aspects of the GINA document are not directly pertinent to this chapter. However, some of the key points of the GINA report that are relevant to pharmacotherapy are highlighted below.

II. Review of NHLBI and GINA Asthma Treatment Guidelines

A. Diagnosis of Asthma

The schema presented for asthma classification and diagnosis is particularly relevant. The GINA document emphasizes the importance of utilizing lung-function measurements in the diagnosis of asthma. The GINA guideline highlights questions that can be used in a clinical setting, which are from the International Union Against Tuberculosis and Lung Disease questionnaire, a validated instrument that has been employed in epidemiologic studies (6).

Traditionally, a diagnosis of asthma is confirmed by a 12% or greater improvement in FEV_1 after inhalation of a β-agonist bronchodilator or after an interval of treatment with systemic or inhaled glucocorticoids. The FEV_1 has been considered the premier endpoint to measure both short-term and long-term asthma clinical trials. However, single measurements of lung function can underestimate asthma severity status unless other symptoms or morbidity indicators are considered, including numbers of acute asthma exacerbations, rescue bronchodilator usage, and quality of life.

Both GINA and NAEPP reports emphasize the importance of objectively confirming asthma, thereby discouraging the common empirical approach to diagnosis and treatment. The usefulness of portable devices that measure peak expiratory flow rates are noted, and these may be available in the primary care setting where spirometry is not. The NHLBI document recommends that PEFR be monitored twice daily for one to two weeks, optimally upon awakening and between 12:00 and 2:00 PM (corresponding to the expected nadir and peak of daily PEFR, respectively) (2). The GINA guidelines suggests that reversibility in PEFR of $\geq 15\%$ supports a diagnosis of asthma, and diurnal variability of $\geq 20\%$ is considered diagnostic of asthma. Serial PEFR measurements are useful in classifying asthma severity. Both NHLB and GINA guidelines identify 20% to 30% variability as consistent with mild persistent asthma, whereas daily variability of $>30\%$ is used to classify patients with moderate and severe persistent asthma. The GINA guideline recommends short-term monitoring of PEFR not only for establishing a diagnosis, but also for monitoring lung function changes associated with exposure to allergen triggers and for responses to any changes in therapy.

In some cases, serial PEFR monitoring can identify improvement in lung function after treatment with a β-agonist or inhaled corticosteroids

(ICS), and help to confirm a diagnosis of asthma. PEFR monitoring is strongly recommended for severe asthmatic patients for aiding in identification of asthma deterioration and for managing exacerbations, especially for those who have poor perception of increases in asthma symptoms. Falsification of data is not unusual, and patient compliance and good technique are essential in obtaining valid and reliable PEFR data (7).

The GINA report notes that diagnosis of asthma in children below the age of five is problematic and can be confounded by other childhood causes of wheezing (e.g., cystic fibrosis, primary immune deficiency, congenital narrowing of intrathoracic airways, and foreign body aspiration) (5). In this group, lung function cannot usually be performed. Wheezing associated with viral infections during infancy is not predictive of childhood asthma (8). The presence of atopy defined by positive aeroallergen skin tests combined with a parental history of asthma is associated with confirmed diagnoses of asthma at age 6 (9). Wheezing during early infancy or before the age of 2 is extremely common and not highly predictive of childhood asthma. The GINA document recognizes that, given the inability to perform lung function before age 5, it is not possible to unequivocally establish a diagnosis of asthma. In such circumstances, the benefits of initiating chronic controller medications to children with persistent wheezing outweigh theoretical concerns about over-treating pediatric patients, some of whom may later be proven not to have asthma (5).

B. Therapeutic Approach: Non-pharmacologic Considerations

The NHLBI report in 1997 is very similar to the GINA document in emphasizing four components of asthma management, including: (i) the use of objective measures of lung function to establish the diagnosis, assess asthma severity, and monitor treatment responses; (ii) control both allergic and non-allergic factors that trigger asthma symptoms and exacerbations; (iii) pharmacologic treatment plans aimed at controlling airways inflammation and treating exacerbations; and (iv) education programs directed at patients (including self-management skills) and families, as well as health care providers.

In addition to recommending asthma drug regimens tailored to asthma severity status, the GINA guidelines stress the importance of non-pharmacologic management and emphasize the need for global initiatives to improve asthma education. Such efforts are directed at improving patient compliance with optimal recommended treatments, which is generally assumed to be the key determinant of favorable outcomes.

The emphasis on education is justified by published data indicating that only 50% of patients are receiving adequate preventive treatments, that 74% of asthma hospitalizations are preventable, and that 90% of fatal asthma events may have been prevented (5). The vast majority of patients dying from asthma had experienced prior hospitalizations and 40% of these occurred within 12 months prior to fatal events (5). Therefore, in an attempt to address this concern, both NHLBI and GINA guidelines have introduced aggressive plans for pharmacologic management of acute asthma exacerbations.

Education

High-risk patients and those who have undergone mechanical ventilation for status asthmaticus should be targeted for self-management education, which is directed at timely recognition and aggressive early interventions for asthma exacerbations. Such programs seek to impart new self-management skills to the patient, which are described in Table 2, and, at the same time, modify behavior patterns.

In addition to the obvious importance of patient education, the authors highlight the importance of widespread and continuing instruction of all segments of diverse groups directly or indirectly involved with some aspect of patient care, including: health care delivery organizations; groups involved with setting health care policy; health care professionals at all levels; families, parents, teachers, and sports coaches.

The framers of the GINA guidelines recognized that their impact will be realized if they are perceived as useful to health care providers in achieving treatment goals for individual patients. Guidelines can be publicized via frequent interactive discussions among health care providers and their peers. Outcomes of the impact of the use of guidelines should be monitored in individual patients during routine physician visits by asking patients if they have continued to experience daytime and nighttime symptoms and how asthma symptoms impact daily activities (e.g., school, work activities, sports, etc.). So far, it appears that issued treatment guidelines have had limited impact on prescribing habits of physicians. In a recent worldwide survey that evaluated adequacy of asthma treatment relative to disease severity, Rabe et al. (10) found that small minorities of patients

Table 2 Basic Principles of Self-Management of Adult Asthma

1. Patients are taught to combine objective assessment of asthma severity (peak-flow recordings) with educated interpretation of key symptoms
2. Patients are taught which medication to use regularly and which medication to use as needed. This may include as needed β-agonist therapy or, for patients with severe asthma, systemic glucocorticoids, high-dose inhaled β-agonist, oxygen therapy, and medical review
3. Self-assessment and self-management are integrated with written guidelines for both the long-term treatment of asthma and the treatment of asthma exacerbations

Source: From Ref. 5.

Table 3 Factors Affecting Compliance

Drug factors
Difficulties with inhaler devices
Awkward regimes (e.g., four times daily or multiple drugs)
Side effects
Cost of medication
Dislike of medication
Distant pharmacies
Non-drug factors
Misunderstanding or lack of instruction
Fears about side effects
Dissatisfaction with health care professionals
Unexpressed/undiscussed fears or concerns
Inappropriate expectations
Poor supervision, training, or follow up
Anger about condition or its treatment
Underestimation of severity
Cultural issues
Stigmatization
Forgetfulness or complacency
Attitudes toward ill health
Religious issues

Source: From Ref. 5.

(9–30%) in various parts of the world, at all severity levels, were receiving long-term preventative treatment; the majority were receiving quick-relief bronchodilators.

Non-compliance

Non-compliance can be defined as failure to take medications as agreed upon by patient and health care provider. The GINA report identifies multiple factors that may influence non-compliance (Table 3), including adverse effects or intolerance to medications, frequency of dosing, lack of instruction, difficulties with inhaler devices, anger about one's condition, poor supervision, complacency, and the high costs of medications. Improving communication between patient and health care provider can enhance compliance with medications (11). Such interactions may increase acceptance of the disease by the patient if they become more informed about asthma-associated risks resulting from under-treatment.

Prevention: Avoidance of Risk Factors

The GINA report recognizes that education about avoidance of allergen triggers is an important part of overall management. There is only limited evidence demonstrating that primary prevention programs implemented during the pre- or postnatal periods can prevent development of asthma. Arshad et al. (12), demonstrated that a program integrating multiple interventions early in life (e.g., environmental control plus early food avoidance) are promising in preventing later development of childhood asthma. However, more studies are needed to confirm this unique observation.

C. Pharmacotherapy for Asthma: Stepwise Approach

Important Caveats

The NAEPP report emphasizes that the stepwise approach should be used to guide but not replace physician decisions regarding treatment of individual patients (2). In rating severity, a patient should be assigned to the most severe step if any one feature of the higher severity category is present. Physicians should follow the strategy of achieving control as quickly as possible (e.g., treating with a burst of oral prednisone, if indicated) and then stepping down to the least medication needed to maintain long-term asthma control. As already mentioned, it is essential to provide patient education in self-management and control of environmental triggers (e.g., allergens). Severely asthmatic patients with acute exacerbations or hospitalizations or poor perception of asthma symptoms should be trained in the use of serial PEFR measurements to aid in early recognition of asthma flareups. This should involve intensive education regarding self-management of acute exacerbations in which patients are provided with a written "action plan." This important aspect of self-management is to facilitate intensification of asthma therapy early, which usually involves timely administration of a burst of systemic corticosteroids. How these strategies lead to favorable clinical outcomes is discussed later in this chapter. Finally, referral to an asthma specialist is recommended for adults and children greater than five years with severe persistent asthma that is difficult to control. Referral is recommended in children ≤ 5 years with moderate or severe asthma and should be considered in mild persistent asthma.

The authors introduce pharmacotherapy for chronic asthma with some thoughtful considerations and caveats. First, individual treatment responses to given regimens may differ significantly from the average response in the asthmatic population at large. Second, treatment decisions are the product of a compromise between physician and patient. Third, the advantages of delivering medications via the inhaled route are emphasized, thereby maximizing local drug delivery and minimizing potential adverse effects.

Physicians and allied health professionals are primarily concerned with relieving asthma symptoms, preventing exacerbations, and improving quality of life. Long-term asthma control is defined in GINA by achieving the following goals: (i) minimal chronic asthma symptoms, including

Table 4 Asthma Stepwise Categories of Disease Severity as Presented in Most Recent Global Initiative for Asthma (GINA) and National Asthma Education and Prevention Program (NAEPP) Reports

---

Step 1: Mild intermittent
   Symptoms less than once a week[a]
   Brief exacerbations
   Nocturnal symptoms not more than twice a month
   • FEV_1 or PEF ≥ 80% predicted
   • PEF or FEV_1 variability < 20%
Step 2: Mild persistent
   Symptoms more than once a week but less than once a day[b]
   Exacerbations may affect activity and sleep
   Nocturnal symptoms more than twice a month
   • FEV_1 or PEF ≥ 80% predicted
   • PEF or FEV_1 variability 20–30%
Step 3: Moderate persistent
   Symptoms daily
   Exacerbations may affect activity and sleep
   Nocturnal symptoms more than once a week
   Daily use of inhaled short-acting 2-agonist
   • FEV_1 or PEF 60–80% predicted
   • PEF or FEV_1 variability > 30%
Step 4: Severe persistent
   Symptoms daily
   Frequent exacerbations
   Frequent nocturnal asthma symptoms
   Limitation of physical activities
   • FEV_1 or PEF ≤ 60% predicted
   • PEF or FEV_1 variability > 30%

---

[a]Symptoms are ≤2 days/wk for mild intermittent in NAEPP 1997 report.
[b]Symptoms are >2 days/wk for mild-persistent asthma in NAEPP 1997 report.
Source: From Refs. 2 and 5.

nocturnal symptoms; (ii) infrequent or no acute exacerbations; (iii) no hospital visits; (iv) little if any requirement for rescue β-agonist; (v) reduction in activity or exercise limitations; (vi) normalization of PEF variability; and (vii) minimal adverse effects attributable to asthma medications (5).

    Both the GINA and NAEPP reports recommend that pharmacotherapy should be customized to asthma severity using a stepwise approach. Asthma medications are increased as a function of disease severity. In the 1991 NAEPP report, three step-categories of asthma disease severity were introduced: mild, moderate, and severe (1). As shown in Table 4, these were expanded in the second report to include the following four graded or "stepwise" categories: mild intermittent, mild persistent, moderate persistent, and severe persistent. These severity classes are defined by frequency of daytime and nocturnal asthma symptoms, FEV_1 and PEFR variability. This classification scheme serves as a useful framework for making stepwise recommendations to achieve pharmacologic control of chronic asthma. The pharmacotherapeutic recommendations and relevant rationale for each category of asthma severity will be discussed below.

D. Pharmacologic Treatment Recommendations

Level of Evidence

Because both the NAEPP and GINA guidelines regarding pharmacotherapy are evidence based, recommendations pertaining to asthma management are often accompanied by ratings of the relative quality of scientific evidence from which they are derived. The GINA document has proposed an asthma severity classification that closely resembles those of the NHLBI guidelines (Table 4). Levels A–D categories of evidence are defined as: Level A—recommendation that is based upon substantial numbers of randomized controlled clinical trials and a rich body of evidence; Level B—recommendation based upon limited numbers of randomized controlled trials; Level C—recommendations based upon observational studies; and Level D—recommendations that are based upon the lowest level of evidence and derived strictly from expert opinion. In contrast to the NAEPP reports, the 2002 GINA report is more diligent about assigning evidence ratings for specific recommendations.

Mild Intermittent (Step 1)

Criteria for this category are presented in Table 4 according to the GINA guideline. In the NAEPP and GINA reports (Table 5), a short-acting β-agonist is recommended for acute relief of occasional bronchospastic symptoms. If symptoms occur more frequently than twice weekly (or greater than once per week, as per GINA), the patient should receive the next step of care (i.e., as recommended for mild persistent). It is recognized that acute severe and even life-threatening acute exacerbations can occur among a small number of high-risk patients with mild intermittent asthma and such patients must be provided with self-management skills and an asthma action plan.

The GINA report goes further than NAEPP in recommending that mild intermittent patients with severe acute exacerbations be stepped up and treated as moderate persistent asthma with long-term controller agents. In a similar fashion, a recent 2002 update of the NAEPP panel report recommends that children experiencing more than three acute exacerbations of asthma per year be considered for initiation of long-term controller medication (3). In the same update, the NAEPP committee recommended initiation of long-term control therapy in infants and young children who had experienced more than three episodes of wheezing within the previous year;

Table 5 Recommended Medications by Level of Severity in Adults—Global Initiative for Asthma (GINA) 2002 Report

Level of severity	Daily controller medications	Other treatment options

Step 1
  Intermittent
  asthma
	None necessary	

Step 2
  Mild persistent
  asthma
	Inhaled glucocorticoid (≤500 μg BDP *or* equivalent)	Sustained-release theophylline, *or* cromone, *or* leukotriene modifier

Step 3
  Moderate
  persistent
  asthma
	Inhaled glucocorticoid 200–1000 μg BDP *or* equivalent) *plus* long-acting inhaled β-agonist	Inhaled glucocorticoid (500–1000 μg BDP *or* equivalent) *plus* long-acting oral β-agonist
		Inhaled glucocorticoid at higher doses (>1000 μg BDP *or* equivalent), *or*
		Inhaled glucocorticoid (500–1000 μg BDP *or* equivalent) *plus* leukotriene modifier *or* sustained release theophylline

Step 4
  Severe persistent
  asthma
	Inhaled glucocorticoid (>1000 μg BDP or equivalent) *plus* long-acting inhaled β-agonist, *plus* one or more of the following, if needed:
	• Sustained-release theophylline
	• Leukotriene modifier
	• Long-acting oral β-agonist
	• Oral glucocorticoid	

All steps: In addition to regular daily controller therapy, rapid-acting inhaled β-agonist should be taken as needed to relieve symptoms, but should not be taken more than 3–4 times a day. Once control of asthma is achieved and maintained for at least three months, a gradual reduction of the maintenance therapy should betried in order to identify the minimum therapy required to maintain control.

Abbreviation: BDP, beclomethasone dipropionate.

if asthma affected sleep and lasted more than one day and the child had known risk factors for development of asthma (i.e., parental asthma history, allergic rhinitis, and peripheral eosinophilia). This new recommendation is analogous to the GINA guidelines for treating young children with mild intermittent asthma and intermittent acute exacerbations. Although the latter recommendations are intuitively rational, they are supported by only a D level of evidence indicating that more long-term studies of the natural history of mild intermittent asthma in early childhood are needed.

Mild Persistent Asthma (Table 5)

Mild persistent asthma (Step 2) is defined by the NAEPP report as symptoms occurring more than twice weekly (or > 1 episode per week according to GINA), nocturnal symptoms more than two times per month, and $FEV_1 \geq 80\%$ predicted and PEF variability of 20% to 30%. Long-term controller medications are indicated according to NAEPP (2002) update. Low-dose inhaled corticosteroids (ICS) (100–400 µg/day budesonide or equivalent) are preferred in adults. Alternative (but not preferred) agents in this group include leukotriene modifiers, sustained-release theophylline, and inhaled cromolyn.

For children five years and younger, a low-dose ICS (via nebulizer, MDI with holding chamber with or without a face mask, or DPI) is the preferred treatment over cromolyn, theophylline, and alternative agents. In the 2002 NAEPP update on treatment of persistent asthma in children ≤ 5 years, the expert panel notes that the latter recommendation is based strictly upon expert opinion (Level D) and is extrapolated from studies in older children, in that adequate controlled clinical trials have not been performed in younger children (3). The treatment recommendations provided by GINA for mild persistent disease are otherwise identical (Table 6).

Moderate Persistent Asthma

According to the NAEPP report, a low dose of ICS combined with a long-acting β-agonist or medium-dose ICS given as monotherapy is preferred treatment for children five years and younger. The recommendation to combine a low-dose ICS with a long acting β-agonist (LABA) in this group is not evidence based; no placebo-controlled studies have been performed to examine this question in this age group. Low-dose ICS combined with either a leukotriene antagonist or theophylline can be considered as alternative but not preferred choices. If asthma is not controlled as reflected by recurrent exacerbations in this age group, low-dose ICS should be stepped up to medium doses combined with a long-acting β-agonist. In this situation, an alternate choice is combining medium doses of ICS with a leukotriene receptor antagonist or theophylline.

In contrast, the GINA guidelines are similar but recommend a moderate dose ICS (400–800 µg budesonide or equivalent), as an initial approach in children (Level A). Other treatment options listed are: an ICS combined with theophylline; an ICS combined with a LABA; high-dose ICS (>800 of budesonide or equivalent); or ICS combined with a leukotriene modifier (Table 6).

Table 6 Recommended Medications by Level of Severity in Children—Global Initiative for Asthma (GINA) 2002 Report

Level of severity	Daily controller medications	Other treatment options
Step 1 Intermittent asthma	None necessary	
Step 2 Mild persistent asthma	Inhaled glucocorticoid (100–400 µg budesonide *or* equivalent)	Sustained-release theophylline, *or* cromone, *or* leukotriene modifier
Step 3 Moderate persistent asthma	Inhaled glucocorticoid Inhaled glucocorticoid (400–800 µg budesonide *or* equivalent)	Inhaled glucocorticoid (< 800 µg budesonide or equivalent) *plus* long-acting inhaled β-agonist, *or* Inhaled glucocorticoid (< 800 µg or equivalent) *plus* sustained release theophylline Inhaled glucocorticoid at higher doses (>800 µg budesonide or equivalent), *or* Inhaled glucocorticoid (< 800 µg or equivalent) *plus* leukotriene modifier
Step 4 Severe persistent asthma	Inhaled glucocorticoid (> 800 µg budesonide or equivalent) *plus* long-acting inhaled β-agonist, *plus* one or more of the following, if needed: • Sustained-release theophylline • Leukotriene modifier • Long-acting inhaled β-agonist • Oral glucocorticoid	

All steps: In addition to regular daily controller therapy, rapid-acting inhaled β-agonist should be taken as needed to relieve symptoms, but should not be taken more than 3–4 times a day. Once control of asthma is achieved and maintained for at least three months, a gradual reduction of the maintenance therapy should be tried in order to identify the minimum therapy required to maintain control.

In adults and children >5 years of age, low to medium doses of ICS combined with LABA are preferred treatment. This is based on excellent evidence in multiple double-blinded controlled studies demonstrating that adding a LABA provides greater control of asthma symptoms and improved lung function versus doubling the ICS dose (13,14). Recent evidence supporting combination therapy was provided by Wallin et al. who reported results of lung biopsy studies performed in asthmatic patients who received either fluticasone propionate (FP) at 1000 mg/day or FP 400 mg/day plus salmeterol for three months. No significant difference was found between the two groups in the numbers of submucosal mast cells or eosinophils. The authors conclude that combination therapy is more effective than doubling ICS doses in improving lung function and asthma control in patients uncontrolled on ICS alone, but combination therapy in lieu of higher ICS doses did not compromise salutary anti-inflammatory effects in the airways (15,16). In the NAEPP 2002 update, alternate recommended approaches in adults include combining medium doses of ICS with a leukotriene inhibitor or theophylline. The GINA documents recommends additional alternative treatment options (not found in the NAEPP report), including: increasing the ICS to higher doses (>1000 µg of BDP); and adding an oral β-agonist to the ICS agent (Table 5).

Severe Persistent Asthma

In children older than five years and adults, high-dose ICS combined with LABA are recommended by the NAEPP for all patients with severe persistent asthma. If indicated, long-term systemic corticosteroids should be instituted to achieve asthma control. Administration of LABA is problematic in young children below the age of five, given the lack of nebulized forms of these drugs. In the United States, children must be mature and coordinated enough to learn how to use a DPI device. NAEPP recommends doses of systemic glucocorticoids not to exceed a total daily prednisone dose of 60 mg or equivalent. All attempts must be made to reduce systemic corticosteroids and maintain control with high-dose ICS.

The GINA report differs in that high dose ICS (>1000 BDP or equivalent ICS dose) combined with LABA are recommended for adults combined with one of the following agents, if indicated: oral corticosteroids, leukotriene antagonists, and sustained release theophylline (Table 5). In children, the GINA guidelines are the same as for adults except that LABA is proposed as one of several options (i.e., in addition to oral corticosteroids, leukotriene antagonists, and theophylline) rather than preferred treatment, as recommended by the NHLBI document (Table 6).

E. Justification for Recommendation of Specific Agents

Both the GINA document of 2002 and the NHLBI-NAEPP report of 1997 present evidence-based rationale for selection of specific agents in both children and adults. Long-term controller medications as defined by GINA include: inhaled corticosteroids, LABA, systemic corticosteroids, long-acting oral β-agonists, sustained-release theophylline, cromolyn sodium, nedocromil, leukotriene-blocking agents, and steroid-sparing agents.

Inhaled Corticosteroids

These are widely recognized as the most effective controller medications and the most effective anti-inflammatory agents. There is excellent evidence (Level A) that these reduce asthma symptoms, improve lung function, reduce airway hyperresponsiveness, decrease frequency of exacerbations, and improve quality of live (2,5). Thus, these are preferred treatments for all levels of persistent asthma. The GINA guidelines point out that the relative potencies of the various agents are difficult to elucidate due primarily to relatively flat dose–response relationships. In other words, there is little additional benefit in asthma outcomes derived from increasing doses beyond 500 µg of beclamethasone diproprionate or an equivalent dose of another ICS agent. At the same time, increasing the ICS dose increases risk of adverse effects. There is excellent evidence (Level A), however, that adding a LABA is more effective than increasing the dose of the ICS. However, there is evidence that the use of high-dose ICS in severe persistent asthma patients reduces the number of acute exacerbations (17). Thus, if necessary, severe patients should be treated with high-dose ICSs in order to prevent exacerbations and to reduce adverse effects associated with use of oral corticosteroids (18).

The NAEPP 1997 report recommended doubling or increasing the doses of inhaled corticosteroids for treatment of mild asthma exacerbations and oral corticosteroids should be administered to patients with moderate and severe asthma exacerbations (2). Increasing ICS dose for mild exacerbations in lieu of using systemic steroids is a controversial strategy that was not supported by a randomized controlled study when the 1997 report was released. It is apparent from the literature that many clinical investigators are not entirely comfortable with this recommendation. However, Levy recently reported in a randomized trial that delivery of high-dose fluticasone (2 mg/day) was as effective as a burst of prednisone in treating adults with acute exacerbations who did not require hospitalization (19). A second study found no significant difference in outcomes between high-dose budesonide (1600 mg/day) versus budesonide (800 mg/day) and methylprednisolone (1 mg/kg) in treating mild-acute asthma exacerbations in children (20). A randomized, double-blind, controlled trial was conducted in 290 patients who were assigned to treatment with either a regular maintenance dose of ICS or were told to double the ICS dose (21). The frequency of treatment failures, defined as requiring subsequent treatment with systemic steroids, unscheduled physician visits, or failure of asthma to return to baseline status, did not differ between treatment arms; both had 40% treatment failure rates. Harrison et al. confirmed these findings in a double-blinded, placebo-controlled study in 390 patients during asthma exacerbations in which subjects were assigned to usual doses or doubling doses or ICS. The endpoint in this study, the need for a subsequent burst of oral prednisolone, did not differ between treatment groups (22). Thus, based on evidence in two well-designed studies, the strategy to manage even mild-acute exacerbations with ICSs should perhaps be reconsidered by the NAEPP panel.

Long-Acting β-Agonists

Excessive use of short-acting β-agonists (i.e., two or more inhaler canisters over three months) have been associated with increased risk of cardiac arrest in patients not using ICSs (23). Thus, the safety of long-term use of LABAs has been scrutinized. Both GINA and NAEPP expert panels endorse the safety of LABAs by stating that there is no evidence that these agents increase airway inflammation and that there is no convincing evidence in the medical literature that LABAs increase asthma exacerbations. The 2002 GINA report states that LABAs do lose their clinical efficacy over time, but acknowledges that the bronchoprotective effect of LABAs for allergen-, methacholine-, and exercise-induced bronchospasm can wane with prolonged usage (5,24). Since introduction of salmeterol, there has been concern over rare reports of severe asthma attacks and possible associations with rare asthma deaths among patients using this agents; such events often occur in patients who are not receiving an ICS (25). Subsequent studies have failed to show a link between chronic use of salmeterol and asthma deaths (26). However, there remains concern as to whether specific patient subgroups have heightened susceptibility to possible paradoxical effects of LABAs related to age or underlying genotype (27). It is emphasized in both documents that a LABA should always be used in conjunction with an anti-inflammatory agent (i.e., ICS). Although not stated specifically, this recommendation implies that there is appropriate concern about the safety of monotherapy with LABA drugs in some patients with persistent asthma.

GINA experts also point out that formoterol is a full β-agonist, whereas salmeterol is a partial agonist, yet the clinical importance of this difference is unclear (5). Because formoterol has a fast onset of action (five minutes) compared with salmeterol, it is better suited for preventing exercise-induced asthma. The LABA drugs are not recommended for treatment of acute asthma symptoms or for exacerbations. There is abundant evidence showing that adding a LABA to moderate or low doses of an ICS is superior to doubling ICS dosage in: improving lung function; reducing asthma symptoms, including nocturnal symptoms and acute exacerbations; reducing utilization of rescue short-acting β-agonist (13). Fixed combinations of an ICS combined with a LABA (e.g., fluticasone propionate + salmeterol, budesonide + formoterol) are as effective as giving the individual drugs concomitantly, but combinations offer the potential benefit of enhancing patient compliance.

Leukotriene Modifiers

These include cysteinyl leukotriene-1 receptor antagonists (i.e., zafirlukast, pranlukast, and montelukast) and zileuton, a 5-lipoxygenase inhibitor. The GINA guidelines note that the role of these drugs in treatment of asthma is being investigated. Although these agents have been shown to have small bronchodilator and anti-inflammatory effects, their overall efficacy for controlling chronic asthma is less than low-dose ICSs. There is evidence (Level B) that leukotriene modifiers improve asthma control in patients not optimally controlled on an ICS, although the effect has been shown to be less than that obtained by adding a LABA (28). The leukotriene modifiers are advantageous for patient compliance in that they can be taken as a tablet. These agents are generally safe. The NAEPP panel mentions that zafirlukast can increase the half-life of warfarin requiring close monitoring and adjustment of warfarin doses, if indicated, in those patients receiving both drugs. Zileuton causes liver toxicity, requiring periodic monitoring of liver tests. Leukotriene modifier agents have been reported to be associated with Churg–Strauss vasculitis in anecdotal case reports, although there is inadequate evidence at this time to establish a causal linkage.

Cromones

These include cromolyn sodium and nedocromil. These are indicated for mild persistent asthma, although they are considered less effective than ICSs (Level B evidence).

Steroid Sparing Therapies

Agents including methotrexate, oral gold, trolandeomycin, cyclosporin, dapsone, and hydroxychloroquine have been studied and shown to have modest benefit in severe persistent asthma. All drugs have significant adverse effects and these drugs should be administered to severe asthmatics (particularly those requiring maintenance doses of oral corticosteroids) under supervision of asthma specialists and only to those patients in whom the benefit outweighs potential risks of these agents. Intravenous gammaglobulin is not recommended by the GINA document due to its high cost and conflicting data pertaining to its oral corticosteroid–sparing activity. Based on a meta-analysis of methotrexate, a small steroid sparing effect was noted (5).

Immunotherapy

The GINA guidelines address the role of specific allergen immunotherapy (IT) in treatment of chronic asthma. When considering controlled clinical studies of allergen IT in asthma, meta-analysis concluded that this modality was effective in asthma (Level A). However, there remain unanswered questions with regard to: which patients will benefit; which specific allergens are most effective; whether or not IT is as effective as other proven modalities such as ICS. Due to the possible risks of injection-related systemic and rare fatal reactions, and long-term inconvenience of IT, the committee concluded that this treatment should be reserved for those patients in whom pharmacologic (including ICS) and environmental interventions have already failed (5). The panel has not yet addressed the possible use of IT for treating mild asthma or for prevention of asthma in childhood. The NAEPP documents have not definitively addressed the role of allergen immunotherapy in asthma treatment.

F. Safey Issues Related to Inhaled and Systemic Corticosteroids

The NHLBI document states that inhaled corticosteroids are the most effective therapy for long-term control of mild, moderate, and severe persistent asthma and are well tolerated at recommended dosages. The overwhelming evidence demonstrating their efficacy far outweighs the small risks of adverse effects. Local adverse effects of ICS include oral candidiasis, dysphonia, reflex cough, or bronchospasm with inhalation. Spacer devices are recommended to prevent dysphonia and oral candidiasis. The key recommendations for reducing the potential adverse effects of ICSs are: (i) administer ICS drugs with holding chambers or spacers; (ii) patients should be instructed to rinse their mouths with tap water after each dose; (iii) use the lowest effective doses; (iv) consider adding a LABA to a low or medium dose of ICS rather than increase ICS dose; (v) monitor growth in children; and (vi) recommend supplemental calcium (1000–1500 mg/day) and vitamin D in postmenopausal women receiving ICS therapy (2).

The GINA document states that, in adults, systemic side effects rarely occur with daily doses of $\leq 500\,\mu$g of BDP or equivalent doses of other ICSs. Higher doses of ICSs are associated with increased risk for bruising, cutaneous laxity, cataracts and glaucoma (in some studies), decreased bone mineral density and adrenal suppression. The expert committee admits that the actual clinical impact of ICS agents on osteoblastic activity and on adrenal suppression has not yet been determined (5). For this reason, specific recommendations for prevention of osteoporosis (in contrast to NAEPP) are not provided.

A major issue has arisen about the possible effects of ICS on reduction in growth velocity in preadolescent children. Presumably concern over adverse growth effects of ICS agents in young children may have a negative impact on physician compliance with published guidelines. The 2002 NAEPP update acknowledges that treatment with low–moderate doses of ICS may reduce growth velocity by 1 cm/yr during the first year of treatment (2). This effect is not believed to continue during subsequent years of treatment, and available evidence indicates that final predicted adult height is attained in children receiving long-term ICS. The committee also reported that long-term observational studies in children receiving ICS therapy for six years failed to show significant effects on bone mineral density or on incidence of subcapsular cataracts or glaucoma. The GINA committee could identify no evidence to support a risk of fracture in young children on ICS agents. However, most of the studies examining growth effect have not been performed in children and infants below the age of six, highlighting the need for future safety studies of ICS therapy in age appropriate subjects (5).

G. Impact of Guidelines on Physicians' Prescribing Patterns

Stafford et al. (29) reported data that reflected prescribing patterns of office-based U.S. physicians. This information was obtained from the National Disease and Therapeutic Index, which tracked trends from 1978 to 2002 in the frequency of asthma visits and patterns of asthma prescriptions. Although annual visits for asthma in the United States increased gradually from 1978 to 1990, the number of physician encounters for asthma had stabilized since 1990. At the same time, use of controller medication increased eight-fold between 1978 and 2002. Utilization of ICSs represented the largest increase in controller medications. An increase was also noted in the ratio of controller-to-reliever medication prescribed. Thus, these data indicate that patterns of asthma pharmacotherapy had changed over 25 years and are perhaps responsible for stabilization in numbers of patient visits since 1990. These prescribing patterns were likely influenced by dissemination of evidence-based guidelines to physicians.

III. Impact of Guidelines on Asthma Outcomes

A. Use of Long-Term Anti-inflammatory Agents

When the NHLBI guidelines were constructed and released in 1991, it was widely assumed that anti-inflammatory controller agents must be initiated early (even in mild persistent asthma) to prevent progressive decline in lung function that would ensue due to unmitigated airways inflammation and subsequent remodeling. This theory was based on retrospective evidence in childhood asthma studies showing that more severe and irreversible airway obstruction was significantly associated with a delay in initiation of an ICS. More recent long-term prospective data from the Childhood Asthma Management Program (CAMP) study collected in asthmatic children treated for five years have failed to show significant differences between placebo, cromolyn, and ICS treated patients in changes in FEV_1 (30). However, the ICS (budesonide) treated group had fewer hospitalizations, urgent visits for asthma, and reduced airway responsiveness compared to nedocromil. Accelerated decline in lung function was significantly associated with low-post bronchodilator FEV_1 at pretreatment baseline, and not related to treatment intervention (31). Based on this study, the purported preventive effect of anti-inflammatory drugs on airway remodeling in uncertain but there are clearly other benefits of ICS drugs that affect long-term disease control. Other investigations of disease outcomes associated with institution of asthma guidelines and/or long-term ICSs are discussed below.

There is good evidence that early institution of ICSs after an asthma diagnosis is established and is associated with reduced risk of subsequent hospitalizations. This was demonstrated in a large nested case control study conducted in Canada for 13,563 newly treated asthmatic subjects in which patients initially prescribed ICSs were compared with those prescribed theophylline for a maximum of 12 months of treatment (32). Those patients prescribed ICSs were 40% less likely to be admitted to the hospital for asthma than patients using theophylline. In this same cohort of patients in the Saskatchewan health system followed between 1977 and 1993, the probability of readmission for asthma was evaluated in relation to whether inhaled corticosteroids were prescribed after initial hospital admission (33). Patients who received regular treatment with ICSs were 40% less likely to be readmitted for asthma. Regular use of inhaled corticosteroids was associated with reductions of 31% in the rate of hospital admissions for asthma (95% confidence interval and 39% in the rate of readmission) (34). This population was also evaluated with possible association between ICS usage and asthma-related deaths (35). After adjustment for covariates, patients receiving one or more metered-dose inhalers of beclomethasone per month were shown to have a significantly lower risk of fatal and near-fatal asthma (odds ratio = 0.1). The mean number of canisters was 1.18 for the patients who died and 1.57 for the controls. The same group of investigators evaluated asthma death related to corticosteroid usage, using a case–control design (36). A dose–response analysis estimated that asthma death rates decreased by 21% with each additional ICS canister used during the previous year (adjusted rate ratio = 0.79). Thus, the beneficial effects in important asthma disease outcomes demonstrated in these studies clearly validate asthma guideline treatment recommendations of long-term use of ICSs in patients with moderate and severe asthma.

Since asthma treatment guidelines were introduced in Japan in the 1990s, the impact of introduction of leukotriene inhibitors and ICSs on asthma mortality was assessed from the period spanning 1987 to 1999 (37). The rate of asthma deaths decreased with increasing use of leukotriene receptor antagonists and inhaled corticosteroids. The rate of asthma deaths was 0.96 per 1 million 25-day treatment courses of inhaled corticosteroids and 0.80 for every 1 million 25-day treatment courses of leukotriene antagonists. This result suggests that the increased use of anti-inflammatory agents in the Japanese health care system may have partially contributed in some way to the decrease in asthma mortality.

Boulet et al. examined a large population of asthma patients who were suboptimally controlled according to Canadian asthma consensus guidelines (38). In separate surveys of patients with uncontrolled asthma and their physicians, 66% of patients and 43% of physicians rated control of asthma symptoms as adequate to very good. These findings indicate that physicians are still not utilizing diagnostic guidelines to assess asthma severity and highlight the need to more effectively disseminate this information to both physicians and their patients. A survey of 445 asthmatic patients in New Zealand used the GINA guidelines as a gold standard for defining asthma control and, on this basis, revealed that 93% of adults and 90% of children were suboptimally controlled (39). Another large survey of parents of children with asthma reported that despite suboptimal control defined by guidelines in 49% of children and under treatment for the level of asthma severity, 89% of parents were satisfied with treatment outcomes (40). Prescription data has also been examined to indirectly assess impact of published guidelines. A three-year survey (1996–1998) of 13,000 patients receiving β-agonist prescriptions in British Columbia revealed a discouraging trend that ICS usage decreased over time (41). As mentioned, a recently published international survey of asthma treatment and severity indicates that only a small minority of patients ($< 30\%$) in all countries surveyed are receiving preventative therapy (10). This suggests that outcomes of treatment and even adherence with physician and guideline directed therapy could be negatively influenced by low parental expectations.

A randomized controlled trial was conducted in 81 general practices in the United Kingdom in which the medical providers were issued abbreviated asthma guidelines. Outcomes were determined by measuring adherence to asthma recommendations among patients. In this brief study, issuance of brief guidelines did not improve adherence to recommendations related to asthma treatment (42). Bender et al. recently reviewed published studies pertaining to outcomes of adherence interventions (43). These authors noted that in 50% of studies experimental interventions do not improve adherence. They acknowledged that a strong physician–patient relationship enhances adherence, highlighting the need for physicians to be familiar enough with evidence-based treatment guidelines to impart important information to their patients with asthma.

Barr et al. (44) assessed adherence to the NAEPP medication guidelines among 5107 elderly female asthma patients. Fifty-seven percent of mild persistent, 55% of moderate persistent, and 32% of severe persistent asthma patients were found to be adherent with asthma medication guidelines. Based on a multivariate analysis, non-adherence was associated with severe asthma, increasing age, lower socioeconomic status, current smoking, earlier onset of asthma, and number of comorbid medical conditions. This study underscores the minimal impact the guidelines have had in the community, which is likely due to ineffective physician education.

Management of Acute Exacerbations

Guideline reports recommend written action plans for moderate or severe asthmatics to guide self-management of acute exacerbations and particularly those who have previously been hospitalized or have undergone mechanical ventilation for near-fatal attacks. The GINA report emphasizes that high-risk patients who have previously received mechanical ventilation are at a 19-fold risk of requiring mechanical ventilation in subsequent attacks (5). A written "action plan" should contain emergency treatment instructions on how to recognize and manage acute exacerbations. Essential components of the action plan should include: instructions on how exacerbations can be recognized by early decrements in lung function (i.e., PEFR); prompt communication with the clinician; prompt and early intensification of therapy, including initiation of a burst of oral corticosteroids; and immediate removal from relevant allergens or irritants (2). Several studies have examined outcomes of implementation of guideline recommendations for managing acute exacerbations, including possible benefits of written action plans. The practice of doubling inhaled corticosteroids doses as opposed to administering oral corticosteroids for acute mild exacerbations has already been addressed earlier in this chapter. The GINA report, recognizing that there is limited evidence to support the latter strategy, recommend systemic steroids for all but the mildest exacerbations. Systemic corticosteroids should be instituted in any patient not showing a prompt response to an inhaled short-acting β-agonist (5).

There is evidence that emergency room physician compliance with published guidelines pertinent to managing acute exacerbations is suboptimal (45,46). There have also been important studies that have evaluated clinical outcomes related to administration of self-management and action plans for managing acute exacerbations. Cote et al. performed an investigation of 98 asthma patients presenting with acute exacerbations (47). Patients were assigned to usual treatment, limited education on a self-action plan by the emergency physician, or a structured educational program emphasizing self-management of asthma exacerbations. At 12 months, only the group receiving structured education was found to have significant improvement in knowledge, willingness to adjust medications, quality of life scores, and peak expiratory flows. The number of unscheduled medical clinic visits for asthma was significantly decreased in the educated group compared to the others. Thus, it appeared that structured educational intervention emphasizing self-management had the greatest impact on patient outcomes. Cowie et al. demonstrated in a prospective study that utilization of a peak-flow based action plan dramatically reduced emergency room visits for acute asthma (48). Adams and coworkers studied 293 patients prospectively, who had moderate or severe asthma. Hospital admissions over a period of 12 months were found to be significantly associated with not possessing a written asthma action plan and lower preferences for autonomy in asthma management decisions (49). Abramson et al. have presented the most convincing evidence supporting the use of asthma actions plans and intensive education in high-risk patients (50). In a case–control study, circumstances of 89 asthma deaths were compared with 322 patients presenting to hospitals with acute asthma. Cases of asthma death were significantly less likely than controls to use a peak flow meter. Furthermore, written action plans were associated with a 70% reduction in the risk of death. The authors concluded that widespread use of written asthma management plans could lead to reductions in asthma mortality.

B. Novel Approaches for Improving Guideline-Directed Treatment Outcomes

Green et al. recently compared treatment outcomes in a group of asthmatics actively managed by using serial sputum eosinophils counts to assess treatment response versus a group managed according to the British asthma treatment guidelines (51). The sputum-managed group had significantly fewer severe asthma exacerbations and asthma hospital admissions than did patients in the guideline managed group, despite the fact that there was no difference in mean doses of ICSs or oral corticosteroids between groups.

A Canadian study evaluated the effectiveness of trained pharmacists in providing asthma education and monitoring compliance (52). Pharmacists participated in providing either enhanced care (asthma education regarding medications, triggers, and self-monitoring) or usual care to 631 asthma patients. After one year, compared to patients receiving usual care, the enhanced care group experienced a 50% reduction in symptom scores, an 11% increase in peak-flow readings, reduced days off work or school, a 50% reduction in use of inhaled β-agonists, and improved overall quality of life. In addition emergency room visits decreased by 75% and medical visits decreased by 75% in the enhanced care group. This study suggests that trained community pharmacists can effectively educate asthmatic patients with regard to treatment and can play a major role in enhancing adherence, thereby improving global outcomes of guideline-directed asthma care.

Outcomes of self-management programs as recommended in GINA guidelines have also been examined. A Dutch study was performed with 193 adults with stable asthma, 98 of whom were instructed on self-management and 95 received usual care (53). Self-management was cost-effective when compared to usual care for all outcomes examined. Janson et al. reported outcomes in a controlled trial of educational self-management intervention conducted in 65 adults with mild to moderate asthma (54). The intervention was a 30-minute education program delivered at biweekly intervals. The intervention group exhibited significant improvements compared to the control group in ICS adherence and self-reported control of asthma. Interestingly, sputum eosinophils declined significantly in the treated group. The authors concluded that education and training in self-management improves adherence with ICSs, a finding validated by concomitant reduction in sputum eosinophilia.

IV. Unresolved Issues and Future Directions

Despite the widespread publicity surrounding the GINA and NAEPP reports within the medical community, their impact in improving asthma treatment has been relatively modest. As already mentioned, published surveys of asthmatic patients in developed countries seem to suggest that asthma pharmacotherapy is suboptimal in many patients, and is not in compliance with evidence-based guidelines. Studies performed by Suissa et al. (34,36) in Canada would suggest that there has been some impact as evidence by more widespread use of ICS agents, which has corresponded to reductions in asthma hospitalizations and mortality. Thus, although progress has been slow, the consequences of guidelines have been beneficial. Educational efforts directed at health care providers and the population at large must be intensified, employing novel approaches that can facilitate better adherence to the principles of asthma guideline-directed treatment.

Other unresolved issues include the undefined roles of approved and yet-to-be approved drugs. The exact role of leukotriene blockers has yet to be defined within the framework of asthma treatment guidelines. Although these drugs are safe, based on available evidence, they are not considered preferred therapy for any asthma severity category in any age group. Yet, these agents have enjoyed tremendous acceptance among physicians and patients alike. This paradoxical phenomenon may have arisen over inflated fears about adverse effects of corticosteroids. On the other hand, researchers may have failed to clearly identify and predict those patient subgroups most likely to exhibit favorable responses. Perhaps pharmacogenomics will permit identifications of subpopulations of asthmatics most likely to respond to this class of drugs.

Concerns over widespread use of LABA agents persist; safety data has identified a small risk. In the future, these will be used exclusively as combination formulations with ICSs. Here again, pharmacogenomics research may help clarify if there are genetically susceptible subgroups of asthmatics at risk for paradoxical responses to the LABA agents. Finally, management of the most severe high-risk asthmatic patients who require high-dose oral corticosteroid therapy remains problematic. Outcomes of guideline-directed and evidence-based therapy aimed at this rare subgroup have not been evaluated. However, there is general consensus that the current armamentarium of agents is not adequate and that more efficacious and safer drugs are needed. In the future, new evidence supporting the roles of novel anti-inflammatory agents and biomodifiers may emerge. Some of these could appear in future updates of GINA or NAEPP asthma guidelines.

References

1. Expert Panel Report: Guidelines for diagnosis and management of asthma. 1991, NIH-NHLBI.
2. Guidelines for the diagnosis and management of asthma: Expert panel report 2. 1997, NIH-NHLBI.
3. National Asthma Education and Prevention Program. Expert Panel Report: guidelines for the diagnosis and management of asthma update on selected topics-2002. J Allergy Clin Immunol 2002; 110(5suppl):S141–219.
4. Global Initiative for Asthma. 1995, NIH-NHLBI.
5. Global Initiative for Asthma. 2002, NIH-NHLBI.
6. Burney PG, Chinn S, Britton JR, Tattersfield AE, Papacosta AO. What symptoms predict the bronchial response to histamine? Evaluation in a community survey of the bronchial symptoms questionnaire (1984) of the International Union Against Tuberculosis and Lung Disease. Int J Epidemiol 1989; 18(1): 165–173.
7. Cote J, Cartier A, Malo JL, Roufeau M, Boulet LP. Compliance with peak expiratory flow monitoring in home management of asthma. Chest 1998; 113(4):968–972.
8. Sporik R, Holgate ST, Cogswell JJ. Natural history of asthma in childhood—a birth cohort study. Arch Dis Child 1991; 66(9):1050–1053.
9. Martinez FD, Wright AL, Taussig LM, Holberg CJ, Halonen M, Morgan WJ. Asthma and wheezing in the first six years of life. The group health medical associates. N Engl J Med 1995; 332(3):133–138.
10. Rabe KF, Adachi M, Lai CK, Soriano JB, Vermeire PA, Weiss KB, Weiss ST. Worldwide severity and control of asthma in children and adults: the global asthma insights and reality surveys. J Allergy Clin Immunol 2004; 114(1):40–47.
11. Cegala DJ, Marinelli T, Post D. The effects of patient communication skills training on compliance. Arch Fam Med 2000; 9(1):57–64.
12. Arshad SH, Bateman B, Matthews SM. Primary prevention of asthma and atopy during childhood by allergen avoidance in infancy: a randomized controlled study. Thorax 2003; 58(6):489–493.
13. Greening AP, Ind PW, Northfield M, Shaw G. Added salmeterol versus higher-dose corticosteroid in asthma patients with symptoms on existing inhaled corticosteroid. Lancet: Allen & Hanburys Limited UK Study Group, 1994; 344(8917):219–224.
14. Woolcock A, Lundback B, Ringdal N, Jacques LA. Comparison of addition of salmeterol to inhaled steroids with doubling of the dose of inhaled steroids. Am J Respir Crit Care Med 1996; 153(5):1481–1488.
15. Wallin A, Sue-Chu M, Bjermer L, Ward J, Sandstrom T, Lindberg A, Lundback B, Djukanovic R, Holgate S, Wilson S. Effect of inhaled fluticasone with and without salmeterol on airway inflammation in asthma. J Allergy Clin Immunol 2003; 112(1):72–78.

16. Masoli M, Holt S, Beasley R. What to do at step 3 of the asthma guidelines-increase the dose of inhaled corticosteroids or add a long-acting beta-agonist drug? J Allergy Clin Immunol 2003; 112(1):10–11.
17. Pauwels RA, Lofdahl CG, Postma DS, Tattersfield AE, O'Byrne P, Barnes PJ, Ullman A. Effect of inhaled formoterol and budesonide on exacerbations of asthma. Formoterol and corticosteroids establishing therapy (FACET) international study group. N Engl J Med 1997; 337(20):1405–1411.
18. Mash B, Bheekie A, Jones PW. Inhaled vs. oral steroids for adults with chronic asthma. Cochrane Database Syst Rev 2000(2):CD002160.
19. Levy ML, Stevenson C, Maslen T. Comparison of short courses of oral prednisolone and fluticasone propionate in the treatment of adults with acute exacerbations of asthma in primary care. Thorax 1996; 51(11):1087–1092.
20. Nuhoglu Y, Bahceciler NN, Barlan IB, Mujdat Basaran M. The effectiveness of high-dose inhaled budesonide therapy in the treatment of acute asthma exacerbations in children. Ann Allergy Asthma Immunol 2001; 86(3):318–322.
21. FitzGerald JM, Becker A, Sears MR, Mink S, Chung K, Lee J. Doubling the dose of budesonide versus maintenance treatment in asthma exacerbations. Thorax 2004; 59(7):550–556.
22. Harrison TW, Oborne J, Newton S, Tattersfield AE. Doubling the dose of inhaled corticosteroid to prevent asthma exacerbations: randomized controlled trial. Lancet 2004; 363(9405):271–275.
23. Lemaitre RN, Siscovick DS, Psaty BM, Pearce RM, Raghunathan TE, Whitsel EA, Weinmann SA, Anderson GD, Lin D. Inhaled beta-2 adrenergic receptor agonists and primary cardiac arrest. Am J Med 2002; 113(9):711–716.
24. Nelson JA, Strauss L, Skowronski M, Ciufo R, Novak R, McFadden ER Jr. Effect of long-term salmeterol treatment on exercise-induced asthma. N Engl J Med 1998; 339(3):141–146.
25. Castle W, Fuller R, Hall J, Palmer J. Serevent nationwide surveillance study: comparison of salmeterol with salbutamol in asthmatic patients who require regular bronchodilator treatment. Bmj 1993; 306(6884):1034–1037.
26. Abramson MJ, Walters J, Walters EH. Adverse effects of beta-agonists: are they clinically relevant? Am J Respir Med 2003; 2(4):287–297.
27. McGraw DW, Almoosa KF, Paul RJ, Kobilka BK, Liggett SB. Antithetic regulation by beta-adrenergic receptors of Gq receptor signaling via phospholipase C underlies the airway beta-agonist paradox. J Clin Invest 2003; 112(4):619–626.
28. Laviolette M, Malmstrom K, Lu S, Chervinsky P, Pujet JC, Peszek I, Zhang J, Reiss TF. Montelukast added to inhaled beclomethasone in treatment of asthma. Montelukast/Beclomethasone additivity group. Am J Respir Crit Care Med 1999; 160(6):1862–1868.
29. Stafford RS, Ma J, Finkelstein SN, Haver K, Cockburn I. National trends in asthma visits and asthma pharmacotherapy, 1978–2002. J Allergy Clin Immunol 2003; 111(4):729–735.
30. Long-term effects of budesonide or nedocromil in children with asthma. The childhood asthma management program research group. N Engl J Med 2000; 343(15):1054–1063.

31. Covar RA, Spahn JD, Murphy JR, Szefler SJ. Progression of asthma measured by lung function in the childhood asthma management program. Am J Respir Crit Care Med 2004; 170(3):234–241.

32. Blais L, Suissa S, Boivin JF, Ernst P. First treatment with inhaled corticosteroids and the prevention of admissions to hospital for asthma. Thorax 1998; 53(12):1025–1029.

33. Blais L, Ernst P, Boivin JF, Suissa S. Inhaled corticosteroids and the prevention of readmission to hospital for asthma. Am J Respir Crit Care Med 1998; 158(1): 126–132.

34. Suissa S, Ernst P, Kezouh A. Regular use of inhaled corticosteroids and the long term prevention of hospitalisation for asthma. Thorax 2002; 57(10): 880–884.

35. Ernst P, Spitzer WO, Suissa S, Cockcroft D, Habbick B, Horwitz RI, Boivin JF, McNutt M, Buist AS. Risk of fatal and near-fatal asthma in relation to inhaled corticosteroid use. Jama 1992; 268(24):3462–3464.

36. Suissa S, Ernst P, Benayoun S, Baltzan M, Cai B. Low-dose inhaled corticosteroids and the prevention of death from asthma. N Engl J Med 2000; 343(5): 332–336.

37. Suissa S, Ernst P. Use of anti-inflammatory therapy and asthma mortality in Japan. Eur Respir J 2003; 21(1):101–104.

38. Boulet LP, Phillips R, O'Byrne P, Becker A. Evaluation of asthma control by physicians and patients: comparison with current guidelines. Can Respir J 2002; 9(6):417–423.

39. Holt S, Kljakovic M, Reid J. Asthma morbidity, control and treatment in New Zealand: results of the Patient Outcomes Management Survey (POMS), 2001. NZ Med J 2003; 116(1174):U436.

40. Kuehni CE, Frey U. Age-related differences in perceived asthma control in childhood: guidelines and reality. Eur Respir J 2002; 20(4):880–889.

41. Lynd LD, Guh DP, Pare PD, Anis AH. Patterns of inhaled asthma medication use: a 3-year longitudinal analysis of prescription claims data from British Columbia, Canada. Chest 2002; 122(6):1973–1981.

42. Baker R, Fraser RC, Stone M, Lambert P, Stevenson K, Shiels C. Randomized controlled trial of the impact of guidelines, prioritized review criteria and feedback on implementation of recommendations for angina and asthma. Br J Gen Pract 2003; 53(489):284–291.

43. Bender B, Milgrom H, Apter A. Adherence intervention research: what have we learned and what do we do next? J Allergy Clin Immunol 2003; 112(3): 489–494.

44. Barr RG, Somers SC, Speizer FE, Camargo CA Jr. Patient factors and medication guideline adherence among older women with asthma. Arch Intern Med 2002; 162(15):1761–1768.

45. Varsano S. (Asthma management in adult emergency departments in Israel in comparison to asthma guidelines). Harefuah 2003; 142(11):722–727,808.

46. Lenhardt R, Malone A, Grant EN, Weiss KB. Trends in emergency department asthma care in metropolitan Chicago: results from the Chicago Asthma Surveillance Initiative. Chest 2003; 124(5):1774–1780.

47. Cote J, Bowie DM, Robichaud P, Parent JG, Battisti L, Boulet LP. Evaluation of two different educational interventions for adult patients consulting with an acute asthma exacerbation. Am J Respir Crit Care Med, 2001; 163(6):1415–1419.

48. Cowie RL, Revitt SG, Underwood MF, Field SK. The effect of a peak flow-based action plan in the prevention of exacerbations of asthma. Chest 1997; 112(6):1534–1538.

49. Adams RJ, Smith BJ, Ruffin RE. Factors associated with hospital admissions and repeat emergency department visits for adults with asthma. Thorax 2000; 55(7):566–573.

50. Abramson MJ, Bailey MJ, Couper FJ, Driver JS, Drummer OH, Forbes AB, McNeil JJ, Haydn Walters E. Are asthma medications and management related to deaths from asthma? Am J Respir Crit Care Med 2001; 163(1):12–18.

51. Green RH, Brightling CE, McKenna S, Hargadon B, Parker D, Bradding P, Wardlaw AJ, Pavord ID. Asthma exacerbations and sputum eosinophil counts: a randomized controlled trial. Lancet 2002; 360(9347):1715–1721.

52. McLean W, Gillis J, Waller R. The BC Community Pharmacy Asthma Study: A study of clinical, economic and holistic outcomes influenced by an asthma care protocol provided by specially trained community pharmacists in British Columbia. Can Respir J 2003; 10(4):195–202.

53. Schermer TR, Thoonen BP, van den Boom G, Akkermans RP, Grol RP, Folgering HT, van Weel C, van Schayck CP. Randomized controlled economic evaluation of asthma self-management in primary health care. Am J Respir Crit Care Med 2002; 166(8):1062–1072.

54. Janson SL, Fahy JV, Covington JK, Paul SM, Gold WM, Boushey HA. Effects of individual self-management education on clinical, biological, and adherence outcomes in asthma. Am J Med 2003; 115(8):620–626.

2

β-Agonists

DAVE SINGH and ASHLEY WOODCOCK

North West Lung Research Centre, South Manchester University Hospitals Trust
Manchester, U.K.

I. Introduction

β-Adrenoreceptors are widely distributed throughout the human body. There are three subtypes: β_1, β_2, and β_3. The function and expression of these receptors varies between tissues with β_2-adrenoreceptors (β_2-AR) being the subtype of importance in the lungs. These receptors play a central role in the regulation of lung function as they are expressed on the surface of bronchial smooth muscle cells. As β-agonists cause smooth muscle relaxation, this class of drug has become extensively prescribed for the treatment of asthma. Among the first β-agonists to be used were adrenaline and isoprenaline. However, the usefulness of these nonselective β-agonists was limited by β_1-AR–mediated cardiac side effects, and this led to the development of highly selective β_2-agonists such as albuterol. The subsequent introduction of other selective short- and long-acting β_2-agonists (SABA and LABA, respectively) has resulted in this class of drug becoming the mainstay of treatment for the symptomatic control of asthma. Recent advances in our understanding of the effects of β_2-agonists has allowed their use in clinical practice to be optimized. This chapter will review the pharmacological properties of β-agonists, and their use in clinical practice.

II. The β_2-Adrenoreceptor

A. Receptor Distribution

The density of β-receptors varies within the lung, with high-expression levels found in the airway epithelium, alveoli, and submucosal glands (1). Importantly, these receptors are also expressed on smooth muscle cells (1,2), as well as inflammatory cells such as mast cells and lymphocytes (3). The majority of pulmonary β-receptors are the β_2-subtype, with a β_2:β_1 ratio of 3:1 (1).

B. Receptor Activation and Signaling

The β_2-adrenoreceptor is a G-protein coupled receptor, with seven transmembrane domains that are connected by intra- and extracellular connecting loops (Fig. 1). It has an extracellular amino terminus and an intracellular carboxyl terminus. The binding sites for ligands lie within the lipophilic transmembrane domains of the receptor. Amino acid residues that are directly involved in binding have been identified, e.g., asp 113, serine 204, and serine 207 (4). It is likely that ligands with different molecular structures can interact with different amino acid residues within the β_2-AR binding site, and this contributes to variations in the pharmacological properties of ligands (5).

The activated β_2-AR binds to cytoplasmic G-proteins (Fig. 2); this coupling process requires several molecular interactions between the intracellular portions of the receptor and G-protein (6). The β_2-AR/G-protein complex activates the enzyme adenyl cyclase, which is responsible for the conversion of ATP to cAMP. This activates protein kinase A, which is able to phosphorylate proteins that are directly involved in the regulation of smooth muscle tone. Additionally, intracellular Ca levels are reduced through a variety of mechanisms. This also contributes to smooth muscle relaxation. There is also evidence that the activated β_2-AR/G-protein complex interacts with cell membrane K channels (7).

For many years β_2-AR and their ligands were thought to interact by a "lock and key" mechanism (Fig. 3A), with agonists that are a suitable shape ("the key") binding to the receptor ("the lock"). This interaction was thought to cause a conformational change in the receptor that was required for effective G-protein coupling. This mechanism was postulated to be a simple "on–off" switch, as there was no receptor activity without an agonist present. As antagonists were thought to act by blocking the agonist-binding site, then agonists and antagonists "competed" for the same receptor molecules (Fig. 3B).

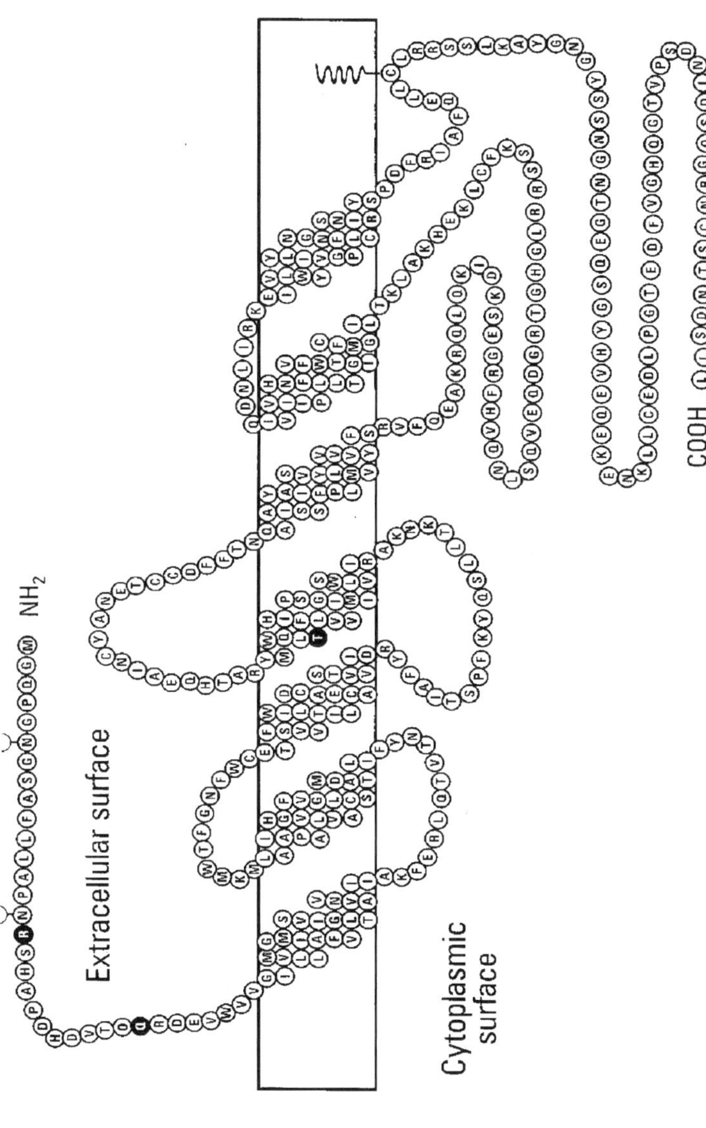

Figure 1 β₂-Adrenoreceptor structure. Transmembrane domains are connected by intra- and extracellular loops. Ligand binding is within the transmembrane domains. *Source:* From Ref. 3.

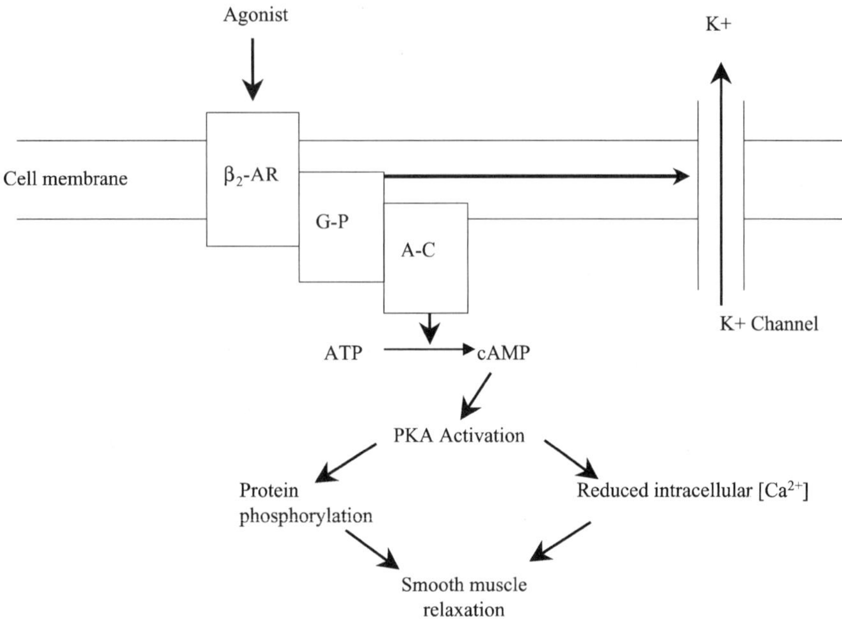

Figure 2 β_2-Adrenoreceptor (β_2-AR) signaling pathways. Agonist binding causes receptor coupling to G-proteins (G-P), which increases adenylate cyclase (A-C) conversion of ATP to cAMP. This activates protein kinase A (PKA), leading to smooth muscle relaxation. The β_2-AR/G-P complex also interacts with potassium channels.

It now appears that the "lock and key" theory was too simplistic, as the β_2-AR is in a state of constant equilibrium between activated and inactivated forms even when there are no ligands present (8,9) (Fig. 4A). The resting equilibrium favors the inactivated form, with only a minority of receptors being active at any given moment. This results in a low-basal level of β_2-AR signaling through G-protein coupling in the absence of agonist binding. β_2-agonists bind to the activated form and stop conversion back to the inactive form (Fig. 4B). This shifts the equilibrium toward the active form, causing increased β_2-AR signal transduction. In contrast, β_2-antagonists bind and stabilize the inactivated form, thus shifting the equilibrium away from the active form. It therefore appears that agonists and antagonists bind to different forms of the β_2-AR. Furthermore, the β_2-AR may exist in equilibrium between many different conformations, each with different levels of signal transduction activity. Partial agonists are either less able to stabilize active conformations, or are specific for conformations with lower basal levels of signal transduction activity compared to full agonists.

Traditionally, the pharmacological effectiveness of β_2-agonists in asthma have been related to the following three factors; local concentration

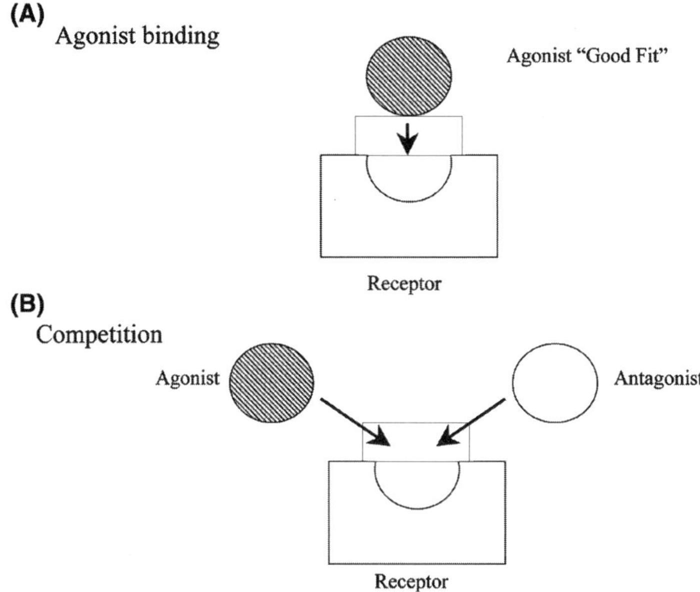

Figure 3 The "lock and key" receptor theory. (A) Agonists have a suitable molecular conformation for receptor binding. (B) Antagonists "compete" for the same binding sites.

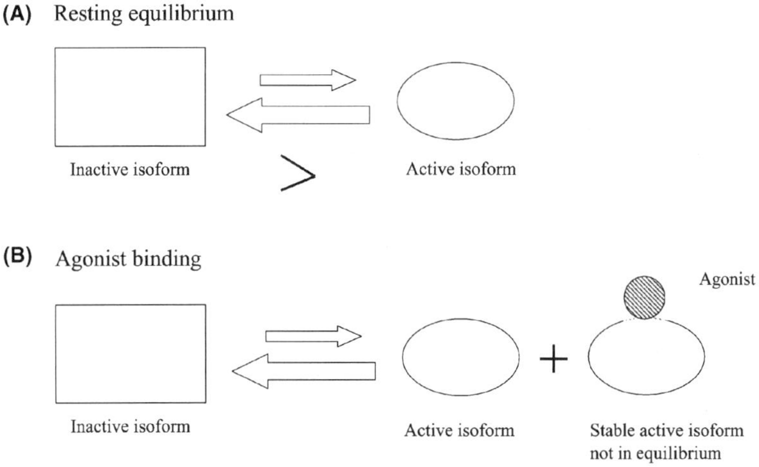

Figure 4 The dynamic model of β_2-adrenoreceptor–ligand interactions. (A) The receptor is in a resting equilibrium that favors an inactive isoform. There is a low-basal level of activity due to the active isoform. (B) Agonist binding stabilizes the active isoform, which is now not in equilibrium. This increases the total number of active receptors, so increasing β_2-adrenoreceptor signaling.

in the lungs, receptor binding affinity, and intrinsic activity. The local concentration is determined by inhaler device characteristics, inhaled particle mass, and lipophilicity. Binding affinity refers to the ability of the ligand to bind to the receptor, while intrinsic activity refers to the degree of stimulation of the receptor due to conformational shape change. Local concentration and binding affinity are undoubtedly of importance in determining the pharmacological effects of inhaled β-agonists. However, the theory of intrinsic activity assumes that β-agonists exert their actions through the "lock and key" mechanism. This theory has now been superceded by evidence that the ability of β-agonists to stabilize active β_2-AR isoforms is an important determinant of pharmacological activity.

C. Receptor Desensitization

Dynamic control mechanisms operate to regulate β_2-AR signal transduction after agonist binding. These may cause desensitization to β-agonist receptor stimulation. Three main control mechanisms have been identified:

1. G-protein-coupled receptor kinase (GRK) phosphorylation of the β_2-AR, which allows binding of β-arrestin to the receptor (10). This is the most rapid and causes uncoupling of the receptor from the G-protein, resulting in reduced signal transduction.
2. Receptor internalization, which involves the endocytosis of cell surface β_2-AR (11).
3. Down-regulation, which is a reduction in the total number of receptors in the cell after prolonged agonist–receptor interaction. This may be due to increased receptor degradation or reduced gene expression (12).

There are differences between cell types in the degree of desensitization caused by β_2-agonists. For example, smooth muscle cells appear to be less prone to desensitization compared to mast cells (13). This may explain why regular treatment with β_2-agonists may cause relatively greater desensitization of bronchoprotection (which is mediated by mast cells) compared to bronchodilation (which is mediated by smooth muscle cells).

III. Pharmacology of β-Agonists

A. Pharmacodynamics

Short-Acting β-Agonists

β-Agonists can only exert their pharmacological effects while bound to the β_2-AR. The duration of action of a β-agonist is therefore related to its ability to remain at the receptor-binding site. This is determined predominantly by the lipophilicity of the molecule. SABA are hydrophilic in nature, and so approach the β_2-AR extracellularly, allowing a rapid onset of action (14). However, diffusion of the ligand into the extracellular compartment occurs easily and results in a relatively short duration of action. SABA therefore cause rapid smooth muscle relaxation, but have a relatively short duration of action.

Long-Acting β-Agonists

LABA are more lipophilic than SABA, and can diffuse into the cell membrane to a greater extent (14–16). This enables interaction with the β_2-AR without rapid diffusion into the extracellular compartment, leading to a longer duration of action.

Two LABA are currently used for the treatment of asthma: salmeterol and formoterol. Salmeterol was designed specifically to be a long-acting bronchodilator by the addition of a long side chain to the albuterol molecule (16,17). This increases the lipophilicity of the molecule. In contrast, formoterol was initially developed as an oral bronchodilator drug, but was observed to be long acting after inhalation (17). Formoterol has a shorter side chain than salmeterol, but greater than albuterol (14,17). Consequently, its lipophilicity is also less than salmeterol, but greater than albuterol. As salmeterol is more lipophilic than formoterol, it diffuses into the cell membrane to a greater extent (14). This difference contributes to a delayed onset of action for salmeterol because of the following reasons:

1. After inhalation, LABA diffuse through the bronchial tissue to the smooth muscle. The greater absorption of salmeterol into cell membranes increases the time to reach the bronchial smooth muscle.
2. When formoterol reaches the bronchial smooth muscle, some of the drug enters the cell membrane and diffuses laterally to the β_2-AR. However, some of the drug is also able to approach the receptor from the extracellular route (similar to the mode of action of SABA), thus allowing a rapid onset of action. In contrast, salmeterol does not bind to the β_2-AR from the extracellular route.

It has been proposed that the long side chain of salmeterol interacts with an "exosite" in the β_2-AR (18). This prevents ligand dissociation, hence promoting a long duration of action. In contrast, the formoterol molecule does not appear to possess a specific stabilizing binding site. The effects of formoterol are highly concentration dependent, both in vitro (19) and in vivo (20). This has been explained by the "depot" hypothesis (14), whereby the effects of formoterol increase as larger doses are delivered into the membrane to form a depot that can diffuse to the β_2-AR.

Salmeterol is less potent (i.e., it has a lower maximal effect) compared to formoterol, both in vitro (19) and in vivo (20). Two possible explanations for this phenomenon were: (i) exosite binding ensures receptor saturation, after which agonist effects do not increase with dose, or (ii) differences in intrinsic activity, i.e., salmeterol is a partial agonist while formoterol is a full agonist (17). These explanations are based on the "lock and key" theory involving competition for the same receptor isoform. However, as reviewed earlier, it is now apparent that different β_2-AR isoforms exist, and pharmacological variations in ligand activity may instead be attributable to their ability to bind to and stabilize isoforms and the level of activity of the bound isoform (9), e.g., salmeterol may be less able to stabilize an active isoform, or may bind to an isoform with a lower level of basal activity compared to formoterol. Further studies are needed to elucidate the isoform-binding properties of salmeterol and formoterol.

B. Pharmacokinetics

β-Agonists are absorbed from both the lungs and gastrointestinal tract. Studies using activated charcoal to block gastrointestinal absorption have shown that the majority of absorption is from the lung fraction (21,22). T_{max} (time to maximal drug concentration) is usually within minutes after inhalation (23,24). β-Agonists undergo first-pass metabolism, resulting in conjugation to inactive forms for excretion either via the urine or feces.

IV. Short-Acting β-Agonists

A. Chirality

β-Agonist preparations consist of two stereoisomers; these racemic mixtures contain active (eutomer) and inactive (distomer) forms (25). This has led to the development of pure R-isomer (active) preparations of albuterol, in the hope that the therapeutic ratio can be improved. However, the difference in bronchodilation between the R-isomer form and the racemic mixture is relatively minor (26), and so the clinical benefit of using preparations containing pure R-isomer have so far been limited.

B. Clinical Effects

Bronchodilation

SABA cause bronchodilation within minutes after administration. In the stable state, maximal bronchodilation is usually achieved 5 to 15 minutes after a single dose (27). The duration of bronchodilation is approximately four to six hours. Desensitization after repeated dosing with SABA can lead to reduced bronchodilation, e.g., the bronchodilator response to albuterol decreases by approximately 20% after four weeks of regular therapy (28).

Bronchoprotection

A single dose of a SABA protects against bronchoconstricting stimuli such as methacholine (29), histamine, and AMP (30). Desensitization after regular SABA treatment reduces this protective effect, e.g., regular treatment with terbutaline for one (31) or two (32) weeks causes a reduction in the magnitude of protection against methacholine.

Adverse Effects

The systemic absorption of SABA can lead to a variety of adverse effects. Cardiac disturbances are among the most common. There is often an increase in heart rate due to (i) direct cardiac β_2-AR stimulation and (ii) peripheral vasodilation triggering a reflex response. Using a metered dose inhaler, the maximum increases in heart rate with albuterol and terbutaline are 8 beats/min. In contrast, fenoterol causes a 29 beats/min increase (33). In clinical practice, significant cardiac arrythmias due to albuterol or terbutaline are uncommon, and are more likely to occur with higher doses (e.g., repeated nebulisation during an acute episode) or preexisting cardiac disease.

SABA may cause tremor (34) or metabolic effects, including hypokalaemia due to K-influx into cells, and hyperglycemia due to increased glyconeolysis (35). These metabolic effects are rarely of clinical significance. However, SABA used at high doses may interact with diuretics to cause hypokalaemia, or increase the likelihood of hyperglycemic episodes in diabetic patients (36). All of these adverse effects decrease in severity after prolonged therapy as desensitization develops.

SABA cause pulmonary vasodilation, which results in increased blood flow to some poorly ventilated areas. The deterioration in ventilation/perfusion matching can result in a temporary reduction in arterial oxygen saturation (37). However, the magnitude of this change is small and so is rarely of clinical significance in the stable state.

C. Clinical Use of SABA

Albuterol was the first β_2-specific bronchodilator to be used for the treatment of asthma. There was initial evidence that regular treatment with this drug over one week improved symptoms and lung function (38). This encouraged clinicians to prescribe albuterol as a regular long-term treatment in order to maximize bronchodilation, and when fenoterol and terbutaline were introduced they were also used in this manner. Fenoterol became widely used in certain countries such as New Zealand. However, it was apparent in the 1970s that its use was associated with an increase in asthma mortality. It is now known that regular treatment with fenoterol increases AHR and so increases exacerbation rates (39). It is now generally accepted that the increase in asthma deaths in New Zealand were due to the inappropriate use of regular SABA, leading to increased AHR, coupled with the under-prescribing of anti-inflammatory medications such as corticosteroids (40). The combination of these factors meant that some patients were at high risk of severe exacerbations. It is also possible that there were cardiac side effects due to fenoterol overuse during these exacerbations. Consequently, fenoterol was withdrawn from the market in New Zealand and there was a subsequent decrease in asthma mortality. This improvement was due to: (i) more appropriate use of SABA "as needed" rather than on a regular basis and (ii) increased prescribing of corticosteroids for anti-inflammatory control.

Clinical trials have subsequently investigated the optimum regime for the long term prescribing of SABA. Large studies have confirmed that regular long-term use of SABA confers no advantages in terms of symptoms and lung function compared to "as needed" use (41,42). Furthermore, the regular use of albuterol provides less bronchoprotection against exercise-induced bronchoconstriction (43), and the effects of inhaled allergen challenges (44,45) compared to "as needed" use. SABA are generally used for the acute relief of symptoms in mild to moderate asthma, rather than continual maintenance therapy. SABA can also be used as prophylaxis against bronchoconstriction in certain situations, e.g., before exercise.

SABA are used for the initial occasional treatment of mild asthma. Persistent symptoms that require regular SABA use indicate the need for the use of regular anti-inflammatory agents, such as corticosteroids. SABA are then used for the treatment of breakthrough symptoms. The frequency of SABA use can be a guide to the effectiveness of anti-inflammatory treatment, e.g., continued regular SABA use indicates inadequate control of airway inflammation. Patients with moderate to severe asthma who remain symptomatic despite maximal anti-inflammatory treatment often require frequent dosing with SABA for symptom control. In such patients, SABA are not only still used "as needed," but are also taken on a regular basis to minimize symptoms.

The choice of drug in clinical practice often depends on the patient's preference and correct use of a particular inhaler device, e.g., terbutaline is available in a turbohaler while albuterol is not. Although inhalers are used by the majority of asthmatics to administer SABA, nebulizers are often prescribed for patients with more severe disease. Typically, nebulizers are charged with the equivalent of 25 or 50 inhaled puffs (2500 or 5000 vs. 100 µg) of SABA. However, the proportion of the administered dose delivered to the lungs from inhalers (using an MDI and spacer) and nebulizers is similar (46). Nevertheless, some patients prefer nebulizers for ease of use and perhaps psychological comfort.

V. Long-Acting β-Agonists

A. Molecular Interactions Between LABA and Corticosteroids

ICS are commonly prescribed for asthmatics with persistent symptoms in order to control inflammation. These drugs bind to the cytoplasmic corticosteroid receptor (GR), which exerts its effects either through (i) interactions with transcription factors, e.g., binding to and hence inactivating NFκB or (ii) translocation to the nucleus and binding to corticosteroid response elements (GREs) in the promotor regions of specific genes, thus increasing mRNA synthesis (47). As LABA are often prescribed in conjunction with ICS, there has been much interest in the possible molecular interactions between these two drugs.

1. *Effects of ICS on β_2-AR function*: the promotor region of the human β_2-AR contains GREs (48). This provides a mechanism for corticosteroids to increase β_2-AR expression, which has been demonstrated in human lungs in vitro (49). Similarly, corticosteroids increase β_2-AR expression in human nasal mucosa in vitro and in vivo (50). It has also been observed that corticosteroids protect against the development of β_2-AR desensitization in mast cells in vitro (51). These findings indicate that ICS may be able to offset the desensitization to LABA after prolonged treatment.
2. *Effects of LABA on GR function*: β-agonists increase protein kinase-A activity, which can result in GR phosphorylation (52). There is also evidence that LABA increase GR nuclear translocation (53). These interactions may result in increased corticosteroid effects. There is in vitro evidence to support the hypothesis that LABA increase corticosteroid effects; the inhibitory effects of corticosteroids on pro-inflammatory cytokine release from perpiheral blood mononuclear cells (54) and smooth muscle cells (55) are enhanced by salmeterol, while this has also been demonstrated for formoterol using epithelial cells (56).

It appears that corticosteroids can reduce LABA desensitization, while LABA can increase corticosteroid effects. These molecular interactions indicate a degree of synergy between these drugs, which may be important clinically.

B. Clinical Effects

Bronchodilation and Bronchoprotection

Formoterol is a more potent bronchodilator than salmeterol in vitro (19). This difference is also evident in vivo (57), as formoterol causes similar bronchodilation compared to salmeterol but at lower doses. Another important difference between these two drugs is the onset of action; formoterol has a faster onset

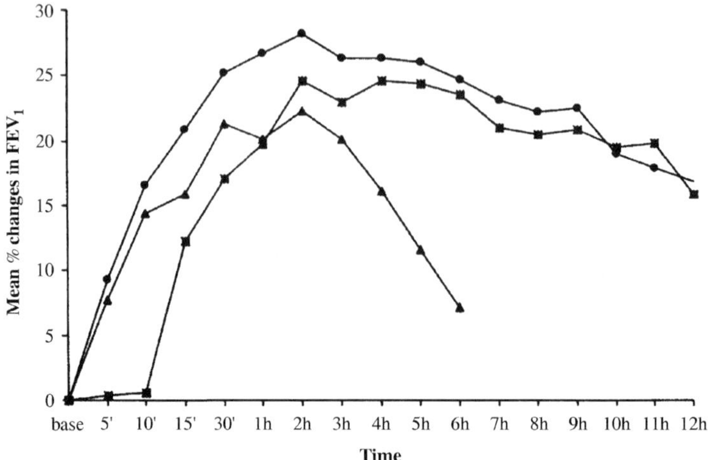

Figure 5   Time course of bronchodilation with short- and long-acting β-agonists. Increase in FEV$_1$ over 12 hours after inhalation of salbutamol 200 μg (*triangles*), salmeterol 50 μg (*squares*) and formoterol 12 μg (*circles*). Formoterol and salbutamol have a faster onset of action compared to salmeterol. The effects of formoterol and salmeterol last for 12 hours. *Source*: From Ref. 27.

with significant smooth muscle relaxation occurring within five minutes (Fig. 5). Using the doses commonly prescribed in clinical practice, the duration of bronchodilation for a single dose of salmeterol or formoterol is similar with therapeutic effects lasting for approximately 12 hours (27,58,59).

LABA protect against bronchoconstricting stimuli such as methacholine, histamine, and AMP (20,32,60–62). For salmeterol, maximal bronchoprotection is achieved after a single dose of 50 μg (20), and increasing the dose further provides no extra bronchoprotection (Fig. 6). A similar level of bronchoprotection is observed after a single 12 μg formoterol dose, but unlike salmeterol, further increases in the dose of formoterol result in greater bronchoprotection. This difference in dose–responsiveness is attributable to the pharmacological differences between the two drugs in their interactions with the β$_2$-AR.

LABA and β$_2$-AR Tolerance

Regular LABA therapy may cause β$_2$-AR desensitization. This effect may manifest as a reduction in bronchodilation or bronchoprotection.

Bronchodilator Tolerance

Studies of regular LABA use for up to one year in duration have shown no deterioration in pulmonary function (58,63,64). This suggests that bronchodilator tolerance during regular LABA therapy is not an important clinical

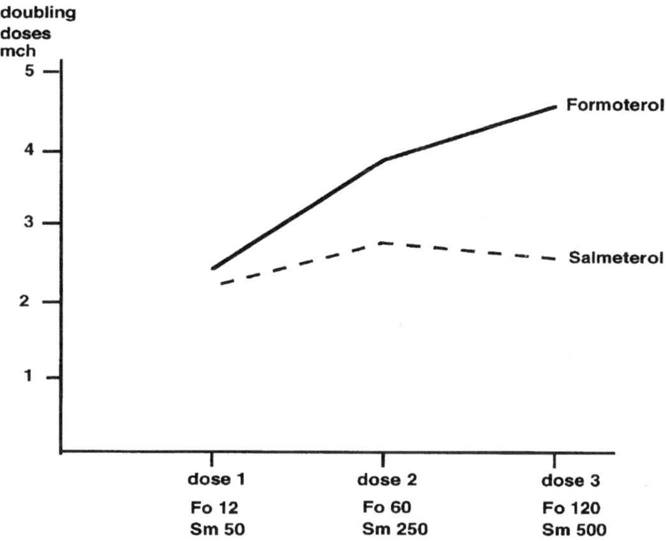

Figure 6 Dose–response effect of formoterol (Fo) and salmeterol (Sm) on PD_{20} methacholine. There was no difference between Fo 12 µg and Sm 50 µg ($p = 0.70$). Higher Fo doses increased PD_{20} values, while there was no change with higher Sm doses. Significant differences between doses two and three in bronchoprotection were observed ($p < 0.01$). *Source*: From Ref. 20.

issue. However, studies assessing tolerance to the effects of a SABA during regular LABA therapy have produced conflicting results. The bronchodilator response to cumulative doses of albuterol were found to be reduced at 36 hours after stopping salmeterol (65) and at 24 hours after stopping formoterol (66). The acute bronchodilator effects of formoterol, itself administered in a cumulative dosing regime, are also reduced after regular dosing with formoterol (67,68). In contrast, other studies have not found the bronchodilator response to albuterol to be blunted during regular LABA therapy (69–71). These studies have been criticized for an inadequate LABA washout period before the assessment of the albuterol response, i.e., the albuterol response was assessed within 12 hours of the last dose of LABA, which would increase the prealbuterol FEV_1, making it difficult to study the bronchodilator response (66). However, it is clear that assessing albuterol within 12 hours of a dose of LABA more accurately simulates the use of SABA in clinical practice. Taken together, these data make it likely that bronchodilator tolerance during regular LABA use is of limited clinical importance.

Tolerance to Bronchoprotection

Regular LABA treatment can reduce the degree of bronchoprotection without a decrease in bronchodilation. For example, salmeterol causes a 10-fold increase in methacholine PC_{20} on the first day of treatment, but this declines to a twofold increase at four and eight weeks despite no change in bronchodilator effect (72). This reduction in bronchoprotection against methacholine can be observed after just two doses of salmeterol (73), and occurs irrespective of the concurrent administration of standard doses of ICS (60,74). Similar loss of bronchoprotection is also observed with salmeterol in AMP (75) and exercise challenge models (76,77), and salmeterol can also reduce the bronchoprotective effect of albuterol (60,74).

Formoterol, in doses ranging from 6 to 24 µg twice daily given to asthma patients already receiving ICS, protects against methacholine-induced bronchoconstriction after the first dose. However, the magnitude of bronchoprotection is significantly reduced after both one and two weeks of treatment (32). The degree of protection afforded by formoterol against AMP is also reduced after one week (78–80).

It is clear that tolerance to bronchoprotection can occur soon after the onset of treatment with either formoterol or salmeterol. An important issue is whether tolerance causes a complete loss of bronchoprotection after prolonged dosing. Larger studies have assessed long-term trends in bronchoprotection loss, and have reassuringly demonstrated that there is still residual bronchoprotection up to 24 weeks (81–83).

Corticosteroid Reversal of LABA Tolerance

Corticosteroids can reverse β_2-AR desensitization, but this effect varies with the route of administration and the dose used. For systemic corticosteroids, it has been demonstrated that high doses completely reverse desensitization (84), but that lower doses cause partial reversal only (66). For high doses of ICS, the degree of reversal may differ for bronchodilation and bronchoprotection. For example, after regular treatment with formoterol, a single budesonide dose of 1600 µg causes partial reversal of tolerance to the albuterol bronchodilator response (66), but complete reversal of bronchoprotection against AMP (78). It should be noted that while high doses of systemic or inhaled corticosteroids can reverse desensitization, conventional ICS doses do not prevent the development of desensitization (60,74).

Anti-inflammatory Effects

Although LABA are used primarily to cause smooth muscle relaxation, in vitro studies have demonstrated that these drugs also have anti-inflammatory effects (85). The potential for LABA to cause airway anti-inflammatory effects in vivo has therefore also been assessed, and the findings of the key studies are summarized in Table 1. Some of these studies have provided conflicting results, due to a variety of factors, including small sample sizes, differences in the severity of disease in the patients studied and the use of different analytical techniques to evaluate samples.

Table 1 Bronchoscopy Studies That Have Investigated the Anti-inflammatory Effects of Salmeterol or Formoterol

Author year	ICS given with LABA	BAL	Mucosal biospy	LABA anti-inflammatory effects
Salmeterol				
Gardiner, 1994	Yes	Yes	No	None
Li, 1999	Yes	Yes	Yes	Decreased eosinophils (biopsy only)
Roberts, 1999	No	Yes	Yes	None
Jeffrey, 2002	No	Yes	Yes	Decreased neutrophils (BAL and biopsy)
Lindqvist, 2003	No	No	Yes	None
Reid, 2003	Yes	Yes	No	Decreased IL-8
Wallin, 2003	Yes	Yes	Yes	Decreased mast cells (biopsy only)
Formoterol				
Wallin, 1999	No	No	Yes	Decreased eosinophils and mast cells
Wilson, 2001	No	No	Yes	Decreased eosinophils

Abbreviation: BAL, bronchoalveolar lavage.

While it has been reported that salmeterol has no effect on airway inflammation (86–88), there is conflicting evidence that this LABA has an antineutrophil effect (89,90). Formoterol, administered without ICS, appears to exert anti-eosinophil effects (91,92). Clinically it is most relevant to study anti-inflammatory effects when LABA and ICS are administered together. In such patients it has been observed that salmeterol added to ICS causes a reduction in mucosal eosinophils (93) and mast cell levels (94). Furthermore, the addition of salmeterol to ICS reduces submucosal angiogenesis (95), suggesting that combination LABA and ICS treatment decreases the degree of airway remodeling in asthma. Further studies are needed to confirm the synergistic anti-inflammatory effects of LABA and ICS in vivo.

Systemic Effects

Formoterol and salmeterol have the capacity to cause side effects due to systemic absorption. In healthy subjects both of these drugs cause dose-dependent increases in heart rate and blood pressure and decreases in plasma glucose and potassium (96). Cardiac monitoring of asthmatic patients reassuringly shows that LABA do not cause clinically significant cardiac events (97,98). The known pharmacological differences between formoterol and salmeterol in their bronchodilator properties is also observed in their systemic effect profiles, i.e., formoterol is more potent and tends to have a faster onset while the duration is longer for salmeterol (96). The duration of systemic effects with LABA is similar to that observed with SABA (35,99). The prolonged bronchodilator effects of LABA relative to their systemic side effects increases their therapeutic index compared to SABA, which have a similar duration for therapeutic and systemic effects. LABA also cause other predictable β-receptor mediated side effects, similar to those observed with SABA, e.g., tremor (97).

C. Clinical Use in Adults

Addition of LABA to ICS Therapy

Inhaled corticosteroids are established as the most effective initial anti-inflammatory treatment for asthmatics with persistent symptoms. The use of LABA monotherapy instead in such patients leads to a loss of asthma control, e.g., there is increased airway inflammation and exacerbation rates for patients treated with salmeterol monotherapy compared to ICS mono-therapy (100). An alternative strategy is to use LABA as an additional therapy in patients who are symptomatic despite taking ICS. Additional LABA therapy in this context has been shown to improve lung function and reduce exacerbations (58,101,102). Before the introduction of LABA, it was common for the dose of ICS to be increased in such patients. However, this can have disappointing results as the dose–response curve for these drugs is relatively flat for the linear segment (103). Using LABA as additional therapy offers advantages over increasing the dose of ICS; LABA provide an alternative mechanism of action (sustained smooth muscle relaxation), which can improve symptoms, and may also allow increased ICS delivery to the peripheral airways. Furthermore, it is possible that LABA and corticosteroids have synergistic anti-inflammatory effects in vivo.

The value of adding a LABA instead of increasing the ICS dose has been investigated in several landmark clinical studies. Greening and coworkers studied 429 mild-asthmatic patients who had persistent symptoms after a run-in period on beclomethasone dipropionate (BDP) 400 µg/day (104). Patients were randomized to receive either an increased steroid dose (1000 µg/day), or the addition of salmeterol (100 µg/day) for six months. While lung function, use of relief medication, and symptoms improved in both groups, the salmeterol group demonstrated the greatest improvements (Fig. 7). A similar study by Woolcock and coworkers (105) involved more severe asthma patients who were symptomatic while being treated with

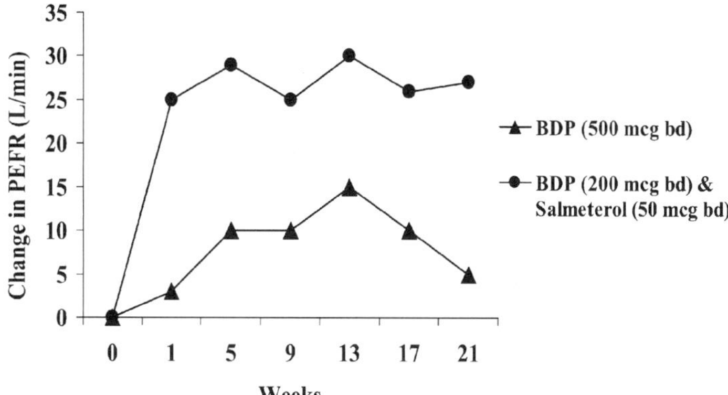

Figure 7 Significant improvements in lung function in asthma patients taking salmeterol with inhaled beclomethasone dipropionate (BDP) compared to doubling the BDP dose without salmeterol. *Source*: From Ref. 104.

BDP 1000 μg/day. Subjects were randomized to one of three treatment arms: addition of salmeterol 100 μg/day, addition of salmeterol 200 μg/day, or a doubling of BDP to 2000 μg/day. Again, the groups receiving LABA therapy had significantly greater improvements in lung function, relief medication use, and symptoms. There was no difference between the effects of the two doses of salmeterol used, as these two salmeterol doses are at the top of the dose–response curve for bronchodilator and bronchoprotective effects (20,97).

The introduction of long-term regular treatment with LABA raised concerns about the possible loss of asthma control in some patients. The basis for this concern was that LABA improve symptoms, which may lead to inadequate doses of ICS being prescribed to control airway inflammation. This has been called "masking" of airway inflammation, and assumes that the effect of LABA is purely bronchodilator in nature, with no synergistic anti-inflammatory activity in conjunction with ICS. This possibility has been investigated during ICS reduction in severe asthmatics; the addition of salmeterol improved lung function and ICS reduction faster compared to placebo, but this was associated with increased sputum eosinophilia (106). However, this phenomenon was not observed in a study involving the reduction of budesonide 1600 to 800 μg daily or 200 μg daily plus formoterol (107). Lung function improved in the formoterol group and overall clinical asthma control and sputum eosinophilia did not differ between the groups. Biopsy studies have also reassuringly demonstrated that LABA therapy in conjunction with ICS does not predispose to worsening airway inflammation (87,94).

The benefits of add-on LABA therapy on asthma control was further investigated in two important studies using formoterol. First, the FACET study investigated the effect of formoterol add-on therapy on exacerbation rates over 12 months (108). The length of this study allowed exacerbation rates to be properly investigated. Symptomatic moderate asthmatics were given budesonide 1600 µg/day for a four-week run-in period, and then randomized to one of four treatments: (i) budesonide 200 µg/day, (ii) budesonide 200 µg and formoterol 18 µg/day, (iii) budesonide 800 µg/day plus placebo, or (iv) budesonide 800 µg and formoterol 18 µg/day. First, the addition of formoterol to either dose of budesonide reduced severe exacerbation rates, and second, the budesonide 800 µg/day group had less severe exacerbations than the budesonide 200 µg/day group (Fig. 8). Lung function over the 12 months showed the greatest improvements in the groups taking both ICS and formoterol, with the greatest increase observed in the budesonide 800 µg/day plus formoterol group. In summary, this study showed that the addition of formoterol to either a low- or medium-ICS dose reduced exacerbations in moderate asthmatics. Optimum control in these patients was achieved with the use of formoterol *plus* the higher dose of ICS.

A second study assessed the use of add-on formoterol therapy in asthmatics with milder disease taking budesonide 200 µg/day (64). The addition of formoterol improved control with fewer exacerbations compared to doubling the ICS dose, but again the maximal reduction in exacerbations was achieved by doubling the dose of budesonide *and* adding in formoterol. A meta-analysis of the use of salmeterol in mild to moderate asthma has

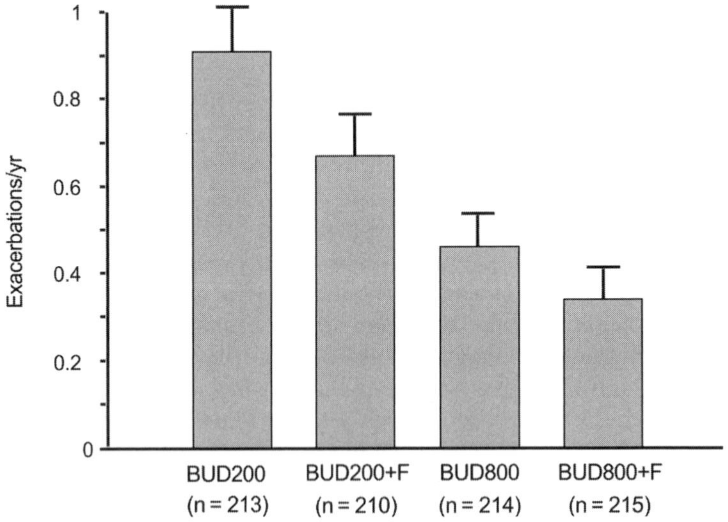

Figure 8 FACET study. Severe exacerbation rates in asthma patients treated with budesonide (200 or 800 µg/day) with and without formoterol for one year. Increasing the budesonide dose and using formoterol both significantly reduced exacerbations ($p < 0.05$). *Source*: From Ref. 108.

confirmed that the introduction of this LABA instead of doubling the ICS dose also reduces exacerbations (109). These studies have changed the use of LABA in asthma; after establishing symptomatic patients on ICS, the next step in pharmacotherapy is now the addition of LABA rather than doubling the dose of ICS.

The Optima study (64) was the first to provide information on the potential benefits in mild asthma in addition to low-dose ICS. This has been further investigated in recent studies; the addition of salmeterol to 200 μg fluticasone propionate per day in comparison to doubling the dose of ICS provides (i) a greater benefit to lung function and symptoms (110,111) (ii) a long-term steroid-sparing effect (112), and (iii) a reduction in exacerbation rates (113). Similarly, the addition of formoterol to budesonide 160 μg/day causes a greater increase in lung function and a reduction in exacerbations compared to doubling the ICS dose (114). While ICS at low doses improve AHR in mild asthma, there may be little effect on pulmonary function (115). The superior clinical effects of combined low-dose ICS/LABA in these patients is due both to a greater improvement in AHR and an increase in pulmonary function. It is interesting to speculate that combined low-dose ICS/LABA may ultimately prove to be the best form of initial pharmacotherapy for patients with symptomatic, persistent asthma. There is evidence of superiority in lung function and symptoms for this approach compared to ICS alone (116), although further studies are required to confirm the potential benefits of this strategy.

LABA Used "As Needed"

The fast onset of action of formoterol (similar to SABA) (27) has led to its use as an "as needed" reliever medication, with the advantage of a long duration of action. Salmeterol, with its slow onset of action, cannot be used for this purpose. Furthermore, formoterol has better dose–response properties than salmeterol, which may be important during repeated dosing when cumulative therapeutic effects may be of clinical benefit.

It is important to consider the safety profile of formoterol as an "as needed" medication, since this may involve cumulative doses that are greater than those given during regular dosing (the maximum dose of formoterol is usually 24 μg as a single dose). The systemic effects of formoterol at higher doses (cumulative doses up to 90 μg) appear to be of similar duration and no worse than for SABA (117).

In a study in asthmatics needing significant SABA therapy (over three inhalations per day) despite regular ICS use, patients randomized to use formoterol "as needed" had fewer severe exacerbations and an improved quality of life score compared to terbutaline (101). Formoterol is also safe and effective when used "as needed" in addition to ICS and regular LABA therapy twice daily (118). The practical advantage of using fewer inhalers, coupled with the long duration of action compared to SABA, may lead to increased usage of formoterol for "as needed" symptom relief in the future. However, data in the context of clinical trials need to be replicated in everyday clinical practice, as there is a potential for patients to take too much formoterol unless appropriately instructed.

Formoterol may also be a useful treatment for acute asthma in the emergency room. High-dose SABA have traditionally been the mainstay of initial bronchodilator treatment in this setting, with inhaled anticholinergics used either concurrently or as second-line treatment. However, formoterol 15 µg repeated to a cumulative dose of 90 µg over three hours produces similar improvements in lung function compared to inhaled terbutaline in acute severe asthma, and has a similar safety profile (119). Additionally, formoterol (cumulative dose 54 µg over one hour) caused a greater increase in lung function than albuterol (cumulative dose 2400 µg), albeit with a greater decrease in serum potassium levels (120). Although these studies suggest that formoterol is potentially an effective bronchodilator for acute severe asthma, further large studies are needed to define the patient group that would respond best to treatment with formoterol, and the doses that can be safely and effectively prescribed.

Single-Inhaler LABA and Corticosteroid Therapy

The increased use of LABA in conjunction with ICS has led to the introduction of "combination" inhalers containing both of these drugs. The currently licensed formulations are salmeterol combined with fluticasone propionate and formoterol with budesonide. There are predictable differences in the onset of bronchodilation of these combination therapies due to the pharmacological properties of the LABA components, i.e., the budesonide/formoterol combination has a faster onset than the fluticasone proprionate/salmeterol combination (121). Combination inhalers provide better asthma control compared to using either the LABA or the ICS component alone. This has been demonstrated for salmeterol across a range of fluticasone doses from 200 to 1000 µg/day (122–124). In symptomatic patients already treated with ICS, the introduction of a LABA using individual component inhalers is known to be a more effective strategy for increasing lung function and reducing exacerbations compared to doubling the dose of ICS (64,104,105,108,109). Using a combination inhaler for LABA introduction provides similar results (114,125). In addition, combination formulations may have greater pharmacological effects compared to the individual components given in separate inhalers, which may be due to "codeposition" in the lungs, thus increasing synergistic effects (126). There are also practical advantages for patients using combination treatments. First, patients receiving long-term treatment may prefer to take one rather than two inhalers. This may explain why fewer patients who were taking a combination inhaler withdrew from a six-month study compared to those taking the individual components (127). Second, combination inhalers improve compliance by ensuring that patients take both medications rather than just the LABA component.

During an exacerbation of asthma, treatment should be intensified. However, there is frequently a delay in the initiation of additional treatment, as many patients seek medical consultation before changing their therapy. The effectiveness of early self-management during an exacerbation using written action plans has been assessed using the budesonide/formoterol combination. The formoterol component allows flexibility in the dosing regime and a rapid onset of bronchodilation. Furthermore, the molecular interactions of ICS and LABA may increase anti-inflammatory activity. Early self-management using an adjustable dosing regime reduces exacerbations compared to fixed dosing LABA/ICS regimes (128,129). The successful implementation of this strategy in clinical practice will depend on adequate patient education, so that patients are able to confidently and effectively vary their own treatment as required.

D. Clinical Use in Children

LABA are known to have similar bronchodilator and bronchoprotective effects in children (130,131) compared to adults. The key issue in clinical practice is whether they should be used in the same way as in adults. It is no surprise that just as in adults LABA alone are less effective than low doses of ICS for the long-term control of asthma in children (132,133). Interest has therefore focused on the potential benefits of the addition of LABA to ICS regimes in children. In mild-asthmatic children, the addition of salmeterol to ICS improves lung function (134). Similar findings have been demonstrated for children with more severe asthma taking higher ICS doses (135). These results provided the impetus for a similar study design to those conducted in adults, i.e., a comparison of adding in a LABA to doubling the dose of ICS (136). Children with moderate asthma (mean FEV_1 86% at entry) were randomized to receive either BDP 400 µg/day, BDP 400 µg/day plus salmeterol, or BDP 800 µg/day for one year. Lung function improved in all three groups, with no difference among the groups at one year. Importantly, there was no difference among these three groups in terms of exacerbations. Further studies in children with different asthma severities are needed to ascertain whether add-on LABA or increasing steroid dosage is the more effective strategy.

The potential benefits of LABA and ICS delivered through a single-inhaler device has also been assessed; it has been demonstrated that BDP 160 per day plus formoterol improves lung function to a greater degree than BDP alone (137). This indicates that for children taking low doses of ICS, the addition of a LABA through a combination inhaler device is an effective and practical option.

VI. Influence of Genotype on β_2-Agonist Effects

ADRB2 is the gene that codes for the β_2-AR. This is a single exon on chromosome-5 with several single base polymorphisms, of which two have been associated with altered clinical outcomes: the substitution of (i) glycine for arginine at position 16 (gly-16 and arg-16, respectively) and (ii) glutamic acid for glutamine at position 27 (glu-27 and gln-27, respectively). Lung tissue has been used in vitro to investigate the role of these genotypes, but conflicting results have been published. For example, it has been reported that the gly-16 genotype is associated with increased β_2-AR desensitization (138,139), but those findings have not been reproduced by other investigators (140). Similarly, the glu-27 genotype has been reported both to protect against desensitization (138,139) and to increase desensitization (141). These differences may be explained by differences in the cell culture and experimental techniques used. Additionally, the possible influence of ADRB2 haplotypes (the combination of alleles at two different sites) on β_2-AR function may have been important.

The importance of these genotypes has been assessed in asthma in vivo. The gly-16 genotype is associated with a reduced bronchodilator response both in children (142) and adults (143). It has been proposed that these findings are due to excessive "endogenous" β_2-AR down-regulation in subjects with the gly-16 genotype, so that inhaled β-agonists have less effect (144). Tan et al. (84) demonstrated that the gly-16 genotype is associated with increased bronchodilator tolerance after regular dosing with formoterol (145). However, the sample size was small, with only four homozygous arg-16 subjects. These findings were not replicated using salmeterol in a placebo-controlled crossover study involving 20 subjects: 10 glu-16 homozygotes and 10 arg-16 homozygotes (146). There was no influence of genotype on bronchodilator response or bronchoprotection after two-weeks treatment. A lack of association between genotype (either at position 16 or 27) and the degree of bronchoprotection was also observed after a single dose of formoterol (147). However, a larger retrospective analysis suggests that the arg-16 genotype is associated with reduced bronchoprotection. Furthermore, in patients with the arg-16 genotype this effect appears to be greater for formoterol compared to salmeterol (61). The conflicting results of these studies can be explained by small sample sizes, differing study designs, and possible haplotype influences. Nevertheless, the existing data suggests that the gly-16 genotype is associated with reduced bronchodilator response, while the arg-16 genotype is associated with reduced bronchoprotection.

The most important issue in clinical practice is the influence of genotypes on long-term asthma control. A retrospective analysis by Taylor et al. (148) demonstrated that in 108 patients being treated with regular ICS and albuterol, only homozygous arg-16 subjects were predisposed to increased

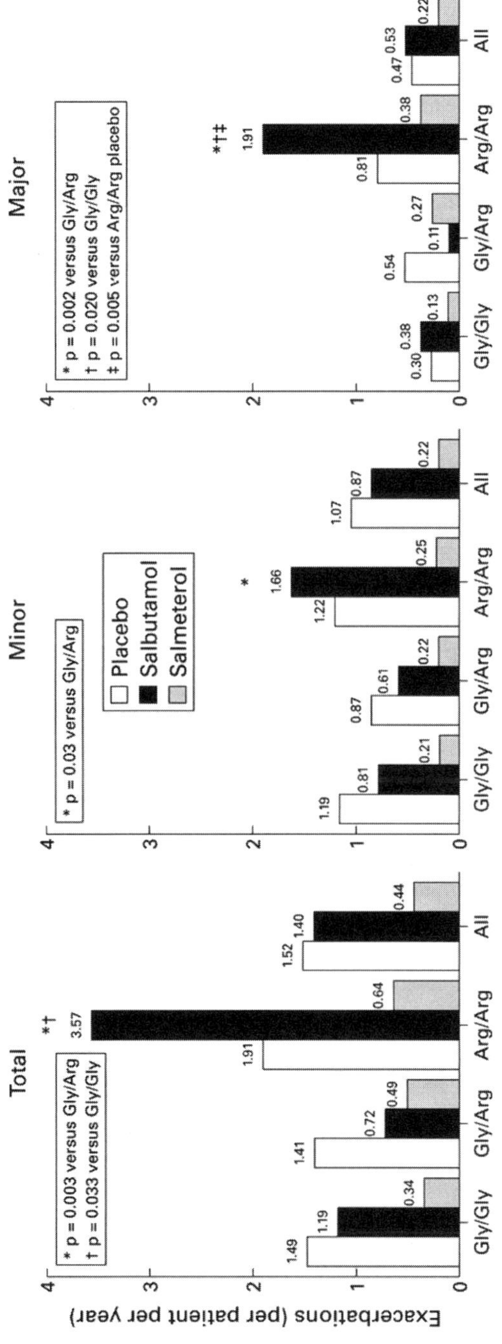

Figure 9 The effect of genotype on exacerbation rates during regular dosing for 24 weeks with salbutamol or salmeterol. Increased exacerbation rates were observed in arg-16 homozygous subjects during regular salbutamol therapy. *Source:* From Ref. 148.

exacerbation rates (Fig. 9). In contrast, there was no difference between genotypes when the same patients were given salmeterol instead of albuterol. A retrospective analysis of 190 patients randomized to receive albuterol regularly or as needed found that there was a decline in lung function, presumably due to desensitization, only in arg-16 homozygotes who took regular treatment (149). This study included genotype assessment of positions 16 and 27, giving nine potential haplotypes. Thus, although the overall study size was large, the number of patients with each haplotype was relatively small. It is clear that further larger studies, preferably prospective in design, are needed to address genotype and haplotype influences on clinical outcomes such as exacerbation rates during long-term β-agonist therapy.

VII. Conclusions

The place of SABA in the symptomatic control of asthma is well established. In contrast, our use of LABA is changing as new insights are gained into mechanisms of action and clinical effects, particularly when used in combination with ICS. The use of LABA and ICS in a single combination inhaler device is increasing, as this is an effective and practical option for patients. The two currently used LABA (formoterol and salmeterol) have different pharmacological properties, which contribute to differences in clinical effects. The pharmaceutical industry is currently developing novel LABA. The pharmacological and clinical profiles of these agents will be of considerable interest.

Abbreviations

AMP	Adenosine monophosphate
BDP	Beclomethasone dipropionate
β_2-AR	β_2-Adrenoreceptor
GR	Glucocorticoid receptor
GRE	Glucocorticoid response element
ICS	Inhaled corticosteroid
LABA	Long-acting β-agonist
SABA	Short-acting β-agonist

References

1. Carstairs JR, Nimmo AJ, Barnes PJ. Autoradiographic visualization of beta-adrenoceptor subtypes in human lung. Am Rev Respir Dis 1985; 132: 541–547.

2. Spina D, Rigby PJ, Paterson JW, Goldie RG. Autoradiographic localization of beta-adrenoceptors in asthmatic human lung. Am Rev Respir Dis 1989; 140:1410–1415.

3. Johnson M. The beta-adrenoceptor. Am J Respir Crit Care Med 1998; 158:S146–S153.

4. Strader CD, Candelore MR, Hill WS, Sigal IS, Dixon RA. Identification of two serine residues involved in agonist activation of the beta-adrenergic receptor. J Biol Chem 1989; 264:13572–13578.

5. Strader CD, Sigal IS, Candelore MR, Rands E, Hill WS, Dixon RA. Conserved aspartic acid residues 79 and 113 of the beta-adrenergic receptor have different roles in receptor function. J Biol Chem 1988; 263: 10267–10271.

6. Dessauer CW, Posner BA, Gilman AG. Visualizing signal transduction: receptors, G-proteins, and adenylate cyclases. Clin Sci (Lond) 1996; 91:527–537.

7. Chiu P, Cook SJ, Small RC, Berry JL, Carpenter JR, Downing SJ, Foster RW, Miller AJ, Small AM. Beta-adrenoceptor subtypes and the opening of plasmalemmal K(+)-channels in bovine trachealis muscle: studies of mechanical activity and ion fluxes. Br J Pharmacol 1993; 109:1149–1156.

8. Onaran HO, Costa T, Rodbard D. Beta gamma subunits of guanine nucleotide-binding proteins and regulation of spontaneous receptor activity: thermodynamic model for the interaction between receptors and guanine nucleotide-binding protein subunits. Mol Pharmacol 1993; 43:245–256.

9. Liggett SB. Update on current concepts of the molecular basis of beta2-adrenergic receptor signaling. J Allergy Clin Immunol 2002; 110:S223–S227.

10. Krupnick JG, Benovic JL. The role of receptor kinases and arrestins in G protein-coupled receptor regulation. Annu Rev Pharmacol Toxicol 1998; 38:289–319.

11. Ferguson SS. Evolving concepts in G protein-coupled receptor endocytosis: the role in receptor desensitization and signaling. Pharmacol Rev 2001; 53:1–24.

12. Hadcock JR, Malbon CC. Down-regulation of beta-adrenergic receptors: agonist-induced reduction in receptor mRNA levels. Proc Natl Acad Sci USA 1988; 85:5021–5025.

13. McGraw DW, Liggett SB. Heterogeneity in beta-adrenergic receptor kinase expression in the lung accounts for cell-specific desensitization of the beta2-adrenergic receptor. J Biol Chem 1997; 272:7338–7344.

14. Anderson GP, Linden A, Rabe KF. Why are long-acting beta-adrenoceptor agonists long-acting? Eur Respir J 1994; 7:569–578.

15. Anderson GP. Formoterol: pharmacology, molecular basis of agonism, and mechanism of long duration of a highly potent and selective beta 2-adrenoceptor agonist bronchodilator. Life Sci 1993; 52:2145–2160.

16. Johnson M, Butchers PR, Coleman RA, Nials AT, Strong P, Sumner MJ, Vardey CJ, Whelan CJ. The pharmacology of salmeterol. Life Sci 1993; 52: 2131–2143.

17. Kips JC, Pauwels RA. Long-acting inhaled beta(2)-agonist therapy in asthma. Am J Respir Crit Care Med 2001; 164:923–932.

18. Green SA, Spasoff AP, Coleman RA, Johnson M, Liggett SB. Sustained activation of a G protein-coupled receptor via "anchored" agonist binding.

Molecular localization of the salmeterol exosite within the 2-adrenergic receptor. J Biol Chem 1996; 271:24029–24035.

19. Naline E, Zhang Y, Qian Y, Mairon N, Anderson GP, Grandordy B, Advenier C. Relaxant effects and durations of action of formoterol and salmeterol on the isolated human bronchus. Eur Respir J 1994; 7:914–920.

20. Palmqvist M, Ibsen T, Mellen A, Lotvall J. Comparison of the relative efficacy of formoterol and salmeterol in asthmatic patients. Am J Respir Crit Care Med 1999; 160:244–249.

21. Bennett JA, Harrison TW, Tattersfield AE. The contribution of the swallowed fraction of an inhaled dose of salmeterol to it systemic effects. Eur Respir J 1999; 13:445–448.

22. Borgstrom L, Nilsson M. A method for determination of the absolute pulmonary bioavailability of inhaled drugs: terbutaline. Pharm Res 1990; 7: 1068–1070.

23. Lecaillon JB, Kaiser G, Palmisano M, Morgan J, Della CG. Pharmacokinetics and tolerability of formoterol in healthy volunteers after a single high dose of Foradil dry powder inhalation via Aerolizer. Eur J Clin Pharmacol 1999; 55:131–138.

24. Newnham DM, McDevitt DG, Lipworth BJ. Comparison of the extrapulmonary beta2-adrenoceptor responses and pharmacokinetics of salbutamol given by standard metered dose-inhaler and modified actuator device. Br J Clin Pharmacol 1993; 36:445–450.

25. Boulton DW, Fawcett JP. Beta2-agonist eutomers: a rational option for the treatment of asthma? Am J Respir Med 2002; 1(5):305–311.

26. Nelson HS, Bensch G, Pleskow WW, DiSantostefano R, DeGraw S, Reasner DS, Rollins TE, Rubin PD. Improved bronchodilation with levalbuterol compared with racemic albuterol in patients with asthma. J Allergy Clin Immunol 1998; 102:943–952.

27. Grembiale RD, Pelaia G, Naty S, Vatrella A, Tranfa CM, Marsico SA. Comparison of the bronchodilating effects of inhaled formoterol, salmeterol and salbutamol in asthmatic patients. Pulm Pharmacol Ther 2002; 15:463–466.

28. Bleecker ER, Tinkelman DG, Ramsdell J, Ekholm BP, Klinger NM, Colice GL, Slade HB. Proventil HFA provides bronchodilation comparable to ventolin over 12 weeks of regular use in asthmatics. Chest 1998; 113:283–289.

29. Creticos PS, Adams WP, Petty BG, Lewis LD, Singh GJ, Khattignavong AP, Molzon JA, Martinez MN, Lietman PS, Williams RL. A methacholine challenge dose–response study for development of a pharmacodynamic bioequivalence methodology for albuterol metered-dose inhalers. J Allergy Clin Immunol 2002; 110:713–720.

30. Taylor DA, Jensen MW, Aikman SL, Harris JG, Barnes PJ, O'Connor BJ. Comparison of salmeterol and albuterol-induced bronchoprotection against adenosine monophosphate and histamine in mild asthma. Am J Respir Crit Care Med 1997; 156:1731–1737.

31. O'Connor BJ, Aikman SL, Barnes PJ. Tolerance to the nonbronchodilator effects of inhaled beta 2-agonists in asthma. N Engl J Med 1992; 327: 1204–1208.

32. Lipworth B, Tan S, Devlin M, Aiken T, Baker R, Hendrick D. Effects of treatment with formoterol on bronchoprotection against methacholine. Am J Med 1998; 104:431–438.

33. Wong CS, Pavord ID, Williams J, Britton JR, Tattersfield AE. Bronchodilator, cardiovascular, and hypokalaemic effects of fenoterol, salbutamol, and terbutaline in asthma. Lancet 1990; 336:1396–1399.

34. Lotvall J, Lunde H, Svedmyr N. Onset of bronchodilation and finger tremor induced by salmeterol and salbutamol in asthmatic patients. Can Respir J 1998; 5:191–194.

35. Bennett JA, Tattersfield AE. Time course and relative dose potency of systemic effects from salmeterol and salbutamol in healthy subjects. Thorax 1997; 52:458–464.

36. Leslie D, Coats PM. Salbutamol-induced diabetic ketoacidosis. Br Med J 1977; 2:768.

37. Williams AJ, Weiner C, Reiff D, Swenson ER, Fuller RW, Hughes JM. Comparison of the effect of inhaled selective and non-selective adrenergic agonists on cardiorespiratory parameters in chronic stable asthma. Pulm Pharmacol 1994; 7:235–241.

38. Shepherd GL, Hetzel MR, Clark TJ. Regular versus symptomatic aerosol bronchodilator treatment of asthma. Br J Dis Chest 1981; 75:215–217.

39. Taylor DR, Sears MR, Herbison GP, Flannery EM, Print CG, Lake DC, Yates DM, Lucas MK, Li Q. Regular inhaled beta agonist in asthma: effects on exacerbations and lung function. Thorax 1993; 48:134–138.

40. Sears MR. The evolution of beta2-agonists. Respir Med 2001; 95:S2–S6.

41. Dennis SM, Sharp SJ, Vickers MR, Frost CD, Crompton GK, Barnes PJ, Lee TH. Regular inhaled salbutamol and asthma control: the TRUST randomised trial. Therapy working group of the national asthma task force and the MRC general practice research framework. Lancet 2000; 355:1675–1679.

42. Drazen JM, Israel E, Boushey HA, Chinchilli VM, Fahy JV, Fish JE, Lazarus SC, Lemanske RF, Martin RJ, Peters SP, Sorkness C, Szefler SJ. Comparison of regularly scheduled with as-needed use of albuterol in mild asthma. Asthma Clinical Research Network. N Engl J Med 1996; 335:841–847.

43. Inman MD, O'Byrne PM. The effect of regular inhaled albuterol on exercise-induced bronchoconstriction. Am J Respir Crit Care Med 1996; 153: 65–69.

44. Cockcroft DW, McParland CP, Britto SA, Swystun VA, Rutherford BC. Regular inhaled salbutamol and airway responsiveness to allergen. Lancet 1993; 342:833–837.

45. Cockcroft DW, O'Byrne PM, Swystun VA, Bhagat R. Regular use of inhaled albuterol and the allergen-induced late asthmatic response. J Allergy Clin Immunol 1995; 96:44–49.

46. Labiris NR, Dolovich MB. Pulmonary drug delivery. Part II: the role of inhalant delivery devices and drug formulations in therapeutic effectiveness of aerosolized medications. Br J Clin Pharmacol 2003; 56:600–612.

47. Barnes PJ. Molecular mechanisms of corticosteroids in allergic diseases. Allergy 2001; 56:928–936.

48. Scott MG, Swan C, Wheatley AP, Hall IP. Identification of novel polymorphisms within the promoter region of the human beta2 adrenergic receptor gene. Br J Pharmacol 1999; 126:841–844.

49. Mak JC, Nishikawa M, Barnes PJ. Glucocorticosteroids increase beta 2-adrenergic receptor transcription in human lung. Am J Physiol 1995; 268: L41–L46.

50. Baraniuk JN, Ali M, Brody D, Maniscalco J, Gaumond E, Fitzgerald T, Wong G, Yuta A, Mak JC, Barnes PJ, Bascom R, Troost T. Glucocorticoids induce beta2-adrenergic receptor function in human nasal mucosa. Am J Respir Crit Care Med 1997; 155:704–710.

51. Chong LK, Drury DE, Dummer JF, Ghahramani P, Schleimer RP, Peachell PT. Protection by dexamethasone of the functional desensitization to beta 2-adrenoceptor-mediated responses in human lung mast cells. Br J Pharmacol 1997; 121:717–722.

52. Adcock IM, Maneechotesuwan K, Usmani O. Molecular interactions between glucocorticoids and long-acting beta2-agonists. J Allergy Clin Immunol 2002; 110:S261–S268.

53. Eickelberg O, Roth M, Lorx R, Bruce V, Rudiger J, Johnson M, Block LH. Ligand-independent activation of the glucocorticoid receptor by beta2-adrenergic receptor agonists in primary human lung fibroblasts and vascular smooth muscle cells. J Biol Chem 1999; 274:1005–1010.

54. Oddera S, Silvestri M, Testi R, Rossi GA. Salmeterol enhances the inhibitory activity of dexamethasone on allergen-induced blood mononuclear cell activation. Respiration 1998; 65:199–204.

55. Pang L, Knox AJ. Synergistic inhibition by beta(2)-agonists and corticosteroids on tumor necrosis factor-alpha-induced interleukin-8 release from cultured human airway smooth-muscle cells. Am J Respir Cell Mol Biol 2000; 23:79–85.

56. Korn SH, Jerre A, Brattsand R. Effects of formoterol and budesonide on GM-CSF and IL-8 secretion by triggered human bronchial epithelial cells. Eur Respir J 2001; 17:1070–1077.

57. Palmqvist M, Persson G, Lazer L, Rosenborg J, Larsson P, Lotvall J. Inhaled dry-powder formoterol and salmeterol in asthmatic patients: onset of action, duration of effect and potency. Eur Respir J 1997; 10:2484–2489.

58. Pearlman DS, Chervinsky P, LaForce C, Seltzer JM, Southern DL, Kemp JP, Dockhorn RJ, Grossman J, Liddle RF, Yancey SW. A comparison of salmeterol with albuterol in the treatment of mild-to-moderate asthma. N Engl J Med 1992; 327:1420–1425.

59. Wallin A, Sandstrom T, Rosenhall L, Melander B. Time course and duration of bronchodilatation with formoterol dry powder in patients with stable asthma. Thorax 1993; 48:611–614.

60. Bhagat R, Kalra S, Swystun VA, Cockcroft DW. Rapid onset of tolerance to the bronchoprotective effect of salmeterol. Chest 1995; 108:1235–1239.

61. Lee DK, Currie GP, Hall IP, Lima JJ, Lipworth BJ. The arginine-16 beta2-adrenoceptor polymorphism predisposes to bronchoprotective subsensitivity in patients treated with formoterol and salmeterol. Br J Clin Pharmacol 2004; 57:68–75.

62. Ketchell RI, Jensen MW, Spina D, O'Connor BJ. Dose-related effects of formoterol on airway responsiveness to adenosine 5′-monophosphate and histamine. Eur Respir J 2002; 19:611–616.

63. Lundback B, Rawlinson DW, Palmer JB. Twelve month comparison of salmeterol and salbutamol as dry powder formulations in asthmatic patients. European Study Group. Thorax 1993; 48:148–153.

64. O'Byrne PM, Barnes PJ, Rodriguez-Roisin R, Runnerstrom E, Sandstrom T, Svensson K, Tattersfield A. Low dose inhaled budesonide and formoterol in mild persistent asthma: the OPTIMA randomized trial. Am J Respir Crit Care Med 2001; 164:1392–1397.

65. Grove A, Lipworth BJ. Bronchodilator subsensitivity to salbutamol after twice daily salmeterol in asthmatic patients. Lancet 1995; 346:201–206.

66. Lipworth BJ, Aziz I. Bronchodilator response to albuterol after regular formoterol and effects of acute corticosteroid administration. Chest 2000; 117:156–162.

67. Newnham DM, Grove A, McDevitt DG, Lipworth BJ. Subsensitivity of bronchodilator and systemic beta 2 adrenoceptor responses after regular twice daily treatment with eformoterol dry powder in asthmatic patients. Thorax 1995; 50:497–504.

68. Newnham DM, McDevitt DG, Lipworth BJ. Bronchodilator subsensitivity after chronic dosing with a formoterol in patients with asthma. Am J Med 1994; 97:29–37.

69. Wilding P, Clark M, Thompson CJ, Lewis S, Rushton L, Bennett J, Oborne J, Cooper S, Tattersfield AE. Effect of long-term treatment with salmeterol on asthma control: a double blind, randomised crossover study. BMJ 1997; 314:1441–1446.

70. Nelson HS, Berkowitz RB, Tinkelman DA, Emmett AH, Rickard KA, Yancey SW. Lack of subsensitivity to albuterol after treatment with salmeterol in patients with asthma. Am J Respir Crit Care Med 1999; 159:1556–1561.

71. Arvidsson P, Larsson S, Lofdahl CG, Melander B, Svedmyr N, Wahlander L. Inhaled formoterol during one year in asthma: a comparison with salbutamol. Eur Respir J 1991; 4:1168–1173.

72. Cheung D, Timmers MC, Zwinderman AH, Bel EH, Dijkman JH, Sterk PJ. Long-term effects of a long-acting beta 2-adrenoceptor agonist, salmeterol, on airway hyperresponsiveness in patients with mild asthma. N Engl J Med 1992; 327:1198–1203.

73. Drotar DE, Davis EE, Cockcroft DW. Tolerance to the bronchoprotective effect of salmeterol 12 hours after starting twice daily treatment. Ann Allergy Asthma Immunol 1998; 80:31–34.

74. Kalra S, Swystun VA, Bhagat R, Cockcroft DW. Inhaled corticosteroids do not prevent the development of tolerance to the bronchoprotective effect of salmeterol. Chest 1996; 109:953–956.

75. Wilson AM, Dempsey OJ, Sims EJ, Lipworth BJ. Evaluation of salmeterol or montelukast as second-line therapy for asthma not controlled with inhaled corticosteroids. Chest 2001; 119:1021–1026.

76. Nelson JA, Strauss L, Skowronski M, Ciufo R, Novak R, McFadden ER Jr. Effect of long-term salmeterol treatment on exercise-induced asthma. N Engl J Med 1998; 339:141–146.

77. Ramage L, Lipworth BJ, Ingram CG, Cree IA, Dhillon DP. Reduced protection against exercise induced bronchoconstriction after chronic dosing with salmeterol. Respir Med 1994; 88:363–368.

78. Aziz I, Lipworth BJ. A bolus of inhaled budesonide rapidly reverses airway subsensitivity and beta2-adrenoceptor down-regulation after regular inhaled formoterol. Chest 1999; 115:623–628.

79. Aziz I, Tan KS, Hall IP, Devlin MM, Lipworth BJ. Subsensitivity to bronchoprotection against adenosine monophosphate challenge following regular once-daily formoterol. Eur Respir J 1998; 12:580–584.

80. Sims EJ, Jackson CM, Lipworth BJ. Add-on therapy with montelukast or formoterol in patients with the glycine-16 beta2-receptor genotype. Br J Clin Pharmacol 2003; 56:104–111.

81. Rosenthal RR, Busse WW, Kemp JP, Baker JW, Kalberg C, Emmett A, Rickard KA. Effect of long-term salmeterol therapy compared with as-needed albuterol use on airway hyperresponsiveness. Chest 1999; 116:595–602.

82. Cloosterman SG, Bijl-Hofland ID, van Herwaarden CL, Akkermans RP, van Den Elshout FJ, Folgering HT, van Schayck CP. A placebo-controlled clinical trial of regular monotherapy with short-acting and long-acting beta(2)-agonists in allergic asthmatic patients. Chest 2001; 119:1306–1315.

83. FitzGerald JM, Chapman KR, Della CG, Stubbing D, Fairbarn MS, Till MD, Brambilla R. Sustained bronchoprotection, bronchodilatation, and symptom control during regular formoterol use in asthma of moderate or greater severity. The Canadian FO/OD1 Study Group. J Allergy Clin Immunol 1999; 103: 427–435.

84. Tan KS, Grove A, McLean A, Gnosspelius Y, Hall IP, Lipworth BJ. Systemic corticosteriod rapidly reverses bronchodilator subsensitivity induced by formoterol in asthmatic patients. Am J Respir Crit Care Med 1997; 156: 28–35.

85. Barnes PJ. Scientific rationale for inhaled combination therapy with long-acting beta2-agonists and corticosteroids. Eur Respir J 2002; 19:182–191.

86. Gardiner PV, Ward C, Booth H, Allison A, Hendrick DJ, Walters EH. Effect of eight weeks of treatment with salmeterol on bronchoalveolar lavage inflammatory indices in asthmatics. Am J Respir Crit Care Med 1994; 150:1006– 1111.

87. Lindqvist A, Karjalainen EM, Laitinen LA, Kava T, Altraja A, Pulkkinen M, Halme M, Laitinen A. Salmeterol resolves airway obstruction but does not possess anti-eosinophil efficacy in newly diagnosed asthma: a randomized, double-blind, parallel group biopsy study comparing the effects of salmeterol, fluticasone propionate, and disodium cromoglycate. J Allergy Clin Immunol 2003; 112:23–28.

88. Roberts JA, Bradding P, Britten KM, Walls AF, Wilson S, Gratziou C, Holgate ST, Howarth PH. The long-acting beta2-agonist salmeterol xinafoate: effects on airway inflammation in asthma. Eur Respir J 1999; 14:275–282.

89. Jeffery PK, Venge P, Gizycki MJ, Egerod I, Dahl R, Faurschou P. Effects of salmeterol on mucosal inflammation in asthma: a placebo-controlled study. Eur Respir J 2002; 20:1378–1385.

90. Reid DW, Ward C, Wang N, Zheng L, Bish R, Orsida B, Walters EH. Possible anti-inflammatory effect of salmeterol against interleukin-8 and neutrophil activation in asthma in vivo. Eur Respir J 2003; 21:994–999.
91. Wallin A, Sandstrom T, Soderberg M, Howarth P, Lundback B, Della-Cioppa G, Wilson S, Judd M, Djukanovic R, Holgate S, Lindberg A, Larssen L, Melander B. The effects of regular inhaled formoterol, budesonide, and placebo on mucosal inflammation and clinical indices in mild asthma. Am J Respir Crit Care Med 1999; 159(1):79–86.
92. Wilson SJ, Wallin A, Della-Cioppa G, Sandstrom T, Holgate ST. Effects of budesonide and formoterol on NF-kappaB, adhesion molecules, and cytokines in asthma. Am J Respir Crit Care Med 2001; 164:1047–1052.
93. Li X, Ward C, Thien F, Bish R, Bamford T, Bao X, Bailey M, Wilson JW, Haydn Walters E. An antiinflammatory effect of salmeterol, a long-acting beta(2) agonist, assessed in airway biopsies and bronchoalveolar lavage in asthma. Am J Respir Crit Care Med 1999; 160:1493–1499.
94. Wallin A, Sue-Chu M, Bjermer L, Ward J, Sandstrom T, Lindberg A, Lundback B, Djukanovic R, Holgate S, Wilson S. Effect of inhaled fluticasone with and without salmeterol on airway inflammation in asthma. J Allergy Clin Immunol 2003; 112:72–78.
95. Orsida BE, Ward C, Li X, Bish R, Wilson JW, Thien F, Walters EH. Effect of a long-acting beta2-agonist over three months on airway wall vascular remodeling in asthma. Am J Respir Crit Care Med 2001; 164:117–121.
96. Guhan AR, Cooper S, Oborne J, Lewis S, Bennett J, Tattersfield AE. Systemic effects of formoterol and salmeterol: a dose-response comparison in healthy subjects. Thorax 2000; 55:650–656.
97. Kemp JP, Bierman CW, Cocchetto DM. Dose-response study of inhaled salmeterol in asthmatic patients with 24-hour spirometry and Holter monitoring. Ann Allergy 1993; 70:316–322.
98. Tranfa CM, Pelaia G, Grembiale RD, Naty S, Durante S, Borrello G. Short-term cardiovascular effects of salmeterol. Chest 1998; 113:1272–1276.
99. Rosenborg J, Bengtsson T, Larsson P, Blomgren A, Persson G, Lotvall J. Relative systemic dose potency and tolerability of inhaled formoterol and salbutamol in healthy subjects and asthmatics. Eur J Clin Pharmacol 2000; 56:363–370.
100. Lazarus SC, Boushey HA, Fahy JV, Chinchilli VM, Lemanske RF Jr, Sorkness CA, Kraft M, Fish JE, Peters SP, Craig T, Drazen JM, Ford JG, Israel E, Martin RJ, Mauger EA, Nachman SA, Spahn JD, Szefler SJ. Asthma Clinical Research Network for the National Heart, Lung, and Blood Institute. Long-acting beta2-agonist monotherapy vs continued therapy with inhaled corticosteroids in patients with persistent asthma: a randomized controlled trial. JAMA 2001; 285:2583–2593.
101. Tattersfield AE, Lofdahl CG, Postma DS, Eivindson A, Schreurs AG, Rasidakis A, Ekstrom T. Comparison of formoterol and terbutaline for as-needed treatment of asthma: a randomised trial. Lancet 2001; 357:257–261.
102. van der Molen T, Postma DS, Turner MO, Jong BM, Malo JL, Chapman K, Grossman R, de Graaff CS, Riemersma RA, Sears MR. Effects of the long acting beta agonist formoterol on asthma control in asthmatic patients using

inhaled corticosteroids. The Netherlands and Canadian Formoterol Study Investigators. Thorax 1997; 52:535–539.

103. Barnes PJ. Efficacy of inhaled corticosteroids in asthma. J Allergy Clin Immunol 1998; 102:531–538.

104. Greening AP, Ind PW, Northfield M, Shaw G. Added salmeterol versus higher-dose corticosteroid in asthma patients with symptoms on existing inhaled corticosteroid. Allen & Hanburys Limited UK Study Group. Lancet 1994; 344:219–224.

105. Woolcock A, Lundback B, Ringdal N, Jacques LA. Comparison of addition of salmeterol to inhaled steroids with doubling of the dose of inhaled steroids. Am J Respir Crit Care Med 1996; 153:1481–1488.

106. Mcivor RA, Pizzichini E, Turner MO, Hussack P, Hargreave FE, Sears MR. Potential masking effects of salmeterol on airway inflammation in asthma. Am J Respir Crit Care Med 1998; 158:924–930.

107. Kips JC, O'Connor BJ, Inman MD, Svensson K, Pauwels RA, O'Byrne PM. A long-term study of the antiinflammatory effect of low-dose budesonide plus formoterol versus high-dose budesonide in asthma. Am J Respir Crit Care Med 2000; 161:996–1001.

108. Pauwels RA, Lofdahl CG, Postma DS, Tattersfield AE, O'Byrne P, Barnes PJ, Ullman A. Effect of inhaled formoterol and budesonide on exacerbations of asthma. Formoterol and Corticosteroids Establishing Therapy (FACET). International Study Group. N Engl J Med 1997; 337:1405–1411.

109. Shrewsbury S, Pyke S, Britton M. Meta-analysis of increased dose of inhaled steroid or addition of salmeterol in symptomatic asthma (MIASMA). BMJ 2000; 320:1368–1373.

110. van Noord JA, Schreurs AJ, Mol SJ, Mulder PG. Addition of salmeterol versus doubling the dose of fluticasone propionate in patients with mild to moderate asthma. Thorax 1999; 54:207–212.

111. Condemi JJ, Goldstein S, Kalberg C, Yancey S, Emmett A, Rickard K. The addition of salmeterol to fluticasone propionate versus increasing the dose of fluticasone propionate in patients with persistent asthma. Salmeterol Study Group. Ann Allergy Asthma Immunol 1999; 82:383–389.

112. Matz J, Emmett A, Rickard K, Kalberg C. Addition of salmeterol to low-dose fluticasone versus higher-dose fluticasone: an analysis of asthma exacerbations. J Allergy Clin Immunol 2001; 107:783–789.

113. Busse W, Koenig SM, Oppenheimer J, Sahn SA, Yancey SW, Reilly D, Edwards LD, Dorinsky PM. Steroid-sparing effects of fluticasone propionate 100 microg and salmeterol 50 microg administered twice daily in a single product in patients previously controlled with fluticasone propionate 250 microg administered twice daily. J Allergy Clin Immunol 2003; 111:57–65.

114. Lalloo UG, Malolepszy J, Kozma D, Krofta K, Ankerst J, Johansen B, Thomson NC. Budesonide and formoterol in a single inhaler improves asthma control compared with increasing the dose of corticosteroid in adults with mild-to-moderate asthma. Chest 2003; 123:1480–1487.

115. Currie GP, Stenback S, Lipworth BJ. Effects of fluticasone vs. fluticasone/salmeterol on airway calibre and airway hyperresponsiveness in mild persistent asthma. Br J Clin Pharmacol 2003; 56:11–17.

116. Pearlman DS, Stricker W, Weinstein S, Gross G, Chervinsky P, Woodring A, Prillaman B, Shah T. Inhaled salmeterol and fluticasone: a study comparing monotherapy and combination therapy in asthma. Ann Allergy Asthma Immunol 1999; 82:257–265.

117. Rabe KF. Formoterol in clinical practice—safety issues. Respir Med 2001; 95:S21–S25.

118. Ind PW, Villasante C, Shiner RJ, Pietinalho A, Boszormenyi NG, Soliman S, Selroos O. Safety of formoterol by Turbuhaler as reliever medication compared with terbutaline in moderate asthma. Eur Respir J 2002; 20:859–866.

119. Malolepszy J, Boszormenyi NG, Selroos O, Larsso P, Brander R. Safety of formoterol Turbuhaler at cumulative dose of 90 microg in patients with acute bronchial obstruction. Eur Respir J 2001; 18:928–934.

120. Boonsawat W, Charoenratanakul S, Pothirat C, Sawanyawisuth K, Seearamroongruang T, Bengtsson T, Brander R, Selroos O. Formoterol (OXIS) Turbuhaler as a rescue therapy compared with salbutamol Pmdi plus spacer in patients with acute severe asthma. Respir Med 2003; 97:1067–1074.

121. Palmqvist M, Arvidsson P, Beckman O, Peterson S, Lotvall J. Onset of bronchodilation of budesonide/formoterol vs. salmeterol/fluticasone in single inhalers. Pulm Pharmacol Ther 2001; 14:29–34.

122. Kavuru M, Melamed J, Gross G, Laforce C, House K, Prillaman B, Baitinger L, Woodring A, Shah T. Salmeterol and fluticasone propionate combined in a new powder inhalation device for the treatment of asthma: a randomized, double-blind, placebo-controlled trial. J Allergy Clin Immunol 2000; 105:1108–1116.

123. Aubier M, Pieters WR, Schlosser NJ, Steinmetz KO. Salmeterol/fluticasone propionate (50/500 microg) in combination in a Diskus inhaler (Seretide) is effective and safe in the treatment of steroid-dependent asthma. Respir Med 1999; 93:876–884.

124. Shapiro G, Lumry W, Wolfe J, Given J, White MV, Woodring A, Baitinger L, House K, Prillaman B, Shah T. Combined salmeterol 50 microg and fluticasone propionate 250 microg in the diskus device for the treatment of asthma. Am J Respir Crit Care Med 2000; 161:527–534.

125. Buhl R, Creemers JP, Vondra V, Martelli NA, Naya IP, Ekstrom T. Once-daily budesonide/formoterol in a single inhaler in adults with moderate persistent asthma. Respir Med 2003; 97:323–330.

126. Nelson HS, Chapman KR, Pyke SD, Johnson M, Pritchard JN. Enhanced synergy between fluticasone propionate and salmeterol inhaled from a single inhaler versus separate inhalers. J Allergy Clin Immunol 2003; 112:29–36.

127. Rosenhall L, Elvstrand A, Tilling B, Vinge I, Jemsby P, Stahl E, Jerre F, Bergqvist PB. One-year safety and efficacy of budesonide/formoterol in a single inhaler (Symbicort Turbuhaler) for the treatment of asthma. Respir Med 2003; 97:702–708.

128. Stallberg B, Olsson P, Jorgensen LA, Lindarck N, Ekstrom T. Budesonide/formoterol adjustable maintenance dosing reduces asthma exacerbations versus fixed dosing. Int J Clin Pract 2003; 57:656–661.

129. Aalbers R, Backer V, Kava TT, Omenaas ER, Sandstrom T, Jorup C, Welte T. Adjustable maintenance dosing with budesonide/formoterol compared with

fixed-dose salmeterol/fluticasone in moderate to severe asthma. Curr Med Res Opin 2004; 20:225–240.

130. Henriksen JM, Agertoft L, Pedersen S. Protective effect and duration of action of inhaled formoterol and salbutamol on exercise-induced asthma in children. J Allergy Clin Immunol 1992; 89:1176–1182.

131. Boner AL, Spezia E, Piovesan P, Chiocca E, Maiocchi G. Inhaled formoterol in the prevention of exercise-induced bronchoconstriction in asthmatic children. Am J Respir Crit Care Med 1994; 149:935–939.

132. Simons FE. A comparison of beclomethasone, salmeterol, and placebo in children with asthma. Canadian Beclomethasone Dipropionate-Salmeterol Xinafoate Study Group. N Engl J Med 1997; 337:1659–1665.

133. Verberne AA, Frost C, Roorda RJ, van der Laag H, Kerrebijn KF. One year treatment with salmeterol compared with beclomethasone in children with asthma. The Dutch Paediatric Asthma Study Group. Am J Respir Crit Care Med 1997; 156:688–695.

134. Meijer GG, Postma DS, Mulder PG, van Aalderen WM. Long-term circadian effects of salmeterol in asthmatic children treated with inhaled corticosteroids. Am J Respir Crit Care Med 1995; 152:1887–1892.

135. Russell G, Williams DA, Weller P, Price JF. Salmeterol xinafoate in children on high dose inhaled steroids. Ann Allergy Asthma Immunol 1995; 75:423–428.

136. Verberne AA, Frost C, Duiverman EJ, Grol MH, Kerrebijn KF. Addition of salmeterol versus doubling the dose of beclomethasone in children with asthma. The Dutch Asthma Study Group. Am J Respir Crit Care Med 1998; 158:213–219.

137. Tal A, Simon G, Vermeulen JH, Petru V, Cobos N, Everard ML, de Boeck K. Budesonide/formoterol in a single inhaler versus inhaled corticosteroids alone in the treatment of asthma. Pediatr Pulmonol 2002; 34:342–350.

138. Green SA, Turki J, Bejarano P, Hall IP, Ligett SB. Influence of beta 2-adrenergic genotypes on signal transduction in human airway smooth muscle cells. Am J Respir Cell Mol Biol 1995; 13:25–33.

139. Green SA, Turki J, Innes M, Ligett SB. Amino-terminal polymorphisms of the human beta 2-adrenergic receptor impart distinct agonist-promoted regulatory properties. Biochemistry 1994; 33:9414–9419.

140. Chong LK, Chowdry J, Ghahramani P, Peachell PT. Influence of genetic polymorphisms in the beta2-adrenoceptor on desensitization in human lung mast cells. Pharmacogenetics 2000; 10:153–162.

141. Moore PE, Laporte JD, Abraham JH, Schwartzman IN, Yandava CN, Silverman ES, Drazen JM, Wand MP, Panettieri RA Jr, Shore SA. Polymorphism of the beta(2)-adrenergic receptor gene and desensitization in human airway smooth muscle. Am J Respir Crit Care Med 2000; 162: 2117–2124.

142. Martinez FD, Graves PE, Baldini M, Solomon S, Erickson R. Association between genetic polymorphisms of the beta2-adrenoceptor and response to albuterol in children with and without a history of wheezing. J Clin Invest 1997; 100:3184–3188.

143. Lima JJ, Thomason DB, Mohamed MH, Eberle LV, Self TH, Johnson JA. Impact of genetic polymorphisms of the beta2-adrenergic receptor on

albuterol bronchodilator pharmacodynamics. Clin Pharmacol Ther 1999; 65: 519–525.

144. Taylor DR, Kennedy MA. Genetic variation of the β2-adrenoceptor, its functional and clinical importance in bronchial asthma. Am J Pharmacogenomics 2001; 1:165–174.

145. Tan S, Hall IP, Dewar J, Dow E, Lipworth B. Association between beta 2-adrenoceptor polymorphism and susceptibility to bronchodilator desensitisation in moderately severe stable asthmatics. Lancet 1997; 350:995–999.

146. Taylor DR, Hancox RJ, McRae W, Cowan JO, Flannery EM, McLachlan CR, Herbison GP. The influence of polymorphism of the β2-adrenoceptor on the development of tolerance to β-agonist. J Asthma 2000; 37:691–700.

147. Lipworth BJ, Hall IP, Tan S, Aziz I, Coutie W. Effects of genetic polymorphism on ex vivo and in vivo function of beta2-adrenoreceptors in asthmatic patients. Chest 1999; 115:324–328.

148. Taylor DR, Drazen JM, Herbison GP, Yandava CN, Hancox RJ, Town GI. Asthma exacerbations during long term beta agonist use: influence of beta(2) adrenoceptor polymorphism. Thorax 2000; 55:762–767.

149. Israel E, Drazen JM, Liggett SB, Boushey HA, Cherniack RM, Chinchilli VM, Cooper DM, Fahy JV, Fish JE, Ford JG, Kraft M, Kunselman S, Lazarus SC, Lemanske RF, Martin RJ, McLean DE, Peters SP, Silverman EK, Sorkness CA, Szefler SJ, Weiss ST, Yandava CN. The effect of polymorphisms of the beta(2)-adrenergic receptor on the response to regular use of albuterol in asthma. Am J Respir Crit Care Med 2000; 162:75–80.

3

Anticholinergic Bronchodilators

NICHOLAS J. GROSS

Loyola University Stritch School of Medicine, VA Hospital
Hines, Illinois, U.S.A.

I. Introduction

Anticholinergic agents were introduced into western medicine early in the 19th century from the Indian subcontinent where they had been used in herbal form for many centuries (1). Atropine and related alkaloids with anticholinergic activity are present in the roots, seeds, and leaves of many plants such as *Datura stramonium* or jimsonweed. In the ayurvedic medical tradition, the leaves of Datura were smoked for the relief of respiratory ailments and this was the form and purpose for which it became widely used in the West. (Indeed "stramonium cigarettes" continued to be used well into the 20th century in both Europe and North America.) Atropine was isolated and discovered to be the active ingredient in such plants by German chemists in the middle of the 19th century, from which time atropine became the standard treatment for "asthma" (2). It was the only bronchodilator available until adrenaline was discovered in the 1920s.

Atropine and other naturally occurring anticholinergic alkaloids have a very narrow therapeutic margin and produce many side effects that make them poorly accepted by patients. Thus, following the discovery of adrenaline and a decade later, the methylxanthines, the use of anticholinergics was largely supplanted. Interest in anticholinergic agents returned in the 1960s when the role of the parasympathetic system in controlling airway tone became understood. Shortly thereafter, synthetic congeners of atropine, which were poorly absorbed and much less prone to produce side effects, were developed.

Today, inhaled anticholinergic agents are mainly used for the symptomatic relief of chronic obstructive pulmonary disease (COPD) (3); however, they also have an adjunctive role in the treatment of asthma.

II. Rationale for Use of Anticholinergic Bronchodilators

A. Autonomic Control of Airways

In humans, almost all of the efferent autonomic nerves in the lungs are branches of the parasympathetic system derived from the vagus nerve, and are cholinergic in action (4). Branches of the vagus nerve travel along the airways and synapse at peribronchial ganglia with short postganglionic nerves, which supply airway smooth muscle cells, mucous glands, and possibly the ciliated epithelial cells, predominantly in the central airways. The release of acetylcholine from varicosities and terminals of the postganglionic nerves activates muscarinic receptors, thereby stimulating smooth muscle contraction, releasing mucus from mucous glands, and possibly accelerating ciliary beat frequency. At rest, a low level of cholinergic, vagal (bronchomotor) tone can be demonstrated in animals. This level of cholinergic activity can be augmented by a variety of stimuli through neural reflex pathways (Fig. 1), resulting in rapid bronchoconstriction and release of mucus from airway mucous glands. Afferent activity can arise from irritant receptors and C fibers located anywhere in the upper and lower airways, and probably also from the esophagus and carotid bodies. Impulses due to receptor stimulation are transmitted along vagal afferents through the brain-stem vagal nuclei to vagal efferents ending mainly in the central airways. Stimuli to which these receptors respond include mechanical irritation; many irritant gases; aerosols; particles; cold, dry air; allergens; and specific mediators such as histamine and some eicosanoids (5,6). The bronchoconstriction that results from these stimuli is inhibitable by atropine. There is, thus, strong experimental evidence that airway caliber is' at least partly under parasympathetic control. There is also clinical evidence that cholinergic bronchomotor tone is increased in both asthma (7) and COPD (8). These data provide the rationale for the use of anticholinergic agents in airways diseases.

By competing with acetylcholine at muscarinic receptors, anticholinergic agents inhibit cholinergic activity, both tonic and phasic, and permit airways to dilate. However, the fact that airflow limitation is seldom completely

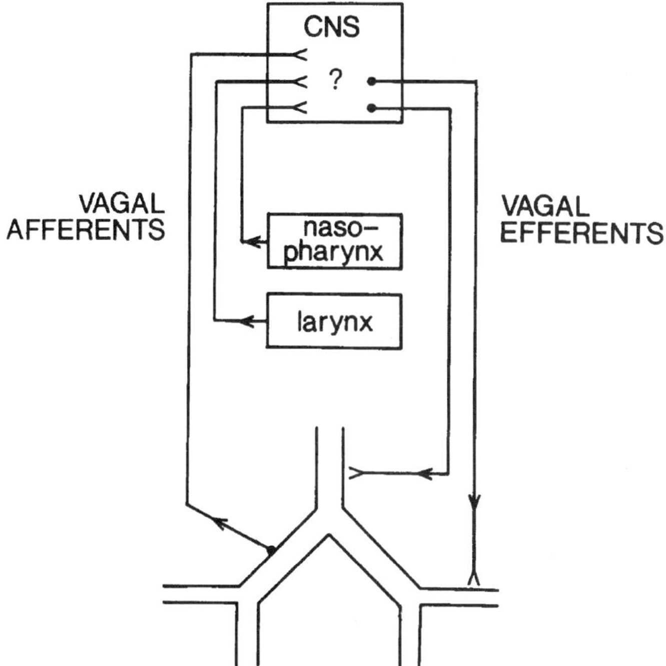

Figure 1 Diagrammatic representation of vagal reflex pathways from irritant receptors through vagal afferents, central nervous system, and vagal efferents to effector cells in the airways. *Source*: From Ref. 3.

reversed by the use of anticholinergic agents in airways diseases suggests that cholinergic vagal activity probably accounts for only a part of the airflow obstruction in patients with asthma or COPD.

Anticholinergic agents do not affect the numerous other mechanisms of airway obstruction in asthma and COPD. They have been shown to have some anti-inflammatory properties in vitro (9,10); however, the relevance of these to their clinical use is uncertain at present.

B. Muscarinic Receptor Subtypes in Airways

At least three muscarinic receptor subtypes, called M1, M2, and M3, are expressed in human lung and they appear to have different physiologic actions (Fig. 2). Current understanding is that M1 receptors, located in peribronchial ganglia, facilitate cholinergic transmission and enhance bronchoconstriction; M3 receptors, located on smooth muscle cells and submucosal glands, mediate smooth muscle contraction and mucus secretion. M2 receptors, located on the postganglionic fibers themselves, are, in contrast, autoreceptors whose stimulation provides feedback inhibition

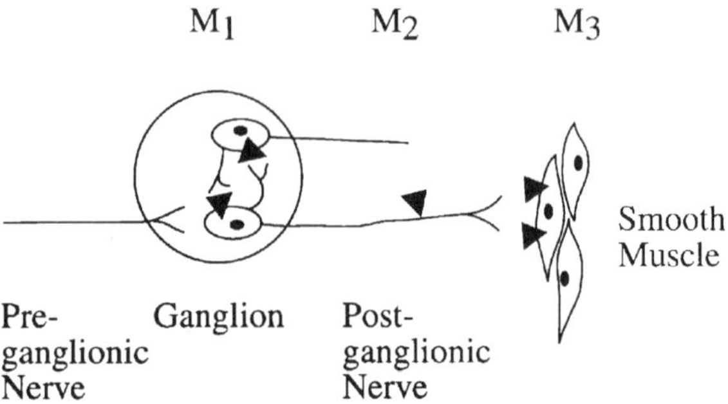

Figure 2 Muscarinic receptor subtypes in airways. M1 receptors are localized to parasympathetic ganglia, M2 receptors to postganglionic cholinergic nerves (autoreceptors), and M3 receptors to airway smooth muscle.

of further acetylcholine release from cholinergic nerves, and thus tend to limit vagally mediated bronchoconstriction (11).

This scheme has clinical implications. Traditional anticholinergics are not selective for muscarinic receptor subtypes and may, therefore, be suboptimal. This provides an opportunity for the development of anticholinergic agents that selectively inhibit M1 and M3 receptor subtypes but spare the M2 receptor. Additionally, M2 receptors are selectively damaged by certain viruses as well as by some eosinophil products, which may contribute to the bronchospasm associated with viral infections and asthma, respectively (12,13).

III. Pharmacology

Atropine-like alkaloids are classified as tertiary or quaternary ammonium compounds, depending on whether the nitrogen atom on the tropane ring is 3-valent or 5-valent, respectively (Fig. 3). All naturally occurring anticholinergic agents such as atropine and scopolamine are tertiary ammonium compounds. They are freely soluble in water and lipids and are well absorbed from mucosal surfaces and the skin. Following administration by the oral or inhalation route, they are rapidly absorbed and widely distributed in the body, cross the blood–brain barrier, enter the breast milk, and counteract parasympathetic activity in almost every system, producing widespread dose-related systemic effects. Atropine, for example, in the dose that results in bronchodilation (1.0–2.5 mg in adults) frequently produces skin flushing, dryness of the mouth, and some tachycardia. In slightly higher doses, it produces blurred vision, urinary retention, and mental effects such as irritability, confusion, and hallucinations. The therapeutic margin of atropine and its natural congeners is thus small, making these agents difficult to use. Tertiary ammonium compounds are no longer

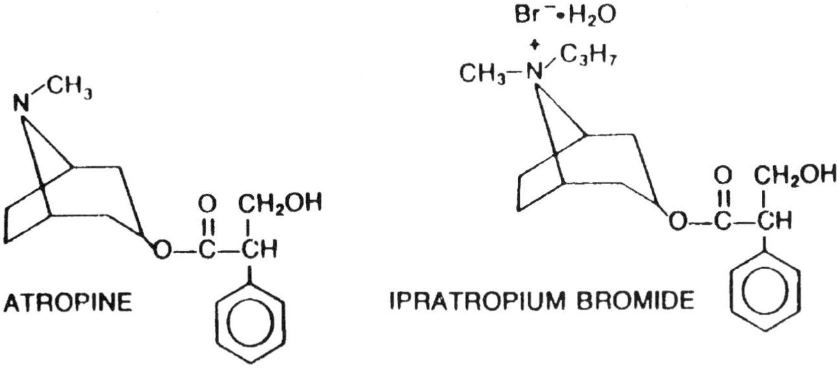

Figure 3 Structures of some anticholinergic agents.

used (or approved in the United States) for the treatment of obstructive lung diseases.

All quaternary ammonium compounds, e.g., ipratropium bromide (Atrovent®), are synthetic. Importantly, the charge associated with the 5-valent nitrogen atom renders these molecules poorly absorbable from mucosal surfaces. Such agents retain their anticholinergic activity at the sites of deposition and will, for example, dilate the pupil if delivered to the eye or dilate the bronchi if inhaled. However, they are not sufficiently absorbed from these sites to produce either significant blood levels or systemic effects, even when delivered in supramaximal doses (14). Quaternary agents can thus be regarded for practical purposes as topical forms of atropine. The group includes, in addition to ipratropium, oxitropium bromide (Oxivent®), atropine methonitrate, glycopyrrolate bromide (Robinul®), and most recently tiotropium bromide (Spiriva®). Tiotropium is of particular interest in that it is functionally selective for the M1 and M3 receptors, sparing the M2 receptor (15–17).

A. Pharmacokinetics

Radiolabeling studies of ipratropium in humans show that, following oral or inhaled doses, the serum levels are very low, with a peak at about one to two hours and a half-life of about four hours. Most of the drug is excreted unchanged in the urine. Following inhalation, the bronchodilator effect is somewhat longer than that of atropine, probably because it is not removed from the airways by absorption. Most of an oral dose is recovered in the feces, a small amount as inactive metabolites in the urine. Very little crosses the blood–brain barrier to reach the central nervous system.

Tiotropium, whose chemical structure is similar to ipratropium and is also lipophilic and very poorly absorbed, has a distribution that is similar to

Table 1 Dissociation Half-Lifes of Ipratropium and Tiotropium on Muscarinic Receptor Subtypes (Hours)

	M1	M2	M3
Ipratropium	0.11	0.035	0.26
Tiotropium	14.6	3.6	34.7

Chinese hamster ovary cells.
Source: From Ref. 18.

ipratropium. However, its unique property is that its duration of action is very long, considerably exceeding that of ipratropium. The in vitro dissociation half-lifes of tiotropium and ipratropium on each muscarinic receptor subtype are shown in Table 1 (18), from which two features are evident. Tiotropium becomes dissociated from the (protective) M2 receptor relatively rapidly as compared to its residence on the M1 and M3 receptors and, more importantly, the half-life of tiotropium on both the M1 and M3 receptors exceeds that of ipratropium by a factor of more than a hundred. The latter indicates the uniquely long duration of action of this agent, consistent with clinical studies that show a duration of bronchodilator effect of more than one day, making it ideally suited for once-daily use.

IV. Clinical Efficacy

A. Dose–Response

The dose–response of anticholinergic agents given by various inhalation methods is provided in a previous review (19). For ipratropium bromide by metered dose inhaler (MDI), the optimal dose in young adults with asthma is 40–80 µg, but in older patients with COPD the optimal dose is much higher, possibly 160 µg, particularly when airways obstruction is severe. By nebulized solution, the optimal dose of ipratropium is 500 µg in adults and 125–250 µg in children. Newer inhalers will employ a dry powder form without propellants, rather than the suspension that is currently used. The optimal dose of the dry powder form may be a little lower than that for the suspension. Thus 10 µg of ipratropium delivered by Turbuhaler® was equipotent to 20 µg delivered by MDI (20). The optimal dose of oxitropium MDI is approximately 200 µg. For less commonly used agents, the optimal doses are as follows: atropine, 0.025–0.04 mg/kg; atropine methonitrate, 0.015–0.02 mg/kg; glycopyrrolate, 0.02 mg/kg. In separate dose-ranging studies (16,21), tiotropium dry powder was administered in doses from 4.5 to 80 µg; all doses of 9 µg and above showed similar improvements in airflow and 18 µg once daily is both the approved dose for clinical use and the dose that has been utilized in all subsequent clinical studies.

B. Protection Against Specific Stimuli

The protection afforded by anticholinergic agents against specific bronchospastic stimuli in a research setting has been reviewed (3). When given in advance of bronchospastic stimuli, anticholinergic agents provide variable degrees of protection. Protection is more or less complete against cholinergic agonists such as methacholine. In asthmatics, they can prevent bronchospasm induced by β-blocking agents and by psychogenic factors. They provide only partial protection against bronchospasm due to most other stimuli, e.g., histamine, prostaglandins, nonspecific dusts and irritant aerosols, exercise, and hyperventilation due to cold, dry air in asthmatic subjects (22,23). Against most of the latter stimuli, adrenergic agents usually provide greater protection. Ipratropium has no prophylactic effect against leukotriene-induced bronchoconstriction (24).

C. Stable Asthma in Adults

A very large number of studies have compared the bronchodilator potential of various anticholinergic agents with that of adrenergic agents in patients with asthma. (There are at present no definitive publications of the effects of tiotropium in asthma, nor is this agent approved in the United States for the treatment of asthma.) While many of these studies are flawed by the fact that they used recommended doses rather than optimal doses, they provide useful information about the comparative actions of these bronchodilators (25). Figure 4, which is typical of most such studies, illustrates many of these points. Ipratropium bromide is slow to reach peak effect, typically 30 to 60 minutes, compared with about 15 minutes for short-acting adrenergic agents. Their peak effect is almost invariably less than that of agents such as albuterol but their duration of action is slightly longer. (Tiotropium bromide is even slower to reach peak effect than ipratropium and is thus not appropriate for occasional use to relieve bronchoconstriction.)

Neither ipratropium nor tiotropium, the only anticholinergic agents available by inhalation in the United States, is indicated for the treatment of asthma by the Food and Drug Administration (FDA). Among asthmatic patients, however, there is substantial variation in responsiveness, and although some patients respond very little to anticholinergic agents, others respond almost as well to them as to adrenergic agents. Ipratropium, either alone or in fixed combination with an adrenergic agent (below), is approved for asthma in some other countries.

It has been difficult to identify subgroups of asthmatic patients who are likely to have the greatest response to anticholinergic therapy. The bronchodilating effect of ipratropium may increase with age, in contrast to the decline in response to albuterol (26). Individuals with intrinsic asthma and those

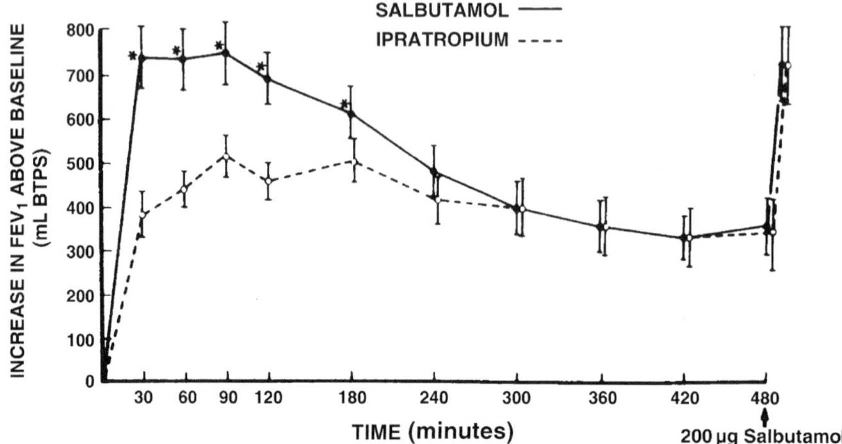

Figure 4   Increase in FEV_1 of 25 patients with asthma after inhalation of 200 µg salbutamol by metered dose inhaler (MDI) or 40 µg ipratropium by MDI on separate days. All patients received an additional dose of salbutamol at 480 minutes. Asterisks denote significant differences ($p < 0.05$). *Source*: From Ref. 25.

with longer duration of asthma may also respond better than individuals with extrinsic asthma (27), although these factors appear to be poor predictors of response. An individual trial remains the best way to identify responsiveness (28).

Recently, attention has focused on the role postnasal drip may play in promoting asthma. Ipratropium nasal spray is commercially available, and effective at reducing rhinorrhea (29), thus, in these patients, it may reduce asthma symptoms.

D.   Stable Asthma in Children

Evidence to support the use of an anticholinergic agent in stable childhood asthma is unclear. Two consensus reports reviewed the published evidence and concluded that although ipratropium was safe for the pediatric population, its benefit compared with an adrenergic agent alone was slight at best (30,31). However, there are reports that the addition of an anticholinergic augmented the bronchodilation due to albuterol alone in children aged 10 to 18 years (32).

There are also scattered reports of ipratropium use in other pediatric conditions such as cystic fibrosis, viral bronchiolitis, exercise-induced bronchospasm, and bronchopulmonary dysplasia, but these do not provide strong and consistent evidence for the benefit of ipratropium over alternative bronchodilators.

E. Acute Severe Asthma (Status Asthmaticus) in Adults

Clinical studies suggest that β_2-adrenergic agonists are more effective bronchodilators in the setting of acute severe asthma, and that an anticholinergic agent should not be used as the sole initial bronchodilator. The question arises whether an anticholinergic agent can add to the bronchodilatation achieved by the adrenergic agent. Rebuck et al. (33) found that the combination of 500 µg nebulized ipratropium with 1.25 mg nebulized fenoterol (a β_2-adrenergic agent available outside the United States) resulted in significantly more bronchodilation over the first 90 minutes of treatment than either agent alone. Moreover, patients with more severe airway obstruction obtained the greatest benefit from the combination. Other studies have addressed this same question and a meta-analysis (34) of 10 such studies (total of 1377 patients) concluded that the addition of ipratropium reduced hospital admissions (relative risk $= 0.73$) and increased FEV_1 by 7.5% (on average 100 mL, 95% CI 50–149 mL) more than groups that received a β_2-adrenergic agent alone. These benefits were both statistically and clinically significant (35).

It seems appropriate to recommend that both classes of bronchodilators be given in acute severe asthma, especially in the early hours of treatment (35) and particularly in patients with more severe airflow obstruction. They can be given separately, or in a fixed combination (e.g., Combivent® by MDI with spacer, or DuoNeb® by nebulization). Conventionally, two to three doses should be given in the first hour of treatment.

F. Acute Severe Asthma in Pediatric Patients

For acute severe asthma in children, two well-conducted trials in the 1980s showed that the addition of ipratropium accelerated the rate of improvement in airflow over albuterol alone (36,37). Subsequent studies (38–43) have yielded conflicting results regarding the efficacy of combined therapy, although some of these studies lacked statistical power. A systematic review (44) of 10 studies concluded that combination therapy with multiple doses of ipratropium was safe, improved lung function, and reduced hospitalization rates, especially in children with severe asthma. As in adult status asthmaticus, therefore, an anticholinergic alone is not recommended in status but the combination of ipratropium with an adrenergic agent is probably more effective than albuterol monotherapy, particularly in severe exacerbations.

G. Stable COPD

Although patients with COPD usually do not exhibit as much response to bronchodilators as do patients with asthma, most are indeed capable of a bronchodilator response (45). A large number of studies have compared anticholinergic agents with other bronchodilators in patients with COPD (46,47). Most show that the anticholinergic agent is a more potent bronchodilator than other agents in COPD (48–50). After large cumulative doses, the anticholinergic agent alone achieves all the available bronchodilatation (51). In this regard, COPD patients contrast sharply with asthmatic patients. In studies where bronchodilator responsiveness was compared between patients with asthma and COPD who had similar baseline airflows, patients with bronchitis had a better response to ipratropium than to adrenergic agents, the reverse being true for patients with asthma [e.g., Fig. 5 (52)]. Why? Possibly because in asthma, airflow obstruction results from airway inflammation that is, at least partially, modified by adrenergic agents but not by anticholinergics; in COPD, the major reversible component is bronchomotor tone, which is best reversed by anticholinergic agents (51).

Accordingly, ipratropium is currently recommended as first-line treatment for stable COPD in most, if not all, current guidelines for COPD (53,54). It should be noted, however, that the clinical utility of ipratropium (and possibly all other bronchodilators) is limited to their short-term relief of symptoms and that they have no demonstrated long-term effect on the natural decline in lung function in COPD (55). Nor is there evidence to suggest that their long-term effect would be different in asthma.

H. Acute Exacerbations of COPD

Four studies comparing the efficacy of bronchodilators in acute exacerbations of COPD have failed to discern a difference among adrenergic agents,

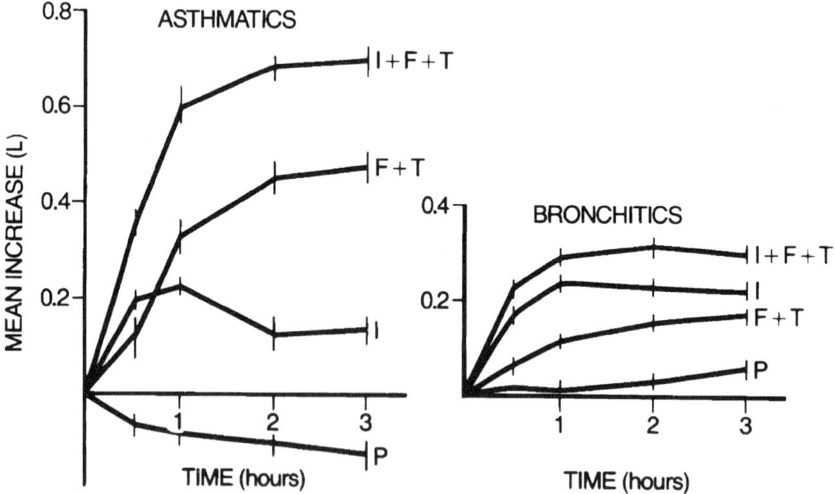

Figure 5 Increase in FEV_1 of 15 patients with asthma (*left panel*) and 15 patients with chronic bronchitis (*right panel*). *Abbreviations*: P, placebo; I, ipratropium 40 μg MDI; F + T, fenoterol 5 mg plus oxtriphylline 400 mg oral. *Source*: From Ref. 52.

anticholinergic agents, or their combination (33,56–58). Current guidelines recommend combination therapy with adrenergic and anticholinergic agents (53,54).

I. Effects on Sleep Quality

Sleep disturbance is common among patients with chronic bronchitis and asthma. Sleep disturbance in children with asthma is associated with psychological problems and impairment of memory (59). Among patients with COPD, 41% reported at least one symptom of disturbed sleep (60), possibly contributing to nocturnal oxygen desaturation, the development of pulmonary hypertension, polycythemia, and cardiac arrhythmias (61,62). A randomized double-blinded study involving 36 patients with moderate to severe COPD showed that ipratropium increased total sleep time, decreased the severity of nocturnal desaturation, and improved the patient's perceptions of sleep quality (63).

J. Combinations with Other Bronchodilators

Combinations of bronchodilators often result in greater bronchodilation than do single agents. Possibly this is partly due to the fact that most clinical studies are performed with recommended rather than optimal doses of the agents. An additional consideration may be that anticholinergic, adrenergic, and methylxanthine agents work by different mechanisms, affect different-sized airways, and have different pharmacodynamic and pharmacokinetic properties, their combination is thus rational. No unfavorable interactions between these three classes of agents have been reported, so the greater bronchodilation achieved by their combination is achieved without increasing the risk of side effects. In practice, it is common to use two or even all of these agents concurrently in airways obstruction, particularly when severe. Fixed combinations in a single-delivery device are more convenient for patient's use and thus likely to lead to greater compliance.

Single MDIs combining different classes of inhaled bronchodilators have been in use since at least the 1950s. Fixed combinations of ipratropium and the β_2-adrenergic agent fenoterol (Berodual® and DuoVent®) have been in wide use outside the United States since the 1980s. The combination of ipratropium and albuterol, both in recommended dosage (Combivent®), has been available for a decade. Clinical trials with this combination in patients with COPD (64–66) suggest that it possesses all the advantages mentioned above, and has been found to be cost-effective (67). Bronchodilation is greater during the first four to five hours after administration, but not much prolonged over that achieved by single agents, and no increase in side effects is incurred. A combination solution of ipratropium bromide and albuterol for nebulization (DuoNeb®) produced similar results (68). The co-administrations of ipratropium with salmeterol (69) or formoterol (70,71) have also been explored.

V. Side Effects

As mentioned above, atropine and its natural congeners are absorbed and produce numerous systemic side effects, which is the principal reason they are no longer used as bronchodilators. Although the quaternary agents currently in use are very poorly absorbed, they have been carefully monitored for atropine-like adverse effects, particularly for effects on the eye (narrow-angle glaucoma) and the urinary tract (urinary retention in males), and effects on respiratory mucus transport. Ipratropium was found to be essentially free of such atropine-like effects after extensive investigation (72). It can, for example, be given to patients with glaucoma without affecting intraocular tension (73) (provided it is not sprayed directly into the eye). It has been found not to affect urinary flow characteristics in older men. Nor has it been found to alter the viscosity and elasticity of respiratory mucus, or mucociliary clearance, as does atropine (74). It has negligible effects on hemodynamics, minute ventilation (75), and the pulmonary circulation (76). Consequently, quaternary anticholinergics do not carry the risk of worsening hypoxemia, as do adrenergic agents (77–79), a theoretical consideration in exacerbations of asthma and COPD. Even massive, inadvertent overdosage of one such agent resulted in trivial effects (14).

In normal clinical use, the only side effects of ipratropium are dryness of the mouth, a brief coughing spell, and paradoxical bronchoconstriction. The latter occurs in perhaps 0.3% of patients and has been variously attributed to hypotonicity of the nebulized solution, idiosyncrasy to the bromine radical, or the benzalkonium preservative (80,81). Paradoxical bronchoconstriction, which may also occur with other anticholinergic agents, warrants withdrawing the drug from that patient. Other than these effects, very extensive investigation and the worldwide use of ipratropium for over two decades demonstrate a remarkably low incidence of untoward reactions. To date, experience with tiotropium has been similar.

VI. Clinical Recommendations

The use of anticholinergic bronchodilators should be limited to the poorly absorbed quaternary forms, e.g., ipratropium, oxitropium (where available), and tiotropium, administered by inhalation. They are sometimes useful in stable asthma as adjuncts to other bronchodilator therapy, and have a demonstrated role in combination with adrenergic agents in the treatment of acute severe asthma, but cannot be recommended as the sole bronchodilator for the latter condition. Their principal indication is the long-term management of stable COPD, where they are probably the most efficacious bronchodilators. Because of their slow onset of action they are best used on a regular, maintenance basis, rather than p.r.n. The usual dose of ipratropium, two puffs of 20 µg each, may be adequate in asthmatics but is probably suboptimal for many patients with COPD (82) and can safely be doubled or quadrupled (83).

References

1. Gandevia B. Historical review of the use of parasympatholytic agents in the treatment of respiratory disorders. Postgrad Med J 1975; 51(suppl 7): 13–20.
2. Courty MA. Treatment of asthma. Edin Med J 1859; 5:665.
3. Gross NJ, Skorodin SM. Anticholinergic, antimuscarinic bronchodilators. Am Rev Respir Dis 1984; 129:856–870.
4. Richardson JB. The innervation of the lung. Eur J Respir Dis 1982; 117(suppl): 13–31.
5. Widdicombe JG. The parasympathetic nervous system in airways disease. Scand J Respir Dis 1979; 103(suppl):38–43.
6. Nadel JA. Autonomic regulation of airway smooth muscle. In: Nadel JA, ed. Physiology and Pharmacology of the Airways. New York: Marcel Dekker, 1980:217–257.
7. Shah PK, Lakhotia M, Mehta S, Jain SK, Gupta GL. Clinical dysautonomia in patients with bronchial asthma. Study with seven autonomic function tests. Chest 1990; 98(6):1408–1413.
8. Gross NJ, Co E, Skorodin MS. Cholinergic bronchomotor tone in COPD. Estimates of its amount in comparison with that in normal subjects (see comments). Chest 1989; 96(5):984–987.
9. Morr H. Immunological release of histamine from human lung. II. Studies on acetylcholine and the anticholinergic agent ipratropium bromide. Respiration 1979; 38:273–279.
10. Sato E, Koyama S, Okubo Y, Kubo K, Sekiguchi M. Acetylcholine stimulates alveolar macrophages to release inflammatory cell chemotactic activity. Am J Physiol 1998; 274:L970–L979.
11. Gross NJ, Barnes PJ. A short tour around the muscarinic receptor. Am Rev Respir Dis 1988; 138(4):765–767.
12. Fryer AD, Jacoby DB. Parainfluenza virus infection damages inhibitory M2 muscarinic receptors on pulmonary parasympathetic nerves in the guinea-pig. Br J Pharmacol 1991; 102(1):267–271.
13. Fryer AD, Jacoby DB. Effect of inflammatory cell mediators on M2 muscarinic receptors in the lungs. Life Sci 1993; 52(5–6):529–536.
14. Gross NJ, Skorodin MS. Massive overdose of atropine methonitrate with only slight untoward effects (letter). Lancet 1985; 2(8451):386.
15. O'Connor BJ, Towse LJ, Barnes PJ. Prolonged effect of tiotropium bromide on methacholine-induced bronchoconstriction in asthma. Am J Respir Crit Care Med 1996; 154(4 Pt 1):876–880.

16. Maesen FP, Smeets JJ, Sledsens TJ, Wald FD, Cornelissen PJ. Tiotropium bromide, a new long-acting antimuscarinic bronchodilator: a pharmacodynamic study in patients with chronic obstructive pulmonary disease (COPD). Dutch Study Group. Eur Respir J 1995; 8(9):1506–1513.

17. Barnes PJ, Belvisi MG, Mak JC, Haddad EB, O'Connor B. Tiotropium bromide (Ba 679 BR), a novel long-acting muscarinic antagonist for the treatment of obstructive airways disease. Life Sci 1995; 56(11–12):853–859.

18. Disse B, Reichl R, Speck G. Ba 679 BR, a novel long-acting anticholinergic bronchodilator. Life Sci 1993; 52(5–6):537–544.

19. Gross NJ, Skorodin M. Anticholinergic agents. In: Jenne JW, Murphy S, eds. Drug Therapy. New York: Marcel Dekker, 1987:615–668.

20. Bollert FG, Matusiewicz SP, Dewar MH, Brown GM, McLean A, Greening AP. Comparative efficacy and potency of ipratropium via Turbuhaler and pressurized metered-dose inhaler in reversible airflow obstruction. Eur Respir J 1997; 10(8): 1824–1828.

21. Littner MR, Ilowite JS, Tashkin DP, Friedman M, Serby CW, Menjoge SS, Witek TJ Jr. Long-acting bronchodilation with once-daily dosing of tiotropium in stable chronic obstructive pulmonary disease. Am J Respir Crit Care Med 2000; 161:1136–1142.

22. Ayala LE, Ahmed T. Is there loss of protective muscarinic receptor mechanism in asthma? Chest 1989; 96(6):1285–1291.

23. Azevedo M, da Costa JT, Fontes P, da Silva JP, Araujo O. Effect of terfenadine and ipratropium bromide on ultrasonically nebulized distilled water-induced asthma. J Int Med Res 1990; 18(1):37–49.

24. Ayala LE, Choudry NB, Fuller RW. LTD4-induced bronchoconstriction in patients with asthma: lack of a vagal reflex. Br J Clin Pharmacol 1988; 26(1): 110–112.

25. Ruffin RE, Fitzgerald JD, Rebuck AS. A comparison of the bronchodilator activity of Sch 1000 and salbutamol. J Allergy Clin Immunol 1977; 59(2):136–141.

26. Ullah MI, Newman GB, Saunders KB. Influence of age on response to ipratropium and salbutamol in asthma. Thorax 1981; 36(7):523–529.

27. Jolobe OM. Asthma vs. non-specific reversible airflow obstruction: clinical features and responsiveness to anticholinergic drugs. Respiration 1984; 45(3):237–242.

28. Brown IG, Chan CS, Kelly CA, Dent AG, Zimmerman PV. Assessment of the clinical usefulness of nebulised ipratropium bromide in patients with chronic airflow limitation. Thorax 1984; 39(4):272–276.

29. Baroody FM, Majchel AM, Roecker MM, Roszko PJ, Zegarelli EC, Wood CC. Ipratropium bromide (Atrovent nasal spray) reduces the nasal response to methacholine. J Allergy Clin Immunol 1992; 89(6):1065–1075.

30. Warner JO, Gotz M, Landau LI, Levison H, Milner AD, Pedersen S. Management of asthma: a consensus statement. Arch Dis Child 1989; 64(7): 1065–1079.

31. Hargreave FE, Dolovich J, Newhouse MT. The assessment and treatment of asthma: a conference report. J Allergy Clin Immunol 1990; 85(6):1098–1111.

32. Vichyanond P, Sladek WA, Sur S, Hill MR, Szefler SJ, Nelson HS. Efficacy of atropine methylnitrate alone and in combination with albuterol in children with asthma. Chest 1990; 98(3):637–642.

33. Rebuck AS, Chapman KR, Abboud R, Pare PD, Kreisman H, Wolkove N. Nebulized anticholinergic and sympathomimetic treatment of asthma and chronic obstructive airways disease in the emergency room. Am J Med 1987; 82(1):59–64.

34. Stoodley RG, Aaron SD, Dales RE. The role of ipratropium bromide in the emergency management of acute asthma exacerbation: a meta-analysis of randomized clinical trials. Ann Emerg Med 1999; 34(1):8–18.

35. Brophy C, Ahmed B, Bayston S, Arnold A, McGivern D, Greenstone M. How long should Atrovent be given in acute asthma? Thorax 1998; 53(5):363–367.

36. Beck R, Robertson C, Galdes-Sebaldt M, Levison H. Combined salbutamol and ipratropium bromide by inhalation in the treatment of severe acute asthma. J Pediatr 1985; 107(4):605–608.

37. Reisman J, Galdes-Sebalt M, Kazim F, Canny G, Levison H. Frequent administration by inhalation of salbutamol and ipratropium bromide in the initial management of severe acute asthma in children. J Allergy Clin Immunol 1988; 81(1):16–20.

38. Storr J, Lenney W. Nebulised ipratropium and salbutamol in asthma. Arch Dis Child 1986; 61(6):602–603.

39. Boner AL, De Stefano G, Niero E, Vallone G, Gaburro D. Salbutamol and ipratropium bromide solution in the treatment of bronchospasm in asthmatic children. Ann Allergy 1987; 58(1):54–58.

40. Ducharme FM, Davis GM. Randomized controlled trial of ipratropium bromide and frequent low doses of salbutamol in the management of mild and moderate acute pediatric asthma. J Pediatr 1998; 133(4):479–485.

41. Schuh S, Johnson DW, Callahan S, Canny G, Levison H. Efficacy of frequent nebulized ipratropium bromide added to frequent high-dose albuterol therapy in severe childhood asthma. J Pediatr 1995; 126(4):639–645.

42. Zorc JJ, Pusic MV, Ogborn CJ, Lebet R, Duggan AK. Ipratropium bromide added to asthma treatment in the pediatric emergency department. Pediatrics 1999; 103(4 Pt 1):748–752.

43. Qureshi F, Pestian J, Davis P, Zaritsky A. Effect of nebulized ipratropium on the hospitalization rates of children with asthma. N Engl J Med 1998; 339(15):1030–1035.

44. Plotnick L, Ducharme F. Should inhaled anticholinergics be added to β2 agonists for treating acute childhood and adolescent asthma? A systematic review. Br Med J 1998; 317:971–977.

45. Gross NJ. COPD: A disease of reversible airways obstruction. Am Rev Respir Dis 1986; 133:725–736.

46. Thiessen B, Pedersen OF. Maximal expiratory flows and forced vital capacity in normal, asthmatic and bronchitic subjects after salbutamol and ipratropium bromide. Respiration 1982; 43(4):304–316.

47. Passamonte PM, Martinez AJ. Effect of inhaled atropine or metaproterenol in patients with chronic airway obstruction and therapeutic serum theophylline levels. Chest 1984; 85(5):610–615.

48. Bleecker ER, Britt EJ. Acute bronchodilating effects of ipratropium bromide and theophylline in chronic obstructive pulmonary disease. Am J Med 1991; 91(4A):24S–27S.

49. Braun SR, McKenzie WN, Copeland C, Knight L, Ellersieck M. A comparison of the effect of ipratropium and albuterol in the treatment of chronic obstructive airway disease (published erratum appears in Arch Intern Med 1990; 150(6):1242). Arch Intern Med 1989; 149(3):544–547.

50. Tashkin DP, Ashutosh K, Bleecker ER, Britt EJ, Cugell DW, Cummiskey JM. Comparison of the anticholinergic bronchodilator ipratropium bromide with metaproterenol in chronic obstructive pulmonary disease. A 90-day multi-center study. Am J Med 1986; 81(5A):81–90.

51. Gross NJ, Skorodin MS. Role of the parasympathetic system in airway obstruction due to emphysema. N Engl J Med 1984; 311(7):421–425.

52. Lefcoe NM, Toogood JH, Blennerhassett G, Baskerville J, Paterson NA. The addition of an aerosol anticholinergic to an oral beta agonist plus theophylline in asthma and bronchitis. A double-blind single dose study. Chest 1982; 82(3): 300–305.

53. Global Initiative for Chronic Obstructive Lung Disease. Executive Summary. www.goldcopd.com.

54. Celli BR, MacNee W, committee members. Standards for the diagnosis and treatment of patients with COPD: a summary of the ATS/ERS position paper. Eur Respir J 2004; 23:932–946.

55. Anthonisen NR, Connett JE, Kiley JP, Altose MD, Bailey WC, Buist AS. Effects of smoking intervention and the use of an inhaled anticholinergic bronchodilator on the rate of decline of FEV1. The lung health study. JAMA 1994; 272(19):1497–1505.

56. Karpel JP, Pesin J, Greenberg D, Gentry E. A comparison of the effects of ipratropium bromide and metaproterenol sulfate in acute exacerbations of COPD. Chest 1990; 98(4):835–839.

57. Patrick DM, Dales RE, Stark RM, Laliberte G, Dickinson G. Severe exacerbations of COPD and asthma. Incremental benefit of adding ipratropium to usual therapy. Chest 1990; 98(2):295–297.

58. Koutsogiannis Z, Kelly A. Does high dose ipratropium bromide added to salbutamol improve pulmonary function for patients with chronic obstructive airways disease in the emergency department? Aust N Z J Med 2000; 30:38–40.

59. Stores G, Ellis AJ, Wiggs L, Crawford C, Thomson A. Sleep and psychological disturbance in nocturnal asthma. Arch Dis Child 1998; 78(5):413–419.

60. Klink M, Quan SF. Prevalence of reported sleep disturbances in a general adult population and their relationship to obstructive airways diseases. Chest 1987; 91(4):540–546.

61. Douglas NJ, Calverley PM, Leggett RJ, Brash HM, Flenley DC, Brezinova V. Transient hypoxaemia during sleep in chronic bronchitis and emphysema. Lancet 1979; 1(8106):1–4.

62. Douglas NJ. Sleep in patients with chronic obstructive pulmonary disease. Clin Chest Med 1998; 19(1):115–125.

63. Martin RJ, Bucher-Bartleson BL, Smith P, Hudgel DW, Lewis D, Pohl G, Koker P, Souhrada JF. Effect of ipratropium bromide treatment on oxygen saturation and sleep quality in COPD. Chest 1999; 115:1338–1345.

64. Petty TL. In chronic obstructive pulmonary disease, a combination of ipratropium and albuterol is more effective than either agent alone. An 85-day

multicenter trial. COMBIVENT Inhalation Aerosol Study Group. Chest 1994; 105(5):1411–1419.

65. Ikeda A, Nishimura K, Koyama H, Izumi T. Bronchodilating effects of combined therapy with clinical dosages of ipratropium bromide and salbutamol for stable COPD: comparison with ipratropium bromide alone. Chest 1995; 107(2):401–405.

66. The COMBIVENT Inhalation Solution Study Group. Routine nebulized ipratropium and albuterol together are better than either alone in COPD. Chest 1997; 112(6):1514–1521.

67. Friedman M, Serby CW, Menjoge SS, Wilson JD, Hilleman DE, Witek TJ Jr. Pharmacoeconomic evaluation of a combination of ipratropium plus albuterol compared with ipratropium alone and albuterol alone in COPD. Chest 1999; 115(3):635–641.

68. Gross N, Tashkin D, Miller R, Oren J, Coleman W, Linberg S. Inhalation by nebulization of albuterol-ipratropium combination (Dey combination) is superior to either agent alone in the treatment of chronic obstructive pulmonary disease. Dey Combination Solution. Study Group. Respiration 1998; 65(5):3 54–362.

69. Van Noord JA, de Munck DRAJ, Bantje ThA, Hop WE, Akveld ML, Bommer AM. Long-term treatment of chronic obstructive pulmonary disease with salmeterol and the additive effect of ipratropium. Eur Respir J 2000; 15:878–885.

70. D'Urzo AD, De Salvo MC, Ramirez-Rivera A, Almeida J, Sichletidis L, Rapatz G, Kottakis J. In patients with COPD, treatment with a combination of formoterol and ipratropium is more effective than a combination of salbutamol and ipratropium. Chest 2001; 119:1347–1356.

71. Sichletidis L, Kottakis J, Marcou D. Bronchodilatory responses to formoterol, ipratropium, and their combination in patients with stable COPD. Int J Clin Pract 1999; 53:185–188.

72. Gross NJ. Ipratropium bromide. N Engl J Med 1988; 319(8):486–494.

73. Watson WT, Shuckett EP, Becker AB, Simons FE. Effect of nebulized ipratropium bromide on intraocular pressures in children. Chest 1994; 105(5):1439–1441.

74. Pavia D, Bateman JR, Sheahan NF, Clarke SW. Effect of ipratropium bromide on mucociliary clearance and pulmonary function in reversible airways obstruction. Thorax 1979; 34(4):501–507.

75. Tobin MJ, Hughes JA, Hutchison DC. Effects of ipratropium bromide and fenoterol aerosols on exercise tolerance. Eur J Respir Dis 1984; 65(6):441–446.

76. Chapman KR, Smith DL, Rebuck AS, Leenen FH. Hemodynamic effects of inhaled ipratropium bromide, alone and combined with an inhaled beta 2-agonist. Am Rev Respir Dis 1985; 132(4):845–847.

77. Ashutosh K, Dev G, Steele D. Nonbronchodilator effects of pirbuterol and ipratropium in chronic obstructive pulmonary disease. Chest 1995; 107(1):173–178.

78. Gross NJ, Bankwala Z. Effects of an anticholinergic bronchodilator on arterial blood gases of hypoxaemic patients with chronic obstructive pulmonary disease. Comparison with a beta-adrenergic agent. Am Rev Respir Dis 1987; 136(5): 1091–1094.

79. Khoukhaz G, Gross NJ. Effects of salmeterol on arterial blood gases in patients with stable chronic obstructive pulmonary disease. Comparison with

albuterol and ipratropium. Am J Respir Crit Care Med 1999; 160(3):1028–1030.

80. Beasley R, Fishwick D, Miles JF, Hendeles L. Preservatives in nebulizer solutions: risks without benefit. Pharmacotherapy 1998; 18(1):130–139.

81. Boucher M, Roy MT, Henderson J. Possible association of benzalkonium chloride in nebulizer solutions with respiratory arrest. Ann Pharmacother 1992; 26(6):772–774.

82. Gross NJ, Petty TL, Friedman M, Skorodin MS, Silvers GW, Donohue JF. Dose response to ipratropium as a nebulized solution in patients with chronic obstructive pulmonary disease. A three-center study. Am Rev Respir Dis 1989; 139(5):1188–1191.

83. Leak A, O'Connor T. High dose ipratropium bromide is it safe? Practitioner 1988; 232(1441):9–10.

4

Inhaled Corticosteroid Therapy in the Management of Asthma in Adults

MATTHEW MASOLI and PHILIPPA SHIRTCLIFFE

Medical Research Institute of New Zealand
Wellington, New Zealand

MARK WEATHERALL

Wellington School of Medicine
and Health Sciences
Wellington, New Zealand

SHAUN HOLT

P3 Research
Wellington, New Zealand

RICHARD BEASLEY

Medical Research Institute of New Zealand
Wellington, New Zealand, and
University of Southampton
Southampton, U.K.

For over three decades inhaled corticosteroids (ICS) have been the most effective disease-modifying therapy available in the management of adult asthma and have represented the mainstay of long-term asthma treatment. This chapter reviews the clinical issues, which are relevant to their optimal use in individual patients with asthma, as well as the public health issues relating to population-based prescribing.

I. Reduction in Airways Inflammation

Corticosteroids not only have a wide range of anti-inflammatory effects in vitro, but also cause a reduction in airways inflammation when inhaled by asthmatic patients (1,2). This evidence comes primarily from bronchial biopsy studies demonstrating that regular treatment with ICS such as beclomethasone dipropionate (BDP), budesonide, and fluticasone propionate (FP) cause a marked reduction in the number of mast cells, T lymphocytes, and eosinophils in the epithelium and submucosa (3–8). There is also a reduction in inflammatory cell activation, as reflected by decreased concentrations of cell-derived mediators in bronchial lavage fluid (9–11).

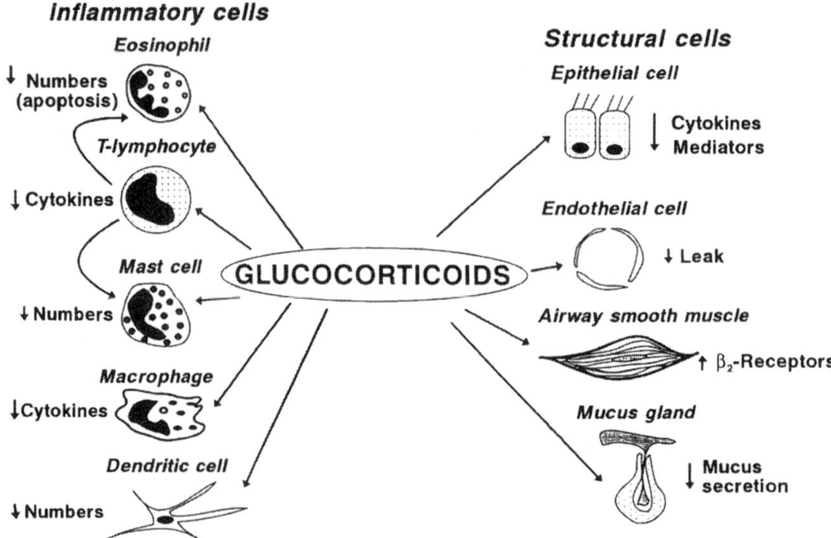

Figure 1 Schematic representation of the anti-inflammatory mechanisms of inhaled corticosteroid therapy. *Source*: From Ref. 1.

At the cellular level, ICS suppress both acute and chronic inflammation, irrespective of the underlying cause, by inhibiting many steps in the inflammatory process (Fig. 1). The disrupted epithelium is restored and the ciliated cell/goblet cell ratio is normalized with long-term treatment (3). There is also some evidence of a reduction in the thickness of the basement membrane, leading to the suggestion that ICS may influence the process of airways remodeling in asthma (6,7). The clinical efficacy of ICS is considered to be primarily due to the reduction in airways inflammation.

II. Reduction in Bronchial Responsiveness

It is well recognized that long-term treatment with ICS leads to a reduction in bronchial hyper-responsiveness (BHR) to different stimuli, including histamine, methacholine, allergen, and exercise (12,13). This occurs within a few weeks of starting treatment, with continued improvement over a period of months (14). For asthmatic individuals, this response means that a lesser degree of bronchoconstriction occurs when exposed to provoking stimuli in their daily lives. On a population level, it indicates that the widespread use of ICS will result in a significant reduction in the proportion of severe asthmatics within a community (15) (Fig. 2).

However, the inability of ICS to reverse the degree of hyper-responsiveness to normal, and the return to previous baseline levels after

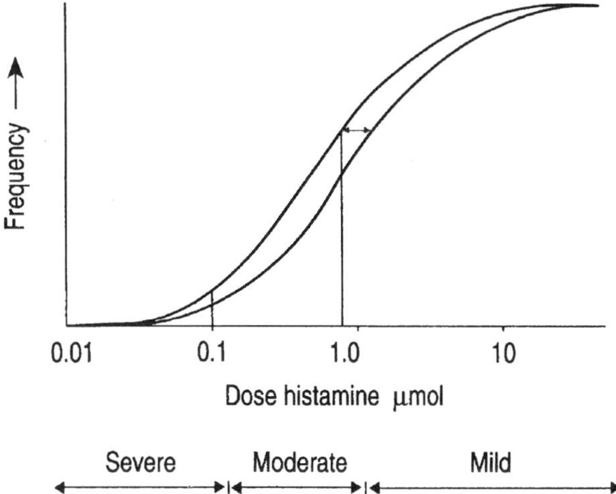

Figure 2 A reduction in bronchial hyper-responsiveness through the use of inhaled corticosteroid therapy will lead to a marked reduction in the proportion of severe asthmatics within an asthmatic population. *Source*: From Ref. 15.

stopping therapy (16,17), indicates that they do not appear to affect the long-term natural history of the disease, i.e., they do not lead to a "cure." Furthermore, these observations indicate that the predominant structural changes associated with remodeling cannot be reversed by ICS therapy. However, there are some data suggesting that ICS limit the maximum degree of airway narrowing in response to provoking stimuli in subjects with mild asthma (18).

III. Clinical Efficacy

Long-term clinical trials have shown that the regular use of ICS leads to a reduction in symptoms such as nocturnal wakening, a reduced requirement for β-agonists, improved lung function, a reduction in the frequency of severe exacerbations, including hospital and intensive care unit (ICU) admissions, and mortality (1,19–22). Importantly, ICS represent the only therapeutic agents used in the long-term management of asthma that reduce the risk of life-threatening attacks, including those leading to hospital or ICU admission (20,23–26), and those that lead to a fatal outcome (21–23,27,28). From a public health perspective, it is these properties that form the basis of the recommendations for the widespread use of ICS in asthma and as such represent the greatest opportunity to reduce the global burden of asthma.

A. Hospital Admissions

The greatest reduction in risk of hospital admission with the regular use of ICS is obtained with the heaviest users of β-agonist drugs, who represent a particular high-risk group of asthmatics. The benefit has been shown to occur within 15 days of starting treatment (20) and to be sustained over the long term, for at least a four-year period (25). It has been calculated that the regular use of ICS therapy could result in a reduction of five hospital admissions and 27 readmissions per 1000 asthma patients treated per year (25).

The clinical significance of the reduction in risk of hospital admission is evident from studies that have observed that a hospital admission identifies patients who are at increased risk of subsequent death from asthma, up to 16-fold greater than an asthmatic without a recent hospital admission (29,30). In addition to the considerable morbidity associated with hospital admissions, the burden in terms of economic cost is also important, due to its major contribution to the total cost of asthma care (31).

B. ICU Admissions

Regular use of ICS also reduces the risk of a life-threatening attack resulting in ICU admission or intubation. A life-threatening attack of this severity is recognized as the strongest risk factor that can be identified for death from asthma (29,30), and following ICU discharge, risks of mortality of 3% to 10% per year have been reported (32,33).

C. Mortality

ICS are the only medications that have been associated with a decrease in the risk of death due to asthma (21–23,27,28). These studies have shown that the protective effects are substantial and that ICS have a relatively greater effect in preventing mortality than reducing the risk of hospitalization. It is likely that the differential impact of ICS on mortality compared with hospital admission rates is due to differences in disease severity. Furthermore, the risk of death is particularly high during the first few months after stopping ICS therapy, an observation that illustrates the importance of continuation of long-term ICS therapy (22).

The benefits in terms of reduced risk of mortality have also been demonstrated in the elderly (23). This observation is important due to the relatively greater risk of mortality in the elderly, compared with younger adults or children and the tendency to under-prescribe ICS in this age group.

IV. Dose–Response Relationships

The most informative approach to the determination of the therapeutic dose range of ICS has been to undertake meta-analyses of clinical studies of specific ICS, which have utilized a similar design (34–38). This approach has provided sufficient power to investigate a comprehensive range of clinical outcomes, including severe exacerbations, which arguably are the most important measure of efficacy, from both an individual asthmatic and public health perspective.

A. Clinical Outcome Measures

The first major meta-analysis of this kind was based on placebo-controlled dose–response studies of the ICS FP in adults and adolescents with asthma (34). This demonstrated that for different outcome measures, including lung function, symptoms, β-agonist use, and exacerbations, at least 90% of the maximum efficacy can be achieved with a dose of FP of around 200 µg/day (Fig. 3). In moderate to severe adult asthmatic patients the maximum effect was achieved with a dose of FP of around 500 µg/day. This meta-analysis challenged the dogma that existed at the time that higher doses were required to achieve the maximal obtainable effect and that there were marked differences in the dose–response relationship for different clinical outcome measures. In particular, the dose of FP required to reduce exacerbations was similar to that required to reduce symptoms and improve lung function.

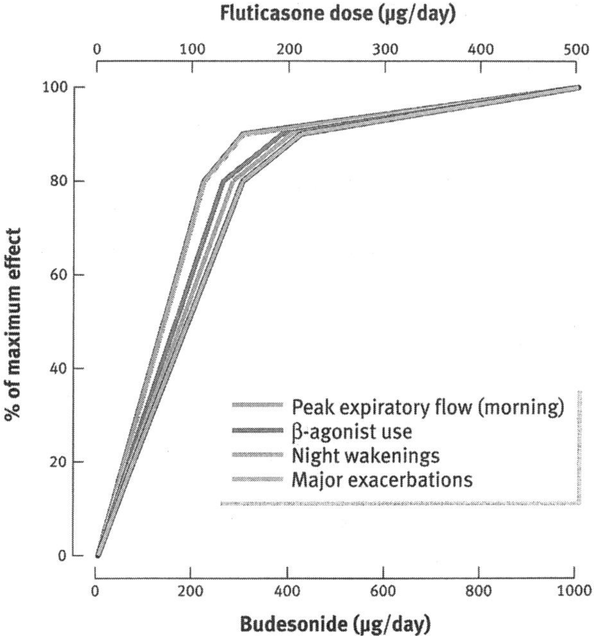

Figure 3 Dose–response curve of fluticasone and budesonide in adult asthma for the major clinical outcomes. *Source*: From Refs. 34, 37.

The major limitation of this meta-analysis was the small number of studies that included FP doses of 1000 µg/day or greater, due to the requirement for the studies to be placebo controlled. This led to a subsequent meta-analysis that specifically focused on comparisons between the dose of 200 µg/day and higher doses to determine whether the 200 µg/day dose regime provided most of the therapeutic benefit as suggested in the original study (35). It was confirmed that most of the therapeutic benefit was achieved with a dose of 200 µg/day, and that the mean further improvement for FEV_1 and morning peak flow resulting from an increase in dose from 200 to $\geq$500 µg/day was 0.07 L (95% CI -0.01 to 0.14) and 5.9 L/min (95% CI -3.0 to 15.3), respectively. The odds ratio for withdrawals with 200 µg/day compared with $\geq$500 µg/day was 1.27 (0.78–2.07).

Similarly in a meta-analysis of eight placebo-controlled trials of FP, no significant differences were noted in magnitude of change in morning peak flow in patients receiving high (500 or 1000 µg/day) or low ($\leq$200 µg/day) doses of FP (36). The time taken to reach either 50% or 100% of the best observed effect was not any longer in the low-dose group, once again demonstrating no reduction in different parameters of efficacy.

A similar meta-analysis with inhaled budesonide has shown that most of the clinical efficacy for the same outcome measures is achieved with a dose of around 400 µg/day (Fig. 3) (37). These findings are comparable with those of FP when their relative potencies are considered [FP vs. budesonide, BDP or triamcinolone (TAA) 2:1]. Consistent findings have also been observed with studies of BDP and TAA in which a plateau in response is observed between 400 and 800 µg/day, depending on the clinical outcome variable (39,40). With regard to mometasone, which has a similar potency to FP (41), the top of the dose–response curve for the major clinical outcome variables is around 400 µg/day (42).

The clinical significance of these dose–response studies is that the therapeutic range for the majority of adult asthmatics lies between 100 and 1000 µg/day of BDP, budesonide, or TAA and 50–500 µg/day of FP or mometasone. As a result, there should be few patients who require doses above this range, as minimal further improvement and clinically significant adverse effects can be expected at higher doses.

This recommendation should be qualified by the recognition that there is considerable interindividual variability in response to ICS in asthma, which means that some patients may obtain a greater clinical benefit at higher doses, just as some patients may obtain the maximum efficacy at lower doses (43). Furthermore, there are some circumstances in which higher doses of ICS may be indicated. These include oral steroid—dependent subjects in whom there is evidence for increasing efficacy up to doses of 2000 µg of FP or equivalent (44–47). There is also preliminary data to suggest that high doses of ICS (e.g., FP 2000 µg/day and budesonide 3200 µg/day) may be as effective as oral steroids in the treatment of moderate to severe exacerbations of asthma (48,49). However, currently there is insufficient evidence to date to recommend the use of such high doses in this situation (50).

B. Mortality

The major clinical outcome measure, which could not be assessed in these ICS dose–response trials, is mortality due to its rare occurrence even in patients with severe asthma. However, it is possible to obtain an indication of the dose–response effect of ICS for reducing the risk of mortality from the epidemiological study of Suissa et al. (22). In this study there was a progressive reduction in risk of mortality with increasing use of ICS, with the rate of death from asthma decreased by 21% with each additional canister of ICS used in the previous year. While these findings primarily relate to compliance and continuity of use of ICS, they also provide a crude assessment of the dose–response relationship in terms of the ability of ICS to reduce the risk of mortality. In the study population over 90% of the prescribed canisters of ICS contained low-dose BDP and as a result it was possible to determine a dose–response relationship in terms of an average daily dose over a prolonged period. Using this approach, the rate of death from asthma among users of ICS decreased by around 20% for each additional 33.3 µg/day of BDP used during the year, up to 335 µg/day of BDP or equivalent. Consistent with the major clinical outcome measures, at least 80% of the maximum obtainable benefit (reduction in mortality) was achieved at around 200 µg of BDP per day (adjusted odds ratio 0.15) (Fig. 4).

As a result, available evidence suggests that low doses of ICS are effective in reducing the risk of death from asthma, with a dose–response similar to that of other major outcome variables such as symptoms, lung function, and severe exacerbations. Furthermore, the observation that the risk of death is particularly high during the first few months after stopping ICS therapy illustrates the importance of compliance with and continuation of long-term ICS therapy to obtain the therapeutic benefits associated with their use.

C. Airways Inflammation

The dose–response relationship for ICS in terms of modifying underlying airways inflammation has also been determined. While most studies have attempted to investigate this issue through measurement of surrogate markers, including inflammatory cells in sputum or exhaled gases, these are indirect indices of uncertain relevance (51,52). A more informative method has been to investigate the nature and magnitude of airways inflammation through the detailed assessment of bronchial biopsies. Utilizing this approach, Wallin et al. (53) found no significant difference in markers of airway inflammation between a dose of 400 µg and 1000 µg/day of FP. This finding was derived from the measurement of submucosal mast cell and eosinophil numbers in bronchial mucosal biopsies after 12 weeks of

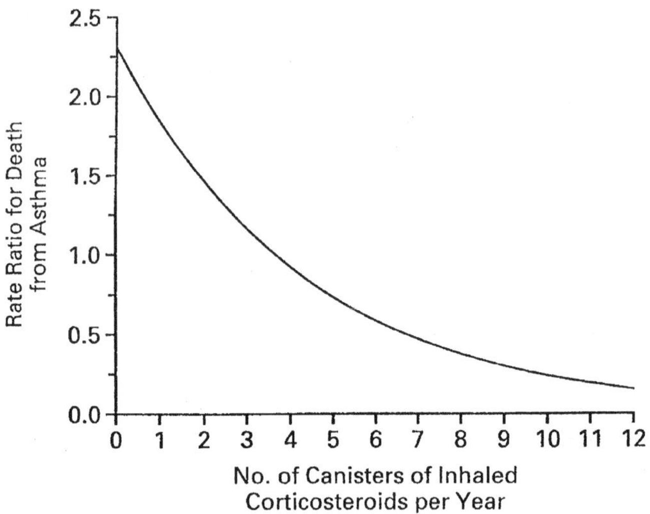

Figure 4 Risk of death from asthma in relation to the number of canisters of inhaled corticosteroids used. The equivalent mean daily dose of ICS was derived: 93% of the prescribed canisters of ICS contained low-dose beclomethasone (200 doses per canister with 50 µg of drug delivered per dose). *Source*: From Ref. 22.

treatment, together with measurement of adhesion molecules and cytokines in the biopsies, and inflammatory cell activation and fibroblastic activity measured in the supernatant of the bronchial wash and bronchoalveolar lavage fluid. These observations are consistent with a similar bronchial biopsy study in which the improvement in lung function and suppression of airways inflammation were optimal at a dose of 500 µg/day of FP with no significant further benefit at 2000 µg/day of FP (54). These studies indicate that the dose–response relationship of ICS for airway anti-inflammatory effects are similar to that for all major clinical outcome measures.

D. Summary

The dose–response relationship for ICS is similar for their effects in reducing airways inflammation and improving clinical outcomes, including reduction in symptoms and rescue β-agonist use, improvement in lung function, and reduction in the frequency and severity of exacerbations, including the risk of mortality. Most of the therapeutic efficacy is obtained at doses of around 400 µg/day of BDP or equivalent, with the mean dose achieving the maximum benefit at around 1000 µg/day. Notwithstanding the considerable individual variability in response to ICS in asthma and the situations in which higher doses are indicated, these findings suggest that reconsideration is required of what are considered "low," "medium," and "high" doses of ICS.

A case can be made for changing the terminology to "moderate" for doses of around 400 µg/day of BDP or equivalent, with "low" and "high" doses represented by doses lower and higher than this moderate dose, respectively.

V. Systemic Side Effects

A number of different systemic adverse effects have been observed with ICS, including reduced bone mineral density and an increased risk of fracture, adrenal suppression, cataracts, easy bruising, and thin skin (55–58). Of these effects, the bone, adrenal, and eye effects are considered to be the most clinically important and represent the primary systemic outcome measures considered in this review. The interpretation of the dose–response studies that have investigated these effects have been limited by inadequate power with small numbers of subjects, use of indirect measures of function or structure, inadequate time periods of study, confounding by previous oral and ICS use, and the lack of placebo-controlled, randomized studies in which more than one dose of ICS has been investigated.

A. Effects on Bone

A number of different methods of assessment have been utilized to determine the effects of ICS on bone, including biochemical markers of bone turnover such as osteocalcin and hydroxyproline, bone mineral density, and the risk of fracture at various sites (59–63). Short-term changes in biochemical markers are of uncertain clinical relevance and the limitations of bone mineral density measurement have been increasingly recognized as well. In particular, there is evidence that the adverse effects of corticosteroids are primarily a consequence of disruption of bone architecture and collagen structure rather than demineralization (64,65) and that the increased risk of fracture with steroid use is only partially due to the reduction in bone mineral density (66). Furthermore, the correlation between corticosteroid use and reduction in bone mineral density is poor and the size of the effect on bone mineral density does not appear to explain the risk of fracture associated with corticosteroid therapy (66). As a result changes in bone mineral density can now be considered to be an indirect marker of the risk of fracture with the use of ICS. A more clinical relevant approach for determining the adverse effects of ICS on bone is the direct assessment of the risk of fracture.

Recently two large population-based case–control studies of ICS and hip fracture have enabled the dose–response relationship of the effects on bone of ICS to be determined (63,67). In the U.K. General Practice Research Database study there was a small dose-dependent increase in the risk of fracture up to a dose of 1600 µg/day, with the risk increasing more markedly at higher doses (63). When adjustment was made for exposure to oral corticosteroids and other confounding factors, the relative risk increased from

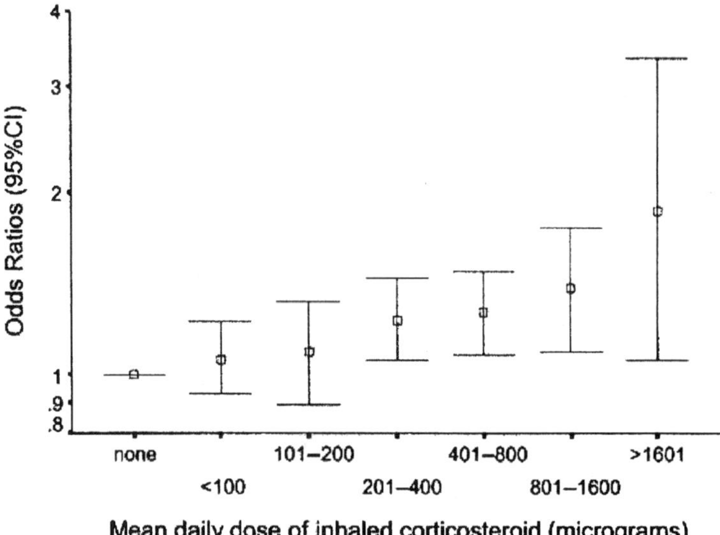

Figure 5   Dose–response relationship between mean daily dose of inhaled corticosteroids and hip fracture (adjusted for exposure to oral corticosteroids). *Source*: From
Ref. 63.

1.39 at the 800–1600 µg dose range with a further increase to 1.87 in the
1.6% of the population prescribed >1600 µg/day (Fig. 5). As 98% of subjects were prescribed either BDP or budesonide, these doses can be considered to relate to BDP or equivalent. The data from this study relates to older
patients, and it could be proposed that the risk may be higher for future gen-
erations who will have been exposed to ICS from an earlier age, although
some of the increase in risk will potentially be offset if courses of oral
steroids are avoided.

Similar risks were observed in a cohort study in which a risk of
non-vertebral fracture of 1.28 was observed in asthmatic patients taking
≥700 µg of ICS per day, compared with a non-asthmatic control group
(68). The other major study, of case-control design, examined the association
of ICS use and risk of fracture from a Canadian population-based cohort (67).
Among subjects followed for over eight years, the rate of hip fracture was only
elevated with daily doses of more than 2000 µg of BDP or equivalent (RR 1.61
95% CI 1.04–2.50). For upper extremity fracture, the rate increased by 12%
with every 1000 µg increase in the daily dose of ICS.

B. Adrenal Effects

The interpretation of studies of the effects of ICS on adrenal function
have proven difficult due to small numbers and insufficient periods to
determine effects of clinical relevance, and the use of single doses or lack of

a placebo-group, thereby preventing the accurate assessment of the dose–response relationship. In addition, most studies have reported single morning plasma cortisol measurements, which is an insensitive and variable measure for detecting adrenal suppression. A preferable method has been to use cosyntropin stimulation tests as a sensitive measure of adrenal suppression (69).

This method was used in the largest dose–response study of adrenal suppression due to budesonide, in which the reduction in cortisol levels after cosyntropin stimulation was 4%, 13%, 11%, and 27% after four weeks treatment with placebo and 800, 1600, and 3200 µg/day of budesonide, compared with a 35% reduction for 10 mg of prednisone (70). The only dose–response study with fluticasone, which examined a comparable dose range, reported reductions in cortisol levels after cosyntopin stimulation of 9%, 21%, 24%, and 24% for 500, 1000, 1500, and 2000 µg/day of fluticasone compared with placebo, and a 35% reduction for 10 mg of prednisone (71). In the comparable study of mometasone, four weeks treatment with 800 and 1600 µg/day of mometasone resulted in a 10% and 21% reduction in 24-hour serum cortisol levels compared with placebo, with a 64% reduction with 10 mg of prednisone (72).

These studies indicate that there is a relatively flat dose–response up to around 1600 µg/day of budesonide (equivalent to around 800 µg of fluticasone or mometasone), although a greater increase in adrenal suppression occurs at higher doses. While this observation is somewhat reassuring in terms of the prescription of ICS within the therapeutic dose–response range for efficacy, it is a concern when the widespread use of excessively high doses of ICS is considered.

C. Cataracts

The importance of ICS increasing the risk of cataracts is evident when the widespread use of ICS in the adult population is considered together with the prevalence of cataracts, which represent the most common cause of blindness in the world (73,74).

The dose–response relationship of ICS and cataracts has recently been defined in the large population-based case–control study based on the U.K. General Practice Research Database (75). Higher doses and longer duration of exposure to ICS were associated with an increased risk of cataract, but there was minimal risk associated with ICS prescribed within the therapeutic dose–response range. After adjustment for systemic steroid use and consultation rate, the relative risk of cataract was 1.18 for the dose range 800–1600 µg/day and 1.69 for the very high-dose range of asthmatic patients taking >1600 µg/day of BDP or equivalent. For the relatively small proportion of people prescribed daily doses of 1600 µg or more, 41% of their risk of cataract could be attributed to ICS use, assuming the association between exposure and cataracts was causal.

These findings are consistent with the clinical studies, which have examined the association between cumulative doses of ICS and risk of cataract (76). In this study, higher cumulative lifetime doses of ICS were associated with higher risks of posterior subcapsular cataracts, with the highest prevalence (27%) found in subjects whose lifetime dose was over 2000 mg of BDP or equivalent, which was associated with a fivefold increased risk.

D. Summary

The dose–response relationships for ICS and risk of fracture, adrenal suppression, and cataracts are generally consistent in showing a small dose-dependent increase in risk up to doses of around 2000 µg/day of BDP or equivalent, with a more marked increase at doses higher than this level. These data can be interpreted in a number of ways. Importantly, it demonstrates that the risk of systemic adverse effects is very low with the use of ICS within the therapeutic dose–response range for clinical efficacy. Conversely, when the widespread use of high-dose ICS beyond the established therapeutic dose–response range is considered, the proportion of patients who are at risk of systemic effects is of concern.

VI. Frequency of Administration

When ICS were first introduced it was recommended they should be taken four times daily. Subsequently it was shown that similar efficacy could be achieved in most patients with a twice-daily regimen (77), although there may be a small benefit with a four-times-daily regimen in those with severe or unstable asthma (78). The twice-daily regimen has major advantages in terms of compliance, and as a result has become the preferred regimen. However, even with a twice-daily regime, less than half of patients are likely to comply with ICS therapy (79). Indeed, it has been reported that one-third of patients prescribed regular ICS actually take them on a "prn" basis (80). One strategy that may be employed to improve compliance is the use of ICS according to a once-daily regime (81). This approach has recently been assessed in mild asthma, for which it has been shown that once-daily treatment may achieve similar control to a twice-daily regimen, and as a result, this regime may be considered for such patients (82–85).

VII. Starting Dose

A number of different approaches have been proposed for starting ICS in a patient with asthma.

- Start with a high dose then step down once control has been achieved (1,86).
- Start with a low dose then step up if required (87).

- Start at the dose considered appropriate for the severity of disease, normally 400 µg/day of BDP or equivalent (88).

These approaches have been the subject of recent research that supports the recommendation of using doses of ICS of around 400 µg/day of BDP or equivalent as initial treatment (89–95). Starting ICS at a higher dose (≥800 µg of BDP or equivalent) with or without a subsequent step-down approach provides minimal additional benefit compared with a standard moderate ICS dose. These findings are consistent with the studies, which have shown that doses of ICS of around 400 µg of BDP or equivalent result in most of the therapeutic benefit as maintenance therapy in adult asthma (34–42). This is reassuring as the alternative start-high regime has the potential risk of patients remaining on unnecessarily high doses if they do not undergo regular medication review, or if such a review led to ongoing use of high doses due to fear of provoking unstable asthma with a dose reduction.

VIII. Back Titration

One of the recommendations of asthma management guidelines is that an attempt is made to reduce the dose of ICS once asthma control has been achieved, a regime referred to as "back titration." This recommendation applies particularly to patients receiving well in excess of the established therapeutic range. This is an important issue as in western countries, many adult patients with asthma are prescribed ICS doses well beyond the top of the dose–response curve (96,97).

Many doctors and patients have been reluctant to reduce the ICS dose, concerned that this might lead to a loss of control; however, there have been numerous studies supporting the efficacy of such an approach. For example, in a general practice-based study in Scotland, adult patients with asthma on a mean baseline dose of around 1400 µg/day of BDP were able to reduce the dose by an average of 350 µg/day without compromising asthma control (98). The regime used in this 12-month randomized, controlled trial was a 50% reduction in dose if the patient met predetermined criteria for asthma control over the previous two-week period. This study also showed that this step-down management approach could be adopted easily by primary care teams, which are responsible for the care of most asthmatic patients.

In the landmark study of the efficacy of initiating treatment with ICS, after two years of budesonide at a dose of 1200 µg/day, maintenance therapy could be given at a reduced dose of 400 µg/day without loss of control (Fig. 6) (16). However, patients whose budesonide was stopped deteriorated to a symptomatic level comparable to that prior to starting ICS. These studies suggest that in many patients, a significant reduction in ICS dose from above 1000 µg/day can be achieved without a loss of control, but that

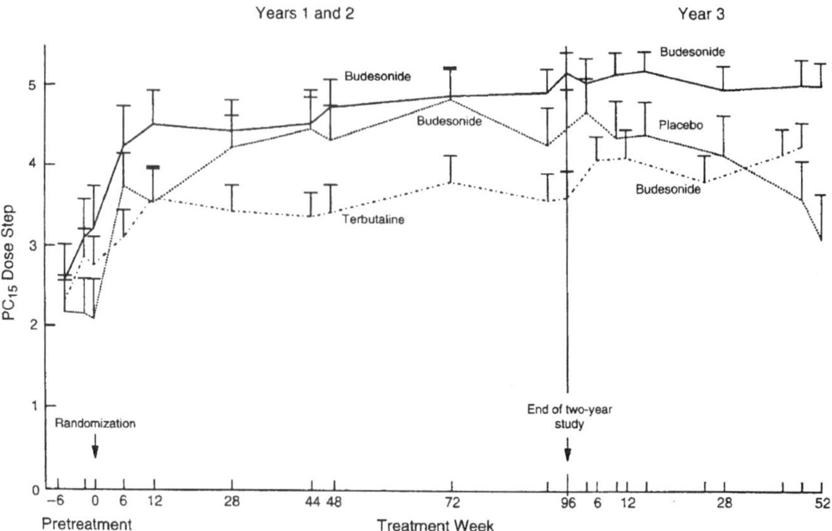

Figure 6 The changes in bronchial hyper-responsiveness associated with treatment regimes: budesonide 1200 μg/day for two years followed by 400 μg/day for one year (—); budesonide 1200 μg/day for two years followed by placebo (. . .); terbutaline for two years followed by budesonide 1200 μg/day for one year (·-·). *Source*: From Ref. 16.

stopping ICS after a prolonged period of good control is likely to lead to unstable asthma in most patients.

An alternative regime to the variable long-term dosing with ICS has been to modify the dose in accordance with the level of BHR in conjunction with optimizing symptoms and lung function (99). This approach has been shown to lead to more effective control of asthma and a greater improvement in chronic airways inflammation than adjustment of the dose based solely on symptoms and lung function. While the repeat assessment of BHR in the long-term assessment and management of asthma is not feasible in routine practice, it does indicate the potential role of monitoring surrogate markers of inflammation in the long-term management of asthma.

IX. Early Intervention

The concept of early intervention with ICS arose with the realization that airways inflammation may be present in patients with clinically mild asthma (100), and that such patients may develop an irreversible component to their airflow obstruction early in the course of the disease (101,102). This led to the question of whether the early introduction of ICS could improve the long-term prognosis, and in particular prevent progressive deterioration of lung function.

The key evidence comes from a long-term study comparing initial treatment with ICS or inhaled β_2-agonist in patients with newly diagnosed mild asthma (14,16). After two years subjects crossed over treatments and were followed for a further year. Patients transferred to ICS therapy (budesonide 1200 µg/day) did not obtain the same degree of improvement in lung function, BHR, or symptoms as those who were treated with ICS at the beginning of the study (Fig. 6).

An alternative approach has been to examine the association between the duration of symptoms prior to initiating treatment with ICS and the magnitude of the clinical response. Following treatment with ICS patients who had experienced symptoms of asthma for less than two years prior to initiation of ICS had better lung function that those who had experienced symptoms for a longer period (103). These studies suggest that early intervention with ICS therapy may lead to a better long-term clinical outcome, including lung function and BHR. As a result, ICS should not be withheld until patients develop moderate or severe asthma, but rather introduced early in the course of the disease, once the patient has developed persistent asthma.

X.　Add-On Therapy with a Long-Acting β-Agonist

It is recommended that if a patient with asthma is inadequately controlled on ICS therapy, a LABA should be prescribed as add-on therapy (Fig. 7) (88,104). However, uncertainty exists as to the optimal ICS dose at which a LABA is needed. This uncertainty is reflected by the British Management Guidelines in which it is recommended that a LABA is added in poorly controlled patients with moderately severe asthma receiving between 200 and 800 µg/day of BDP or equivalent (88). This recommendation is based on clinical trials that have shown a dose–response relationship for ICS within this therapeutic range (34–42), and efficacy with adding a LABA to ICS within (and beyond) this range (105–110).

In the MIASMA meta-analysis of nine studies, the addition of the LABA salmeterol was significantly more effective than increasing (at least doubling) the baseline dose of ICS, which ranged from 400 to 1000 µg of BDP or equivalent (105). While demonstrating the efficacy of this approach, it did not determine whether there was a differential response to the addition of LABA therapy across the ICS therapeutic range. In contrast, the FACET study investigated a lower comparative ICS dose and demonstrated that the addition of the LABA formoterol to 200 µg/day of budesonide resulted in a lesser reduction in severe exacerbations (the primary outcome variable) than the higher 800 µg/day budesonide dose (106). This finding was in some respects not surprising as 200 µg of budesonide achieves only about half the maximum obtainable benefit, whereas 800 µg/day is

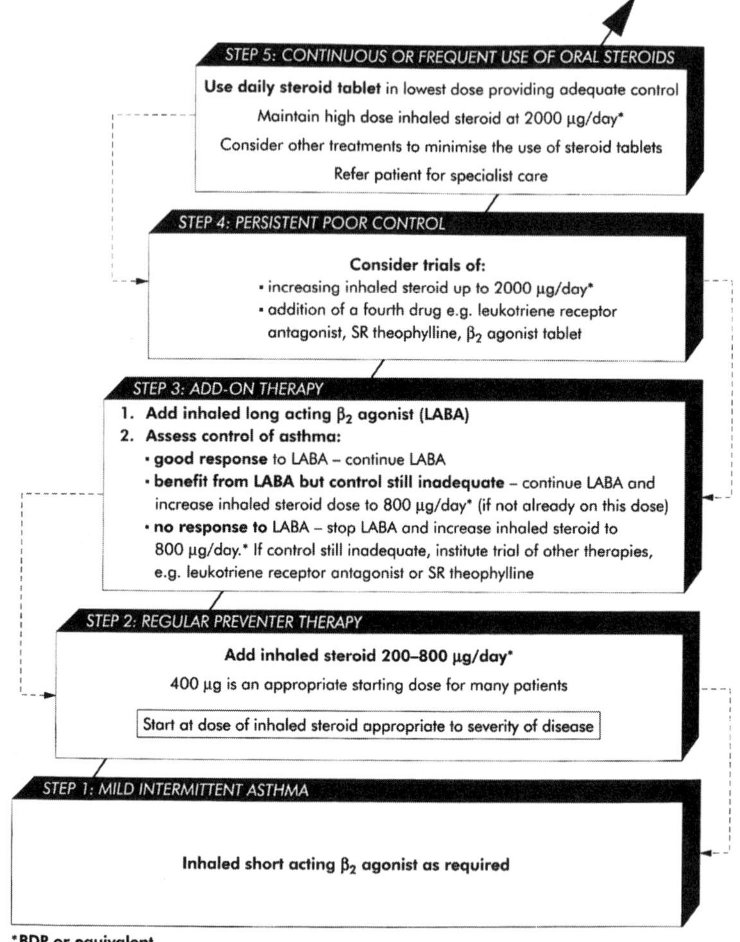

Figure 7 British Thoracic Society guidelines on asthma management: summary of the stepwise approach to asthma management in adults based on inhaled corticosteroid therapy. *Source*: From Ref. 88.

close to the top of the dose–response curve (37). As a result, an increase to this higher budesonide dose was likely to achieve a greater reduction in severe exacerbations than the addition of LABA therapy to the lower dose.

It would seem logical that in a patient with unstable asthma, a LABA should be added at a dose of ICS at which most of the therapeutic benefit has already been obtained, rather than at a lower dose or a dose at or beyond the top of the dose–response curve. This has recently been investigated in a meta-analysis of studies, which have compared the clinical benefit of adding salmeterol in patients not controlled on a dose of BDP of

400 µg/day or equivalent with increasing the dose of ICS by at least twofold (111). This analysis showed that the addition of salmeterol was superior to increasing the dose of ICS for all major clinical outcome measures. For the primary outcome variables of withdrawals due to asthma and moderate or severe exacerbations, subjects receiving salmeterol had a 35% to 50% reduced risk compared with high-dose ICS therapy. As a result, it can be recommended that 400 µg/day of BDP or equivalent represents a suitable level at which to add a LABA in a patient with asthma not well controlled with ICS therapy. If a patient remains poorly controlled despite the addition of a LABA, an increase in the dose of ICS in combination with the LABA would be an appropriate next step. Conversely, in patients with asthma controlled on high-dose ICS therapy, it is possible to markedly reduce the ICS dose through the addition of a LABA while maintaining overall asthma control (112,113).

The opportunity exists to prescribe the combination of ICS and LABA therapy from separate inhalers or from a single combination inhaler (114). The main advantage of a single combination inhaler is that it ensures that the patient cannot take the LABA as sole therapy, which would inevitably lead to a clinically significant loss of asthma control (115,116). In addition, it has now been demonstrated that there is improved compliance with ICS therapy through the use of a combination inhaler. This evidence comes from a recent HMO-based study, which monitored patient medication refill persistence over a 12-month period (117). The use of FP in a combination inhaler with salmeterol was at least two-thirds higher than the prescription of FP from a single inhaler, either as sole therapy or in combination with additional therapy such as salmeterol in a separate inhaler. This greater compliance was associated with a significantly lower use of short-acting β-agonist therapy, suggesting an overall improvement in asthma control. There is also some evidence to suggest that, in the case of salmeterol and fluticasone, when administered from a single combination inhaler, there may be increased clinical efficacy over concurrent use from separate inhalers (118).

Two regimens have been proposed for the use of combination ICS/ LABA therapy. The standard regime is the use of a fixed dose twice daily with the option of different dose combinations for patients of differing asthma severity. The alternative is an adjustable dosing regime in which patients step up or step down their therapy depending on changes in asthma control. Pending long-term studies comparing these approaches, it is likely that the regime chosen will depend on patient and doctor preference.

XI. Alternative Add-On Therapy

The option to add a LABA to ICS therapy in symptomatic patients may be limited due to cost or availability, and as a result it is necessary to consider alternatives. Low-dose theophylline represents one option resulting in additional efficacy when used as add-on therapy with low to high doses of ICS (119–121). When used in this way it is likely to result in both bronchodilator and anti-inflammatory effects. However, a recent systematic review suggests that the efficacy of this approach is relatively less than the addition of a LABA, while being associated with greater side effects (122).

The main other option is to add a leukotriene receptor antagonist (LTRA) drug (123). The addition of an LTRA is likely to result in variable benefit when added to ICS (124–126). At least two studies have reported similar efficacy with the addition of a LABA or LTRA to ICS in terms of severe exacerbations (127,128), although this has not been confirmed in other studies (129,130), and outcome variables such as lung function and symptoms consistently favor the addition of a LABA.

XII. Incorporation with an Asthma Self-Management Plan System of Care

The asthma self-management plan system of care represents an approach whereby patients are given the ability to recognize worsening asthma, and are provided with written guidelines for the appropriate medical response (131). Asthma self-management plans have been shown to be effective in the treatment of asthma, leading to significant reductions in morbidity and improved outcomes (132–134). ICS therapy forms the basis of long-term management within this system, with patients taking twice-daily ICS as regular therapy (in addition to an inhaled short-acting β-agonist as required) and being instructed to increase the dose (or initiate therapy) for worsening asthma (Table 1).

There is conflicting evidence as to whether the instruction to increase the dose of ICS during an exacerbation contributes to the improvement in asthma control noted with this system of care, and whether any such improvement is due to the pharmacological effect of the higher dose, or through changes in patient behavior such as improved compliance (135–137). Available evidence suggests that patients are more compliant with ICS therapy because their self-management plan stresses its importance, in part through the instruction to double the dose of ICS in unstable asthma (137). This interpretation is supported by the study of Lahdensuo et al. (133), in which the group following a self-management plan had strikingly better asthma control than the group on standard management, despite almost identical prescribed doses of ICS throughout the 12-month study period. Improved compliance with ICS therapy, through implementation of the plan (which included the provision to double the dose of ICS in unstable asthma) seems the most likely explanation for the improvement in outcome seen. Indirect evidence for this effect also comes from the Harrison et al. study (135), in which there was a

Table 1 Prototype Asthma Self-Management Plan Based on Inhaled Corticosteroid Therapy

Step	Peak flow	Symptoms	Action[a]
1	80–100% best	Intermittent/few	Continue regular inhaled corticosteroids; use inhaled beta agonist for relief of symptoms
2	60–80% best	Waking at night with asthma; symptoms of a "cold"	Increase the dose of inhaled corticosteroid or start if not currently taking
3	40–60% best	Increasing breathlessness or poor response to frequent use of bronchodilator	Start oral corticosteroids and contact a doctor
4	<40% best	Severe attack of asthma	Call emergency doctor or ambulance urgently

[a]At all stages, take beta agonist for relief of symptoms.

similar fivefold decrease in the number of courses of prednisone simply with the instruction to double the dose of ICS therapy in worsening asthma, for both placebo and active ICS "doubling" groups. Compliance with ICS therapy is poor in clinical practice; self-management has the potential to improve this.

XIII. Other Issues

A. Potency vs. Efficacy

Potency reflects biological activity per unit weight, whereas efficacy reflects the maximum biological activity of a drug; this difference is important when comparative doses of different ICS are considered. Clinical studies suggest that FP and mometasone are about twice as potent as BDP, budesonide, or TAA (42,138). This means that FP or mometasone are likely to achieve the same therapeutic effect at half the dose of BDP, budesonide, or TAA, but that at high doses, the different ICS will have a similar maximum effect.

B. Spacers/Inhaler Devices

A proportion of patients fail to coordinate actuation with inhalation when using a standard metered dose inhaler (MDI) and greater deposition in the airways can be achieved through the use of a spacer device (139). For this reason spacers are recommended for most asthmatics receiving corticosteroid therapy delivered by MDI, and certainly those on high doses. Technique is still important with spacers. For example, multiple actuations before inhalation and a delay between actuation and inhalation may reduce the proportion of drug inhaled. Frequent washing with a mild detergent, rinsing in warm water, and then air-drying are also recommended to reduce the accumulation of static electricity (which attracts drug particles), which occurs with plastic spacers.

Over recent years there has been a proliferation of pressurized aerosol and dry powder devices, in part due to the phasing out of the chlorofluoro-carbon-containing MDIs. Although it has become extraordinarily difficult to be familiar with the properties of each device and the dose equivalence when compared with the standard MDI device, it is necessary that prescribers are aware of this information in relation to the devices they commonly use.

C. Emergency Treatment of Severe Asthma

A clinical situation that has recently been investigated is the use of high doses of ICS in the emergency treatment of severe attacks of asthma (48–50). The rationale for such an approach includes the delivery of steroid directly to the airways, lower systemic side effects, and a greater efficacy in reducing BHR compared with oral steroids. A systematic review of the seven trials that have investigated this indication identified that inhaled steroids may reduce hospital admission rates by about half in patients with acute severe asthma (50). In con-trast, ICS did not achieve clinically important changes in pulmonary function or symptom scores. Furthermore, it was unclear if there was a benefit of ICS when used in addition to systemic corticosteroids. As a result, further research is required to determine the effects of ICS in acute severe asthma, in particular comparing the use of ICS with oral steroids, the dose–response relationship, and whether ICS have efficacy when used in addition to oral corticosteroids. In the meantime it would be reasonable to prescribe repeated high doses of ICS in the situation of severe asthma if for some reason oral steroids were not available.

D. Oral Steroid Reduction

The original study of the efficacy of BDP demonstrated its ability to achieve a reduction of oral steroids in patients with severe steroid-dependent asthma (47). Since then ICS therapy across a wide dose range has been shown to be effective in reducing the dose of oral steroids in patients requir-ing continuous oral steroid treatment (44–46,140–142). While clinicians have predominantly focused on this ability of such high doses of ICS to allow oral steroid reduction or withdrawal, these results also suggest that ICS may have greater effectiveness in the control of asthma than oral prednisone in patients with chronic severe disease. This interpretation is consistent with the greater efficacy of very high doses of ICS (FP 2000 µg/day) in improving BHR to both methacholine and AMP than oral steroids (30 mg/day prednisolone) (143).

E.　Steroid Resistance

There is a very small subgroup of patients who do not respond clinically to the beneficial effects or experience adverse systemic effects of high doses of systemic and/or inhaled steroids, despite having marked airway variability and being responsive to inhaled bronchodilators (144,145). In the workup of such a patient it is important not only to determine that they fail to respond to high-dose oral and inhaled steroids, but also that they do not have another diagnosis such as paradoxical vocal cord dysfunction or COPD. Reduced responsiveness to high doses of inhaled or oral steroids is considerably more common than steroid resistance. This subgroup of patients who deteriorate when the dose of oral steroids is reduced is referred to as "steroid-dependent." In this group, underlying causes such as provoking or sensitizing factors associated with occupational or allergen exposure should be investigated.

Another important factor that reduces responsiveness to ICS therapy is tobacco smoking (146). Tobacco smoking markedly reduces the improvements in lung function, BHR, and sputum eosinophils otherwise achieved by ICS therapy in nonsmoking asthmatics (147,148). Smoking also impairs the efficacy of short-term oral steroid treatment in asthma, with partial recovery of responsiveness in ex-smokers (149). These observations are important not only in terms of its clinical implications but also with respect to the mechanisms of action of ICS in asthma. It has been proposed that tobacco smoking may reduce histone deacetylase-2 expression and activity in the airway wall and alveolar macrophages, thereby reducing the effect of ICS (150).

F.　Pregnancy

The recommendation to use ICS for the management of moderate or severe asthma during pregnancy is based on studies that have established both their safety and efficacy in this situation (88). The largest epidemiological study undertaken to date, based on the Swedish Medical Birth Register, reported that mothers who used budesonide during pregnancy gave birth to infants of normal gestational age, birth weight, and length, with no increased rate of stillbirths or multiple births (151). There is also evidence that the use of BDP or budesonide during pregnancy is not associated with an increase in major congenital malformations (152,153).

In contrast, uncontrolled asthma is associated with many maternal and fetal complications, including hypertension, pre-eclampsia, complicated labor, intrauterine growth restriction, preterm birth, and perinatal mortality (154–157). However, ICS therapy has been shown to decrease the risk of an acute attack of asthma in pregnancy (158) and the risk of readmission following an asthma exacerbation (159). As a result, pregnancy can be considered as an indication to optimize ICS therapy to reduce the risk of unstable asthma and its complications.

XIV. Summary

ICS are the first-line anti-inflammatory therapy in the treatment of adult asthma. ICS therapy is the only class of medication that can reduce the risk of life-threatening attacks and mortality from asthma, in addition to reducing symptoms and improving lung function and quality of life. Their therapeutic dose range is 100–1000 µg/day of BDP, budesonide, or TAA; 50–500 µg/day of FP or mometasone. Doses in excess of this range are not recommended for routine use as they are likely to result in clinically significant systemic side effects without further increase in efficacy. Instead, in those patients with poorly controlled asthma despite 400–1000 µg BDP or equivalent, it is recommended that a long-acting β-agonist is added, preferably in a combination inhaler device.

There is evidence that the early introduction of ICS therapy in persistent asthma leads to an improved outcome when compared with a delay in treatment until more severe disease has developed. In stable patients on higher doses of ICS it is worth back-titrating the dose as a substantial dosage reduction can often be achieved. Finally, the greatest benefits with long-term ICS are likely to be achieved when their use is incorporated within the structure of an asthma self-management plan system of care.

References

1. Barnes PJ, Pedersen S, Busse W. Efficacy and safety of ICS: new developments. Am J Respir Crit Care Med 1998; 157(3 Pt 2):S1–S39.
2. Kamada AK, Szefler SJ. Glutocorticoids in asthma and rhinitis. In: Busse WW, Holgate ST, eds. Asthma and Rhinitis. 2nd ed. Oxford: Blackwell Science, 2000:1569–1581.
3. Laitinen LA, Laitinen A, Haahtela T. A comparative study of the effects of an inhaled corticosteroid, budesonide, and a beta 2-agonist, terbutaline, on airway inflammation in newly diagnosed asthma: a randomized, double-blind, parallel-group controlled trial. J Allergy Clin Immunol 1992; 90(1):32–42.
4. Djukanovic R, Wilson JW, Britten KM, Wilson SJ, Walls AF, Roche WR, Howarth PH, Holgate ST. Effect of an inhaled corticosteroid on airway inflammation and symptoms in asthma. Am Rev Respir Dis 1992; 145(3): 669–674.
5. Olivieri D, Chetta A, Del Donno M, Bertorelli G, Casalini A, Pesci A, Testi R, Foresi A. Effect of short-term treatment with low-dose inhaled fluticasone propionate on airway inflammation and remodeling in mild asthma: a placebo-controlled study. Am J Respir Crit Care Med 1997; 155(6):1864–1871.

6. Trigg CJ, Manolitsas ND, Wang J, Calderon MA, McAulay A, Jordan SE, Herdman MJ, Jhalli N, Duddle JM, Hamilton SA, Devalia JL, Davies RJ. Placebo-controlled immunopathologic study of four months of inhaled corticosteroids in asthma. Am J Respir Crit Care Med 1994; 150(1):17–22.

7. Jeffery PK, Godfrey RW, Adelroth E, Nelson F, Rogers A, Johansson SA. Effects of treatment on airway inflammation and thickening of basement membrane reticular collagen in asthma. A quantitative light and electron microscopic study. Am Rev Respir Dis 1992; 145(4 Pt 1):890–899.

8. Burke C, Power CK, Norris A, Condez A, Schmekel B, Poulter LW. Lung function and immunopathological changes after inhaled corticosteroid therapy in asthma. Eur Respir J 1992; 5(1):73–79.

9. Duddridge M, Ward C, Hendrick DJ, Walters EH. Changes in bronchoalveolar lavage inflammatory cells in asthmatic patients treated with high dose inhaled beclomethasone dipropionate. Eur Respir J 1993; 6(4):489–497.

10. Adelroth E, Rosenhall L, Johansson SA, Linden M, Venge P. Inflammatory cells and eosinophilic activity in asthmatics investigated by bronchoalveolar lavage. The effects of antiasthmatic treatment with budesonide or terbutaline. Am Rev Respir Dis 1990; 142(1):91–99.

11. Wilson JW, Djukanovic R, Howarth PH, Holgate ST. Inhaled beclomethasone dipropionate downregulates airway lymphocyte activation in atopic asthma. Am J Respir Crit Care Med 1994; 149(1):86–90.

12. Colasurdo GN, Larsen GL. Airway hyperresponsiveness. In: Busse WM, Holgate ST, eds. Asthma and Rhinitis. 2nd ed. Oxford: Blackwell Scientific Press, 2000:1248–1260.

13. Barnes PJ. Effect of corticosteroids on airway hyperresponsiveness. Am Rev Respir Dis 1990; 141(2 Pt 2):S70–S76.

14. Haahtela T, Jarvinen M, Kava T, Kiviranta K, Koskinen S, Lehtonen K, Nikander K, Persson T, Reinikainen K, Selroos O, et al. Comparison of a beta 2-agonist, terbutaline, with an inhaled corticosteroid, budesonide, in newly detected asthma. N Engl J Med 1991; 325(6):388–392.

15. Mitchell EA. Is current treatment increasing asthma mortality and morbidity? Thorax 1989; 44:81–84

16. Haahtela T, Jarvinen M, Kava T, Kiviranta K, Koskinen S, Lehtonen K, Nikander K, Persson T, Selroos O, Sovijarvi A, et al. Effects of reducing or discontinuing inhaled budesonide in patients with mild asthma. N Engl J Med 1994; 331(11):700–705.

17. Vathenen AS, Knox AJ, Wisniewski A, Tattersfield AE. Time course of change in bronchial reactivity with an inhaled corticosteroid in asthma. Am Rev Respir Dis 1991; 143(6):1317–1321.

18. Bel EH, Timmers MC, Zwinderman AH, Dijkman JH, Sterk PJ. The effect of inhaled corticosteroids on the maximal degree of airway narrowing to methacholine in asthmatic subjects. Am Rev Respir Dis 1991; 143(1):109–113.

19. Barnes PJ. Inhaled glucocorticoids for asthma. N Engl J Med 1995; 332: 868–875.

20. Blais L, Ernst P, Boivin J-F, Suissa S. Inhaled corticosteroids and the prevention of readmission to hospital for asthma. Am J Respir Crit Care Med 1998; 158:126–132.

21. Ernst P, Walter O, Spitzer MD, Suissa S, Cockcroft D, Habbick B, Horwitz RI, Boivin J-F, McNutt M, Buist AS. Risk of fatal and near-fatal asthma in relation to inhaled corticosteroid use. JAMA 1992; 268:3462–3464.

22. Suissa S, Ernst P, Benayoun S, Baltzan M, Cai B. Low-dose inhaled corticosteroids and the prevention of death from asthma. N Engl J Med 2000; 343:332–336.

23. Sin DD, Tu JV. Inhaled corticosteroid therapy reduces the risk of rehospitalization and all-cause mortality in elderly asthmatics. Eur Respir J 2001; 17: 380–385.

24. Blais L, Suissa S, Boivin J-F, Ernst P. First treatment with inhaled corticosteroids and the prevention of admissions to hospital for asthma. Thorax 1998; 53: 1025–1029.

25. Suissa S, Ernst P, Kezouh A. Regular use of inhaled corticosteroids and the long term prevention of hospitalisation for asthma. Thorax 2002; 57:880–884.

26. Donahue JG, Weiss ST, Livingston JM, Goetsch MA, Greineder DK, Platt R. Inhaled steroids and the risk of hospitalization for asthma. JAMA 1997; 277: 887–981.

27. Lanes SF, Rodriguez LAG, Huerta C. Respiratory medications and risk of asthma death. Thorax 2002; 57:683–686.

28. Abramson MJ, Bailey MJ, Couper FJ, Driver JS, Drummer OH, Forbes AB, McNeil JJ, Walters EH. Are asthma medications and management related to deaths from asthma? Am J Respir Crit Care Med 2001; 163:12–18

29. Rea HH, Scragg R, Jackson R, Beaglehole R, Fenwick J, Sutherland DC. A case-control study of deaths from asthma. Thorax 1986; 41:833–839.

30. Crane J, Pearce N, Burgess C, Woodman K, Robson B, Beasley R. Markers of risk of death and readmission in the 12 months following a hospital admission in asthma. Int J Epidemiol 1992; 21:737–744.

31. Weiss KB, Sullivan SD. The health economics of asthma. In: Busse W, Holgate S, eds. Asthma and Rhinitis. 2nd ed. Cambridge, MA: Blackwell Scientific, 2000:1786–1792.

32. Molfino NA, Nannini LJ, Rebuck AS, Slutsky AS. The fatality-prone asthmatic patient: follow-up study after near fatal attacks. Chest 1992; 101:621–623.

33. Wasserfallen J-B, Schaller M-D, Feihl F, Perret CH. Sudden asphyxic asthma: a distinct entity? Am Rev Respir Dis 1990; 142:108–111.

34. Holt S, Suder A, Weatherall M, Cheng S, Shirtcliffe P, Beasley R. Dose-response relation of inhaled fluticasone propionate in adolescents and adults with asthma: meta-analysis. BMJ 2001; 323(7307):253–256.

35. Masoli M, Weatherall M, Holt S, Beasley R. Clinical dose-response relationship of fluticasone propionate in adults with asthma. Thorax 2004; 59:16–20.

36. Szefler SJ, Bousher HA, Pearlman DS, Togia A, Liddle R, Furlong A, Shah T, Knobil K. Time to onset of effect of fluticasone propionate in patients with asthma. J Allergy Clin Immunol 1999; 103:780–788.

37. Masoli M, Holt S, Weatherall M, Beasley R. Dose-response relationship of inhaled budesonide in adult asthma: a meta-analysis. Eur Respir J 2004; 23:1–7.

38. Bousquet J, Ben-Joseph R, Messonnier M, Alemao E, Gould AL. A meta-analysis of the dose-response relationship of inhaled corticosteroids in adolescents and adults with mild to moderate persistent asthma. Clin Ther 2002; 24:1–20.

39. Busse WW, Brazinsky S, Jacobson K, Stricker W, Schmitt K, Vanden Burgt J, Donnell D, Hannon S, Colice GL. Efficacy response of inhaled beclomethasone dipropionate in asthma is proportional to dose and is improved by formulation with a new propellant. J Allergy Clin Immunol 1999; 104:1215–1222.

40. Welch MJ, Levy S, Smith JA, Feiss G, Farrar JR. Dose-ranging study of the clinical efficacy of twice-daily triamcinolone acetonide inhalation aerosol in moderately severe asthma. Chest 1997; 112:597–606.

41. O'Connor B, Bonnaud G, Haahtela T, Luna JM, Querfurt H, Wegener T, Lutsky BN. Dose-ranging study of mometasone furoate dry powder inhaler in the treatment of moderate persistent asthma using fluticasone propionate as an active comparator. Ann Allergy Asthma Immunol 2001; 86(4):397–404.

42. Sharpe M, Jarvis B. Inhaled mometasone: a review of its use in adults and adolescents with persistent asthma. Drugs 2001; 61:1325–1350.

43. Szefler SJ, Martin RJ, King TS, Boushey HA, Cherniack RM, Chinchilli VM, Craig TJ, Dolovich M, Drazen JM, Fagan JK, Fahy JV, Fish JE, Ford JG, Israel E, Kiley J, Kraft M, Lazarus SC, Lemanske RF Jr, Mauger E, Peters SP, Sorkness CA. Significant variability in response to inhaled corticosteroids for persistent asthma. J Allergy Clin Immunol 2002; 109:410–418.

44. Nelson HS, Busse WW, de Boisblanc BP, Berger WE, Noonan MJ, Webb DR. Fluticasone propionate powder: oral corticosteroid-sparing effect and improved lung function and quality of life in patients with severe chronic asthma. J Allergy Clin Immunol 1999; 103(2 Pt 1):267–275.

45. Fish JE, Karpel JP, Craig TJ, Bensch GW, Noonan M, Webb DR, Silverman B, Schenkel EJ, Rooklin AR, Ramsdell JW, et al. Inhaled mometasone furoate reduces oral prednisone requirements while improving respiratory function and health-related quality of life in patients with severe persistent asthma. J Allergy Clin Immunol 2000; 106(5):852–860.

46. Miyamoto T, Takahashi T, Nakajima S, Makino S, Yamakido M, Mano K, Nakashima M, Tollemar U, Selroos O. A double blind placebo-controlled steroid-sparing study with budesonide turbuhaler in Japanese oral steroid-dependent asthma patients. Respirology 2000; 5:231–240.

47. Morrow Brown H, Storey G, George WHS. Beclomethasone dipropionate: a new steroid aerosol for the treatment of allergic asthma. BMJ 1972; 1:585–590.

48. Levy ML, Stevenson C, Maslen T. Comparison of short courses of oral prednisone and fluticasone propionate in the treatment of adults with acute exacerbations of asthma in primary care. Thorax 1996; 51:1087–1092.

49. Fitzgerald JM, Shragge D, Haddon J, Jennings B, Lee J, Bai T, Pare P, Kassen D, Grunfeld A. A randomized controlled trial of high dose inhaled budesonide versus oral prednisone in patients discharged from the emergency department following an acute asthma exacerbation. Can Respir J 2000; 7:61–67.

50. Edmonds ML, Camargo CA Jr, Pollack CV Jr, Rowe BH. Early use of inhaled corticosteroids in the emergency department treatment of acute asthma. Cochrane Database Syst Rev Cochrane Library 2002; 2:1–29.

51. Gershman N, Wong H, Liu J, Fahy J. Low and high dose fluticasone propionate in asthma: effects during and after treatment. Eur Respir J 2000; 15:11–18.

52. Jatakanon A, Kharitonov S, Lim S, Barnes PJ. Effect of differing doses of inhaled budesonide on markers of airway inflammation in patients with mild asthma. Thorax 1999; 54:108–114.

53. Wallin A, Sue-Chu M, Bjermer L, Ward J, Sandström T, Lindberg A, Lundbäck B, Djukanović R, Holgate S, Wilson S. Effect of inhaled fluticasone with and without salmeterol on airway inflammation in asthma. J Allergy Clin Immunol 2003; 112:72–78.

54. O'Sullivan S, Cormican L, Murphy M, Poulter LW, Burke CM. Effects of varying doses of fluticasone propionate on the physiology and bronchial wall immunopathology in mild-to-moderate asthma. Chest 2002; 122:1966–1972.

55. Leone FT, Fish JE, Szefler SJ, West SL. Systematic review of the evidence regarding potential complications of inhaled corticosteroid use in asthma. Chest 2003; 124:2329–2340.

56. Kamada AK, Szefler SJ, Martin RJ, Boushey HA, Chinchilli VM, Drazen JM, Fish JE, Israel E, Lazarus SC, Lemanske RF. Issues in the use of inhaled corticosteroids. Am J Respir Crit Care Med 1996; 153:1739–1748.

57. Lipworth BJ, Wilson AM. Dose response to inhaled corticosteroids: benefits and risks. Sem Respir Crit Care Med 1998; 19:625–646.

58. Sorkness CA. Comparisons of systemic activity and safety among different inhaled corticosteroids. J Allergy Clin Immunol 1998; 102:S52–S64.

59. Teelucksingh S, Padfield PL, Tibi L, Gough KJ, Holt PR. Inhaled corticosteroids, bone formation, and osteocalcin. Lancet 1991; 338(8758):60–61.

60. Kerstjens HA, Postma DS, van Doormaal JJ, van Zanten AK, Brand PL, Dekhuijzen PN, Koeter GH. Effects of short-term and long-term treatment with inhaled corticosteroids on bone metabolism in patients with airways obstruction. Thorax 1994; 49(7):652–656.

61. Wong CA, Walsh LJ, Smith CJP, Wisniewski AF, Lewis SA, Hubbard R, Cawte S, Green DJ, Pringle M, Tattersfield AE. Inhaled corticosteroid use an bone mineral density in patients with asthma. Lancet 2000; 355:1399–1403.

62. Toogood JH, Sorva R, Puolijoki H. Review of the effects of inhaled steroid therapy on bone. Int J Risk Saf Med 1994; 5:1–14.

63. Hubbard RB, Smith CJP, Smeeth L, Harrison TW, Tattersfield AE. Inhaled corticosteroids and hip fracture: a population-based case-control study. Am J Respir Crit Care Med 2002; 166:1563–1566.

64. Verstraeten A, Dequeker J. Vertebral and peripheral bone mineral content and fracture incidence in postmenopausal patients with rheumatoid arthritis: effect of low dose corticosteroids. Ann Rheum Dis 1986; 45(10):852–857.

65. Luengo M, Picado C, Del Rio L, Guanabens N, Montserrat JM, Setoain J. Vertebral fractures in steroid dependent asthma and involutional osteoporosis: a comparative study. Thorax 1991; 46(11):803–806.

66. Walsh LJ, Lewis SA, Wong CA, Cooper S, Oborne J, Cawte SA, Harrison T, Green DJ, Pringle M, Hubbard R, Tattersfield AE. The impact of oral corticosteroid use on bone mineral density and vertebral fracture. Am J Respir Crit Care Med 2002; 166:691–695.

67. Suissa S, Baltzan M, Kremer R, Ernst P. Inhaled and nasal corticosteroid use and the risk of fracture. Am J Respir Crit Care Med 2004; 169:83–88.

68. Van Staa TP, Leufkens HGM, Cooper C. Use of inhaled corticosteroids and risk of fractures. J Bone Miner Res 2001; 16:581–588.

69. Lipworth BJ, Seckl JR. Measures for detecting systemic bioactivity with inhaled and intranasal corticosteroids. Thorax 1997; 52:476–482.

70. Aaronson D, Kaiser H, Dockhorn R, Findlay S, Korenblat P, Thorsson L, Källén A. Effects of budesonide by means of the Turbuhaler on the hypothalamic-pituitary-adrenal axis in asthmatic subjects: a dose-response study. J Allergy Clin Immunol 1998; 101:312–319.

71. Kellerman D, Stricker W, Howland W, Sorkness C, Dockhorn R, Galant S, Vargas R, Hamedani A, Liao E. Effects of inhaled fluticasone propionate (FP) on the HPA axis of patients with asthma. Eur Respir J 1996; 9(suppl 23):162s.

72. Affirme MB, Kosoglou T, Thonoor CM, Flannery BE, Herron JM. Mometasone furoate has minimal effects on the hypothalamic-pituitary-adrenal axis when delivered at high doses. Chest 2000; 118:1538–1546.

73. World Health Organization Office of Information. Blindness and Visual Disability. Part 2: Major causes worldwide. WHO Fact Sheet 143, Geneva: WHO 1997.

74. Dolin P. Epidemiology of cataract. In: Johnson GJ, Minassian DC, Weale R, eds. The Epidemiology of Eye Disease. London: Chapman & Hall, 1998:103–118.

75. Smeeth L, Boulis M, Hubbard R, Fletcher AE. A population based case-control study of cataract and inhaled corticosteroids. Br J Ophthalmol 2003; 87:1247–1251.

76. Cumming RG, Mitchell P, Leeder SR. Use of inhaled corticosteroids and the risk of cataracts. N Engl J Med 1997; 337:8–14.

77. Meltzer EO, Kemp JP, Welch MJ, Orgel HA. Effect of dosing schedule on efficacy of beclomethasone dipropionate aerosol in chronic asthma. Am Rev Respir Dis 1985; 131(5):732–736.

78. Toogood JH, Baskerville JC, Jennings B, Lefcoe NM, Johansson SA. Influence of dosing frequency and schedule on the response of chronic asthmatics to the aerosol steroid, budesonide. J Allergy Clin Immunol 1982; 70(4):288–298.

79. Chemelik F, Doughty A. Objective measurements of compliance in asthma treatment. Ann Allergy 1994; 73:527–532.

80. Leflein J. Once daily use of inhaled corticosteroids: a new regimen in the treatment of persistent asthma. Allergol Int 2000; 49:7–17.

81. Eisen S, Miller D, Woodward R, Spitznagel E, Przybeck T. The effect of prescribed daily dose frequency on patient medication compliance. Arch Int Med 1990; 150(9):1881–1884.

82. Kemp JP, Berkowitz RB, Miller SD, Murray JJ, Nolop K, Harrison JE. Mometasone furoate administered once daily is as effective as twice-daily administration for treatment of mild-to-moderate persistent asthma. J Allergy Clin Immunol 2000; 106(3):485–492.

83. Gagnon M, Cote J, Milot J, Turcotte H, Boulet LP. Comparative safety and efficacy of single or twice daily administration of inhaled beclomethasone in moderate asthma. Chest 1994; 105(6):1732–1737.

84. Masoli M, Weatherall M, Holt S, Beasley R. Budesonide once versus twice-daily administration: meta-analysis. Respirol 2004; 9(4):528–534.

85. Hyland M. Rationale for once daily therapy in asthma: compliance issues. Drugs Supplement 1999; 58(suppl 4):1–6.
86. National Asthma Council. Asthma Management Handbook. 2002.
87. New Zealand Guidelines Group. Best practice evidence-based guideline: the diagnosis and treatment of adult asthma. New Zealand Guidelines Group, September 2002:101.
88. British Thoracic Society and Scottish Intercollegiate Guidelines Network. British Guideline on Asthma Management: a national clinical guideline. Thorax 2003; 58 (suppl 1):i1–i94.
89. Campbell LM, Gooding TN, Aitchison WR, Smith N, Powell JA. Initial loading (400 micrograms twice daily) versus static (400 micrograms nocte) dose budesonide for asthma management. Int J Clin Prac 1998; 52(6):361–368, 370.
90. Chanez P, Karlstrom R, Godard P. High or standard initial dose of budesonide to control mild-to-moderate asthma? Eur Respir J 2001; 17(5):856–862
91. Lorentzson S, Boe J, Eriksson G, Persson G. Use of inhaled corticosteroids in patients with mild asthma. Thorax 1990; 45(10):733–735.
92. Miyamoto T, Takahashi T, Nakajima S, Makino S, Yamakido M, Mano K, Nakashima M, Tollemar U, Selroos O. A double-blind, placebo-controlled dose-response study with budesonide Turbuhaler in Japanese asthma patients. Respirol 2000; 5(3):247–256.
93. O'Byrne P, Cuddy L, Taylor DW, Birsh S, Morris J, Syrotuik J. Efficacy and cost benefit of inhaled corticosteroids in patients considered to have mild asthma in primary care practice. Can Respir J 1996; 3:169–175.
94. Sheffer AL, LaForce C, Chervinsky P, Pearlman D, Schaberg A. Fluticasone propionate aerosol: efficacy in patients with mild to moderate asthma. J Fam Pract 1996; 42(4):369–375.
95. van der Molen T, Meyboom-de Jong B, Mulder HH, Postma DS. Starting with a higher dose of inhaled corticosteroids in primary care asthma treatment. Am J Respir Crit Care Med 1998; 158(1):121–125.
96. Black PN, Lawrence BJ, Goh KH, Barry MS. Differences in the potencies of inhaled steroids are not reflected in the doses prescribed in primary care in New Zealand. Eur J Clin Pharmacol 2000; 56:431–435.
97. Antonicelli L, Bucca C, Neri M, de Benedetto F, Sabbatani P, Bonifazi F, Eichler H-G, Zhang Q, Yin DD. Asthma severity and medical resource utilisation. Eur Respir J 2004; 23:723–729.
98. Hawkins G, McMahon AD, Twaddle S, Wood SF, Ford I, Thomson NC. Stepping down inhaled corticosteroids in asthma: randomised controlled trial. BMJ 2003; 326:1115–1120.
99. Sont JK, Willems LNA, Bel EH, van Krieken HJM, Vandenbroucke JP, Sterk JP and the AMPUL Study Group. Clinical control and histological outcome of asthma when using airway hyperresponsiveness as an additional guide to long-term treatment. Am J Respir Crit Care Med 1999; 159:1043–1051.
100. Beasley R, Roche WR, Roberts JA, Holgate ST. Cellular events in the bronchi in mild asthma and after bronchial provocation. Am Rev Respir Dis 1989; 139:806–817.
101. Brown PJ, Greville HW, Finucane KE. Asthma and irreversible airflow obstruction. Thorax 1984; 39(2):131–136.

102. Peat JK, Woolcock AJ, Cullen K. Rate of decline of lung function in subjects with asthma. Eur J Respir Dis 1987; 70(3):171–179.

103. Selroos O, Pietinalho A, Lofroos AB, Riska H. Effect of early vs late intervention with inhaled corticosteroids in asthma. Chest 1995; 108(5):1228–1234.

104. Global Initiative for Asthma. Global strategy for asthma management and prevention NHLBI/WHO Workshop Report. National Institutes of Health, National Heart, Lung and Blood Institute, 2002.

105. Shrewsbury S, Pyke S, Britton M. Meta-analysis of increased dose of inhaled steroid or addition of salmeterol in symptomatic asthma (MIASMA). BMJ 2000; 320:1368–1373.

106. Pauwels RA, Lofdahl C-G, Postma DS, Tattersfield AE, O'Byrne P, Barnes PJ, Ullman A. Effect of inhaled formoterol and budesonide on exacerbations of asthma. New Engl J Med 1997; 337:1405–1411.

107. Baraniuk J, Murray JJ, Nathan RA, Berger WE, Johnson M, Edwards LD, Srebro S, Rickard KA. Fluticasone alone or in combination with salmeterol vs triamcinolone in asthma. Chest 1999; 116:625–632.

108. Greening A, Ind P, Northfield M, Shaw G. Added salmeterol versus higher dose corticosteroid in asthma patients with symptoms on existing inhaled corticosteroid. Lancet 1994; 344:219–224.

109. Matz J, Emmett A, Rickard K, Kalberg C. Addition of salmeterol to low-dose fluticasone versus higher-dose fluticasone: an analysis of asthma exacerbations. J Allergy Clin Immunol 2001; 107:783–789.

110. O'Byrne P, Barnes P, Rodriguez-Roisin R, Runnerstrom E, Sandstrom T, Svensson K, Tattersfield A. Low dose inhaled budesonide and formoterol in mild persistent asthma (OPTIMA). Am J Respir Crit Care Med 2001; 164: 1392–1397.

111. Masoli M, Weatherall M, Holt S, Beasley R. Moderate dose inhaled corticosteriods plus salmeterol vs. higher doses of inhaled corticosteroids in symptomatic asthma. Thorax (in press).

112. Bloom J, Calhoun W, Koenig S, Yancey S, Reilly D, Edwards L, Stauffer J, Dorinsky P. Fluticasone propionate/salmeterol 100/50 µg is inhaled steroid sparing in patients who require fluticasone propionate 250 µg for asthma stability. Am J Respir Crit care Med 2003; 167(7):A891.

113. Busse W, Koenig SM, Oppenheimer J, Sahn SA, Yancey SW, Reilly D, Edwards LD, Dorinsky PM. Steroid-sparing effects of fluticasone propionate 100 microg and salmeterol 50 microg administered twice daily in a single product in patients previously controlled with fluticasone propionate 250 microg administered twice daily. J Allergy Clin Immunol 2003; 111(1):57–65.

114. Barnes PJ. Scientific rationale for inhaled combination therapy with long-acting β_2-agonoists and corticosteroids. Eur Respir J 2002; 19:182–191.

115. Lazarus SC, Boushey HA, Fahy JV, Chinchilli VM, Lemanske RF Jr, Sorkness CA, Kraft M, Fish JE, Peters SP, Craig T, Drazen JM, Ford JG, Israel E, Martin RJ, Mauger EA, Nachman SA, Spahn JD, Szefler SJ. Asthma Clinical Research Network for the National Heart, Lung, and Blood Institute. Long-acting beta2-agonist monotherapy vs continued therapy with inhaled corticosteroids in patients with persistent asthma: a randomized controlled trial. JAMA 2001; 285(20):2583–2593.

116. Lemanske RF Jr, Sorkness CA, Mauger EA, Lazarus SC, Boushey HA, Fahy JV, Drazen JM, Chinchilli VM, Craig T, Fish JE, Ford JG, Israel E, Kraft M, Martin RJ, Nachman SA, Peters SP, Spahn JD, Szefler SJ. Inhaled corticosteroid reduction and elimination in patients with persistent asthma receiving salmeterol: a randomized controlled trial. JAMA 2001; 285(20):2594–2603.

117. Stoloff SW, Stempel DA, Meyer J, Stanford RH, Carranza Rosenzweig JR. Improved refill persistence with fluticasone propionate and salmeterol in a single inhaler compared with other controller therapies. J Allergy Clin Immunol 2004; 113:245–251.

118. Nelson HS, Chapman KR, Pyke SD, Johnson M, Pritchard JN. Enhanced synergy between fluticasone propionate and salmeterol inhaled from a single inhaler versus separate inhalers. J Allergy Clin Immunol 2003; 112:29–36.

119. Evans DJ, Taylor DA, Zetterstrom O, Chung KF, O'Connor BJ, Barnes PJ. A comparison of low-dose inhaled budesonide plus theophylline and high-dose inhaled budesonide for moderate asthma. N Engl J Med 1997; 337(20): 1412–1418.

120. Lim S, Jatakanon A, Gordon D, Macdonald C, Chung KF, Barnes PJ. Comparison of high dose inhaled steroids, low dose inhaled steroids plus low dose theophylline, and low dose inhaled steroids alone in chronic asthma in general practice. Thorax 2000; 55(10):837–841.

121. Ukena D, Harnest U, Sakalauskas R, Magyar P, Vetter N, Steffen H, Leichtl S, Rathgeb F, Keller A, Steinijans VW. Comparison of addition of theophylline to inhaled steroid with doubling of the dose of inhaled steroid in asthma. Eur Respir J 1997; 10(12):2754–2760.

122. Wilson AJ, Gibson PG, Coughlan J. Long-acting beta agonists versus theophylline for maintenance treatment of asthma. Cochrane Database Syst Rev 2000; 2:1–29.

123. Ducharme FM. Inhaled glucocorticoids versus leukotriene receptor antagonists as single agent asthma treatment: systematic review of current evidence. BMJ 2003; 326:621–625.

124. Laviolette M, Malmstrom K, Lu S, Chervinsky P, Pujet JC, Peszek I, Zhang J, Reiss TF. Montelukast added to inhaled beclomethasone in treatment of asthma. Montelukast/Beclomethasone Additivity Group. Am J Respir Crit Care Med 1999; 160(6):1862–1868.

125. Price DB, Hernandez D, Magyar P, Fiterman J, Beeh KM, James IG, Konstantopoulos S, Rojas R, van Noord JA, Pons M, Gilles L, Leff JA. Randomised controlled trial of montelukast plus inhaled budesonide versus double dose inhaled budesonide in adult patients with asthma. Thorax 2003; 58:211–216.

126. Robinson DS, Campbell D, Barnes PJ. Addition of leukotriene antagonists to therapy in chronic persistent asthma: a randomised double-blind placebo-controlled trial. Lancet 2001; 357:2007–2011.

127. Bjermer L, Bisgaard H, Bousquet J, Fabbri LM, Greening AP, Haahtela T, Holgate ST, Picado C, Menten J, Balachandra Dass S, Leff JA, Polos PG. Montelukast and fluticasone compared with salmeterol and fluticasone in protecting against asthma exacerbation in adults: one year, double blind, randomised, comparative trial. BMJ 2003; 327:891–896.

128. Fish JE, Israel E, Murray JJ, Emmett A, Boone R, Yancey SW, Rickard KA. Salmeterol powder provides significantly better benefit than montelukast in asthmatic patients receiving concomitant inhaled corticosteroid therapy. Chest 2001; 120:423–430.

129. Nelson HS, Busse WW, Kerwin E, Church N, Emmett A, Rickard K, Knobil K. Fluticasone propionate/salmeterol combination provides more effective asthma control than low-dose inhaled corticosteroid plus montelukast. J Allergy Clin Immunol 2000; 106:1088–1095.

130. Busse W, Nelson H, Wolfe J, Kalberg C, Yancey SW, Rickard KA. Comparison of inhaled salmeterol and oral zafirlukast in patients with asthma. J Allergy Clin Immunol 1999; 103(6):1075–1080.

131. Fishwick D, D'Souza W, Beasley R. The asthma self-management plan system of care: What does it mean, how is it done, does it work, what models are available, what do patients want and who needs it? Patient Educ Couns 1997; 32:S21–S33

132. Gibson PG, Coughlan J, Wilson AJ, Abramson M, Bauman A, Hensley MJ, Walters EH. Self-management education and regular practitioner review for adults with asthma. Cochrane Database Syst Rev Cochrane Library 2000; 2:1–44.

133. Lahdensuo A, Haahtela T, Herrala J, Kava T, Kiviranta K, Kuusisto P, Peramaki E, Poussa T, Saarelainen S, Svahn T. Randomised comparison of guided self-management and traditional treatment of asthma over one year. BMJ 1996; 312:748–752.

134. Ignacio-Garcia JM, Gonzalez-Santos P. Asthma self-management education program by home monitoring of peak expiratory flow. Am J Respir Crit Care Med 1995; 151:353–359.

135. Harrison TW, Oborne J, Newton S, Tattersfield AE. Doubling the dose of inhaled corticosteroid to prevent asthma exacerbations: randomised controlled trial. Lancet 2004; 363:271–275.

136. Foresi A, Morelli MC, Catena E. Low-dose budesonide with the addition of an increased dose during exacerbations is effective in long-term asthma control. Chest 2000; 117(2):440–446.

137. Masoli M, Beasley R. Asthma exacerbations and inhaled corticosteroids. Lancet 2004; 363:1236 (letter).

138. Adams N, Bestall JM, Jones PW. Fluticasone versus beclomethasone or budesonide for chronic asthma. Cochrane Database Syst Rev Cochrane Library 2002; 2:1–82.

139. O'Callaghan C, Barry P. Spacer devices in the treatment of asthma. BMJ 1997; 314(7087):1061–1062.

140. Noonan M, Chervinsky P, Busse W, Weisberg S, Pinnas J, De Boisblanc B, Boltansky H, Pearlman D, Repsher L, Kellerman D. Fluticasone propionate reduces oral prednisone use while it improves asthma control. Am J Ther 1996; 3:497–505.

141. Lauresen LC, Taudorf E, Weeke B. High-dose inhaled budesonide in treatment of severe steroid-dependent asthma. Eur J Respir Dis 1986; 68:19–28.

142. Hummel S, Lehtonen L. Comparison of oral-steroid sparing by high-dose and low-dose inhaled steroid in maintenance treatment of severe asthma. Lancet 1992; 340:1483–1487.

143. Meijer RJ, Kerstjens HA, Arends LR, Kauffman HF, Koeter GH, Postma DS. Effects of inhaled fluticasone and oral prednisolone on clinical and inflammatory parameters in patients with asthma. Thorax 1999; 54:894–899.

144. Lane SJ, Lee TH. Glucocorticoid-resistant asthma. In: Holgate ST, Boushey HA, Fabbri LM, eds. Difficult Asthma. London: Martin Dunitz, 1999: 389–411.

145. Lee TH, Leung DYM. Glucocorticoid-insensitive bronchial asthma. In: Busse WW, Holgate ST, eds. Asthma and Rhinitis. 2nd ed. Oxford: Blackwell Science, 2000:1582–1590.

146. Kerstjens HA, Brand PL, Hughes MD, Robinson NJ, Postma DS, Sluiter HJ, Bleecker ER, Dekhuijzen PN, de Jong PM, Mengelers HJ, et al. A comparison of bronchodilator therapy with or without inhaled corticosteroid therapy for obstructive airways disease. Dutch Chronic Non-Specific Lung Disease Study Group. N Engl J Med 1992; 327(20):1413–1419.

147. Chalmers GW, Macleod KJ, Little SA, Thomson LJ, McSharry CP, Thomson NC. Influence of cigarette smoking on inhaled corticosteroid treatment in mild asthma. Thorax 2002; 57:226–230.

148. Meijer RJ, Postma DS, Kauffman HF, Arends LR, Koeter GH, Kerstjens HAM. Accuracy of eosinophils and eosinophil cationic protein to predict steroid improvement in asthma. Clin Exper Allergy 2002; 32:1096–1103.

149. Chaudhuri R, Livingston E, McMahon AD, Thomson L, Borland W, Thomson NC. Cigarette smoking impairs the therapeutic response to oral corticosteroids in chronic asthma. Am J Respir Crit Care Med 2003; 168: 1308–1311.

150. Barnes PJ, Ito K, Adcock IM. Corticosteroid resistance in chronic obstructive pulmonary disease: inactivation of histone deacetylase. Lancet 2004; 363:731–733.

151. Norjavaara E, Gerhardsson de Verdier M. Normal pregnancy outcomes in a population-based study including 2968 pregnant women exposed to budesonide. J Allergy Clin Immunol 2003; 111:736–742.

152. Schatz M, Zeiger RS, Harden K, Hoffman CC, Chilingar L, Petitti D. The safety of asthma and allergy medications during pregnancy. J Allergy Clin Immunol 1997; 100(3):301–306.

153. Kallen B, Rydhstroem H, Aberg A. Congenital malformations after the use of inhaled budesonide in early pregnancy. Obstet Gynecol 1999; 93(3):392–395.

154. Fitzsimons R, Greenberger PA, Patterson R. Outcome of pregnancy in women requiring corticosteroids for severe asthma. J Allergy Clin Immunol 1986; 78(2):349–353.

155. Perlow JH, Montgomery D, Morgan MA, Towers CV, Porto M. Severity of asthma and perinatal outcome. Am J Obstet Gynecol 1992; 167(4 Pt 1): 963–967.

156. Schatz M, Zeiger RS, Hoffman CP. Intrauterine growth is related to gestational pulmonary function in pregnant asthmatic women. Kaiser-Permanent Asthma and Pregnancy Study Group. Chest 1990; 98(2):389–392.

157. Demissie K, Breckenridge MB, Rhoads GG. Infant and maternal outcomes in the pregnancies of asthmatic women. Am J Respir Crit Care Med 1998; 158(4): 1091–1095.

158. Stenius-Aarniala BS, Hedman J, Teramo KA. Acute asthma during pregnancy. Thorax 1996; 51(4):411–414.

159. Wendel PJ, Ramin SM, Barnett-Hamm C, Rowe TF, Cunningham FG. Asthma treatment in pregnancy: a randomized controlled study. Am J Obstet Gynecol 1996; 175(1):150–154.

5

Optimal Management of Asthma: Leukotriene Modifiers

MICHAEL E. WECHSLER

Pulmonary and Critical Care Division, Department of Medicine,
  Brigham and Women's Hospital and Harvard Medical School
Boston, Massachusetts, U.S.A.

I. Introduction

The optimal management of asthma involves control of symptoms, prevention of variable obstruction to airflow, decrease of bronchial hyperresponsiveness, and reversal of the underlying inflammation involved in its pathogenesis. The ideal asthma therapy has a rational scientific basis, is effective in decreasing symptoms and maintaining lung function, is safe, is easy to administer, and meets the expectations of patients who take the drug. Over the last decade, leukotriene modifiers have emerged as one of the few new therapeutic options for asthma that meets each of these criteria. Leukotriene modifiers include both cysteinyl leukotriene receptor antagonists (such as zafirlukast, montelukast, and pranlukast) and 5-lipoxygenase (5-LO) inhibitors (such as zileuton). They are the first asthma therapies to evolve from our understanding of the pathophysiology of the disease: They specifically target a pathway of pathogenesis, rather than nonspecifically mediating inflammation and controlling symptoms. In this chapter, we discuss the attributes of these medications that make them an excellent therapy for asthma and the roles of these agents in the context of other asthma treatment modalities.

II. Historical Perspectives and the Rational Scientific Basis for Leukotriene Modifiers in Asthma

A. Historical Perspectives

Leukotrienes are so named because they were initially isolated from leukocytes and because their carbon backbone contained three double bonds in series, constituting a triene. However, these molecules were recognized as distinct biological entities several decades before they were chemically defined and purified in the late 1970s. Their role in asthma pathogenesis was first implicated in 1938 after Feldberg and Kellaway noted that cobra venom caused a slow-onset, sustained contraction of smooth muscle in Guinea pig lung perfusate (1). Two years later, they became known as the slow-reacting substances of anaphylaxis (SRS-A), when Kellaway and Trethewie revealed that the time course of this contraction was distinct from that caused by histamine (2). A role in asthma was further suggested in the 1960s when SRS-A was found to be released from lung fragments of a subject with asthma who was exposed to allergen (3) and in the 1970s, when Drazen and Austen demonstrated the effect of intravenous SRS-A administration on pulmonary mechanics in Guinea pigs (4). By 1980, SRS-A was finally chemically characterized as a mixture of three specific cysteinyl leukotriene products derived from the metabolism of arachidonic acid by the 5-LO pathway, whose chemical structures were elucidated as 5(S)-hydroxy-6(R)-glutathionyl-7, 9-*trans*-11, 14-*cis*-eicosatetraenoic acid and its cysteinyl-glycyl and cysteinyl congeners (leukotriene C4, D4, and E4, respectively) (5).

B. Leukotriene Biosynthesis

Leukotrienes are fatty acids and members of a larger group of biomolecules known as eicosanoids, which also encompasses cyclooxygenase products such as prostaglandins, thromboxanes, and prostacyclin and the products of 12- or 15-lipoxygenase (the lipoxins) and 5- and 15-lipoxygenase (5,6). Leukotrienes are synthesized in mast cells, eosinophils, and alveolar macrophages (7–9), all of which have been implicated as critical effector cells in the pathobiology of asthma. Airway epithelial cells (10,11) and pulmonary vascular endothelial cells (12) may also produce leukotrienes via transcellular metabolism (13,14). Leukotriene synthesis is initiated following trauma, infection, inflammation, and a variety of stimuli, including the activation of mast cell antigen-specific IgE bound to Fc receptors (15,16); hyperventilation of cold, dry air (17); aspirin ingestion by aspirin-intolerant individuals (18–20); hypoxia (21); hyperoxia (22); and exposure to platelet-activating factor (23). In these circumstances, cytosolic phospholipase A2 selectively cleaves arachidonic acid from perinuclear cell membranes, which is converted sequentially to 5-hydroperoxyeicosatetraenoic acid (5-HPETE) and then to leukotriene A4 (LTA4) (5,6-oxido-7,9-*trans* 11,

14-*cis*-eicosatetraenoic acid) by a catalytic complex consisting of 5-LO and the 5-LO activating protein (FLAP), which binds arachidonic acid and is critical to leukotriene synthesis (24) (Fig. 1). LTA4 is unstable and may be transformed through the action of the enzyme LTA4 epoxide hydrolase in polymorphonuclear leukocytes into LTB4, which is involved in eosinophil and neutrophil chemotaxis. Alternatively, in the presence of LTC4 synthase, glutathione is adducted to the C6 position of LTA4 in eosinophils, mast cells, and alveolar macrophages to yield the molecule known as leukotriene C4 (LTC4). The glutamic acid moiety of LTC4 is cleaved by γ-glutamyltranspeptidase to form the active entity leukotriene D4 (LTD4) whose glycine moiety may be cleaved by a variety of dipeptidases, resulting in the formation of leukotriene E4 (LTE4). LTC4, LTD4, and LTE4 are all known as the cysteinyl leukotrienes, as each one contains a cysteine.

Leukotrienes exert their biologic activities by binding to specific receptors that have been characterized functionally through comparisons of the activity of various agonists and antagonists. While leukotriene B4 (LTB4) binds to the B-leukotriene receptor (BLT), a G-protein-coupled

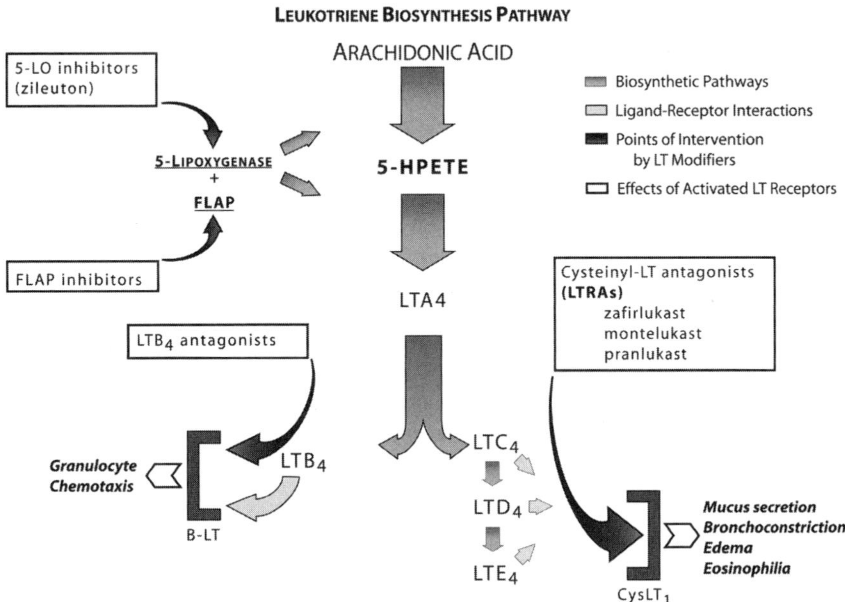

Figure 1 Leukotriene biosynthesis, effects, and points of therapeutic interruption. Leukotrienes are synthesized from arachidonic acid via the action of 5-LO and FLAP and help mediate airway inflammation. Leukotriene modifiers include both 5-LO inhibitors and cysteinyl leukotriene antagonists. FLAP inhibitors and LTB4 antagonists are currently under investigation. *Source*: Adapted from Ref. 196.

receptor cell surface protein that predominantly transduces chemotaxis and cellular activation (25–28), the cysteinyl leukotrienes bind to two distinct receptors that have been identified pharmacologically as *CysLT*1 and *CysLT*2. Previously known as the LTD4 receptor LTRD, *CysLT*1 is a 45-kDa membrane protein found in airway smooth muscle. Stimulation of this receptor by phosphoinositide-stimulated signal transduction causes smooth muscle constriction (29–32). LTD4 is the preferred ligand, but LTC4 and LTE4 also bind to this receptor, albeit with less biopotency (33–36). The *CysLT*2 receptor was previously known as the LTC4 receptor or LTRc. Stimulation of this pulmonary vascular smooth muscle receptor results in smooth muscle constriction and chemotaxis.

C. Biologic Effects of Leukotrienes: Rationale for a Role in Asthma

Since elucidating the structure and biosynthetic pathway of leukotrienes, researchers have further demonstrated their potency in smooth muscle constriction in both human and animal models, in vitro and in vivo, and have shown that 5-LO products stimulate smooth muscle proliferation (37–39). For example, inhaled LTC4 and LTD4 resulted in potent airway obstruction as manifest by decreased specific airway conductance (S_{Gaw}) (40), and Bisgaard et al. (41) demonstrated that asthmatic subjects were 100 to 1000 times more responsive to LTD4 than controls. Subsequent studies demonstrated that prior inhalation of leukotrienes caused an increase in airway responsiveness to both histamine and methacholine that lasted as long as one week. 5-LO products may also cause tissue edema (42,43) and stimulate smooth muscle proliferation (44–46) as well as eosinophil and neutrophil recruitment and activation (47–50). Invoked as causative agents in a host of inflammatory conditions such as inflammatory bowel disease, psoriasis, rheumatoid arthritis, and glomerulonephritis (51), leukotrienes are particularly implicated in the airway inflammatory pathway of asthma. For instance, cysteinyl leukotrienes have been shown to be potent mucus secretagogues and to modulate the activity of several components of the immune system. Furthermore, a variety of physical, chemical, and immunological stimuli (including activation of mast cell antigen-specific IgE bound to Fc receptors; hyperventilation of cold, dry air; and aspirin ingestion by aspirin-intolerant individuals) (52–54) activate many of the critical effector cells implicated in asthma pathobiology (mast cells, eosinophils, and alveolar macrophages) to produce leukotrienes (55–58).

Despite their rapid metabolism and degradation, leukotrienes have been identified in plasma, nasal and bronchoalveolar lavage (BAL) fluids, and urine. LTC4 and LTD4 have been found in greater levels in the plasma and BAL fluids of patients with stable asthma than in controls (59). Lam et al. (60) identified LTC4 and LTB4 in the sputum of patients with asthma, but not in that of patients with other lung diseases. Following endobronchial allergen challenge of normal subjects, BAL LTC4 levels are increased, as are urine LTE4 levels (61–63). Urine LTE4 levels are also increased among many (but not all) patients having spontaneous asthma attacks (64) and in subjects with nocturnal asthma (65), exercise-induced asthma, and aspirin-induced asthma (66,67). At baseline, urinary LTE4 levels are approximately sixfold higher in aspirin-sensitive than in aspirin-tolerant asthmatics; this aspirin-sensitive population also has increased levels of LTC4 in nasal lavage and demonstrates a fourfold increase in urinary LTE4 six hours after aspirin challenge; similar findings are not seen in aspirin-tolerant asthmatics (68,69).

As asthma pathogenesis is characterized by many features attributable to the actions of leukotrienes—namely, bronchoconstriction, hyper-responsiveness, increased microvascular permeability with tissue edema, hypersecretion of mucus, and eosinophil recruitment—and because leukotrienes have been recovered in greater quantities in the plasma, urine, sputum, exhaled breath condensate, and BAL fluid of asthmatics than in controls (70–73), several medications directed at the 5-LO pathway were developed over the last decade to treat asthma. Currently, one 5-LO inhibitor and three distinct cysteinyl leukotriene receptor antagonists are available throughout the world as treatment for asthma.

III. Leukotriene Modifiers Are Effective in Several Types of Asthma

A number of agents developed to interrupt the 5-LO pathway are available in many countries around the world as treatments for asthma (Fig. 1). Initial studies with these drugs focused on their ability to decrease leukotriene production (as measured by urinary leukotriene production) (74) and inhibit bronchoconstriction induced by inhalation of leukotrienes such as LTD4 (75–79). Because all of these studies demonstrated that each of the leukotriene modifiers had a substantial impact on either leukotriene synthesis or CysLT1 receptor–mediated bronchoconstriction, as well as on many of the mediators of inflammation produced in asthma by eosinophils, alveolar macrophages, and lymphocytes (80), these drugs were subsequently tested in cohorts of asthmatics in a variety of settings: (1) laboratory-induced asthma, (2) asthmatic bronchoconstriction and airway inflammation, and (3) chronic persistent asthma.

A. Laboratory-Induced Asthma

Laboratory-induced asthma includes asthma that is induced by challenge with cold air, exercise, aspirin, or antigen.

Cold Air–Induced Asthma

When asthmatic subjects hyperventilate cold, dry air, bronchospasm is often induced by a mechanism thought to be similar to that responsible for exercise-induced asthma. Israel and colleagues demonstrated that zileuton attenuated the bronchoconstrictor response to cold air (81). Similarly, Fischer et al. (82) demonstrated that regular treatment with zileuton for 13 weeks improved airway responsiveness to cold air–induced airway obstruction for as long as 10 days after completion of treatment, suggesting that inhibition of leukotriene generation can improve airway hyper-responsiveness. In addition, zafirlukast has been shown to similarly attenuate both cold-induced response as well as exercise-induced bronchoconstriction. These observations led to the proposal that the cooling and drying of airways provoked by these challenges results in leukotriene generation, which, in turn, results in bronchoconstriction. However, the variable response to leukotriene modifiers among some subjects challenged by cold air and the variable urinary leukotriene production in response to exercise (83) suggest that cold-air or exercise-induced bronchospasm is not leukotriene mediated in all such subjects.

Exercise-Induced Asthma

Exercise-induced bronchoconstriction occurs in approximately 80% of asthma patients (84); although there have been negative studies, several studies demonstrate increased levels of urinary leukotrienes following exercise (85,86). Several different leukotriene modifiers have been shown to inhibit the maximal bronchoconstrictor response after exercise by up to 70% (87–92). In 30% to 50% of subjects receiving these drugs, this response was completely inhibited, while in others, time to recovery of normal lung function was significantly shortened. While the bronchoprotective effect of β-agonists in exercise-induced asthma is lost with recurrent use (93), leukotriene modifiers maintain their bronchoprotective effects over many weeks of treatment (94). Edelman et al. (95) compared montelukast with salmeterol in a double-blind, placebo-controlled study of 191 adults with exercise-induced bronchoconstriction. Patients treated with montelukast had sustained improvement in symptoms, and 67% had a maximal decrease in FEV_1 of less than 20% throughout the eight weeks of the study. The bronchoprotective effect of salmeterol decreased significantly, and only 46% of patients had less than a 20% decrease in FEV_1 at the end of the study period.

Aspirin-Induced Asthma

Aspirin-induced asthma affects 5% to 8% of asthmatics and may cause life-threatening bronchospasm as well as dermal, nasoocular, and gastrointestinal symptoms. Patients with this susceptibility have elevated levels of urinary leukotrienes at baseline and even higher levels following aspirin challenge (18). An increase in the number of cells that are immunopositive for LTC4 synthase in bronchial biopsies suggests that this enzyme is involved in the pathogenesis of this syndrome (96). The physiological effects of aspirin challenge in aspirin-sensitive patients pretreated with zileuton is almost completely blocked, as such patients failed to develop any clinically significant adverse effects and urinary LTE4 levels were reduced by 68% (19). Dahlen et al. (97) subsequently demonstrated that administration of the cysteinyl leukotriene receptor antagonist montelukast to subjects with aspirin-sensitive asthma resulted in improved lung function even in the absence of aspirin provocation; the magnitude of FEV_1 improvement increased while urinary leukotriene levels decreased. These data suggest that the bronchospasm related to aspirin-sensitive asthma is mediated by leukotrienes and that leukotriene modifiers are the treatment of choice for these patients. However, while these agents are effective therapy for these individuals and modulate the response to subclinical doses of anti-inflammatory agents, they may not completely prevent the response to higher doses of aspirin or other anti-inflammatory agents in some highly sensitive subjects. For example, one patient developed an anaphylactic response to ibuprofen despite treatment with zafirlukast (98) and another patient receiving montelukast had an anaphylactic response to diclofenac (99).

Allergen-Associated Asthma

Leukotrienes have also been implicated in the bronchoconstriction and airway hyper-responsiveness characteristic of the early and late response in allergen-induced asthma. Urinary leukotrienes are elevated during the early asthmatic response, and a number of leukotriene receptor antagonists have been shown to inhibit bronchoconstriction during this response by as much 84% (100–103). However, one study with zileuton showed no significant response, and other studies with 5-LO inhibitors have had mixed results. Furthermore, these drugs have demonstrated only limited efficacy in the late response (104,105) and none of the agents studied to date has completely prevented the bronchoconstrictor response (particularly of the late response) elicited by antigen stimulation. While it appears that leukotrienes play a partial role in modulating the asthmatic allergic response, other mediators are clearly involved. Interestingly, patients with allergen-induced bronchospasm who were treated with both an antihistamine (loratidine) and a leukotriene receptor antagonist (zafirlukast) had almost complete inhibition of the early and late phase response (106).

B. Asthmatic Bronchoconstriction and Airway Inflammation

A major attribute of any asthma medication is its ability to counteract the spontaneous reversible bronchoconstriction that may develop in patients with mild to moderate asthma who withhold bronchodilator therapy. To assess the role of leukotrienes in the spontaneous airway narrowing of asthma, several leukotriene modifiers have been administered to patients with varying degrees of asthma, and spirometry has been performed. Each of the leukotriene modifiers has produced acute bronchodilatation and improvement in airway function within one to three hours. While the magnitude of bronchodilatation is often not as great as that with β-agonist therapy, FEV_1 is generally increased by 5% to 30%; the bronchodilator effect is also greater in patients with greater degrees of airway obstruction. Furthermore, the effects of the leukotriene modifier were additive to the effect of the β-agonist, suggesting that distinct contractile mechanisms are involved in each response (107–112). Because similar studies of non-asthmatic subjects have shown no reversal of airway tone, the reversal of asthmatic bronchoconstriction by leukotriene modifiers suggests that a significant component of asthmatic bronchoconstriction and basal airway tone in patients with asthma is mediated by the effect of leukotrienes produced by ongoing leukotriene synthesis by 5-LO at the CysLT1 receptor.

Leukotriene modifiers also have a significant preventive effect on bronchial hyper-responsiveness and airway inflammation (113). In one study, pranlukast given orally for one week to patients with stable asthma produced a small but significant reduction in bronchial hyper-responsiveness to methacholine (114). In another study, pranlukast given twice daily was associated with improvement in clinical symptoms, as well as improved histamine reactivity by bronchial challenge at 12 and 24 weeks after treatment. In a crossover trial, 21 patients received montelukast and the inhaled corticosteroid trimacinolone; both of these agents resulted not only in significant improvement in peak expiratory flow, but also in comparable significant improvements in methacholine and AMP responsiveness (115). Hence, cysteinyl leukotrienes are involved in hyper-responsiveness in chronic asthma and in allergen challenge–induced asthma.

Two important markers of airway inflammation, sputum eosinophils and exhaled nitric oxide (NO), are both affected by treatment with leukotriene modifier. Pranlukast caused a significant reduction in activated eosinophils in bronchial biopsy specimens by decreasing bone marrow eosinophilopoiesis and airway chemotactic and eosinophilopoietic cytokines, including eotaxin and interleukin-5 (116). Furthermore, both zafirlukast and montelukast significantly reduce sputum as well as peripheral blood eosinophil counts in conjunction with an improvement in peak flow and a suppression of sputum eosinophilic cationic protein production (117,118). Several studies show that leukotriene modifiers effectively reduce levels of exhaled NO, even in infants and in children with asthma aged two to five (119–125).

How do leukotriene modifiers affect airway remodeling, the airway structural changes that occur in patients with asthma in response to persistent inflammation resulting in airway wall thickening, subepithelial fibrosis, and hyperplasia of mucus glands, myofibroblasts, smooth muscle, and vasculature? To date, there have been no studies assessing the ability of leukotriene modifiers to affect remodeling. However, Henderson and colleagues used an acute-murine model of human asthma to show that specific inhibitors of 5-LO and FLAP that prevent leukotriene formation block airway mucus release and infiltration by eosinophils, indicating the importance of leukotrienes in these features of allergic pulmonary inflammation (126). They subsequently used a chronic model of allergic airway inflammation in mice with subepithelial fibrosis and found that montelukast significantly reduced the airway eosinophil infiltration, mucus plugging, smooth muscle hyperplasia, and subepithelial fibrosis in Ovalbumin (OVA)-sensitized/challenged mice, suggesting an important role for cysteinyl leukotrienes in the pathogenesis of chronic allergic airway inflammation with fibrosis and a potentially important role for leukotriene modifiers in preventing key features of airway remodeling (127).

C. Chronic Stable Asthma

In addition to their anti-inflammatory effects and benefits in patients with a variety of lab-induced models of asthma, leukotriene modifiers have significant efficacy in patients with chronic persistent asthma, compared with placebo, both as monotherapy and as add-on therapy to other controllers.

Leukotriene Modifiers as Monotherapy

Multiple studies have shown that, when asthma patients who used inhaled β-agonists as their only asthma medication were treated with a leukotriene modifier (pranlukast, zafirlukast, montelukast, or zileuton), asthma improved such that they had improvement in airway obstruction, decreased need for rescue treatment with β-agonists, relief of asthma symptoms, and decreased frequency of asthma exacerbations that required systemic corticosteroid therapy (111,112,128,129).

In studies of four to six weeks duration, patients with moderate asthma (mean FEV_1 of 65% predicted) treated only with β-agonists were given placebo in a single-blind manner for a run-in period of 7 to 14 days, followed by an active treatment period of four to six weeks (followed in some cases by a withdrawal period). In most of the trials, during the first month of treatment, the FEV_1 improved significantly by 10% to 15% and the degree of improvement was statistically significant with active agent compared with placebo. Improvement encompassed decreases in asthma symptoms, nighttime awakenings, and β-agonist use and increases in morning and evening peak flow rates. In the trials with zileuton (112) and zafirlukast (128), patients receiving higher doses of either drug had a significantly greater increase in FEV_1 than did patients receiving placebo; patients receiving lower doses had an increase of intermediate magnitude.

Long-term studies with each of the leukotriene modifiers have had similar findings. For instance, when 401 patients were randomized in a double-blind fashion to three months of therapy with placebo or with one of two doses of zileuton, there was a significant increase in FEV_1 with zileuton compared with placebo (16% with zileuton 600 mg four times a day vs. 8% with placebo), a significant decrease in asthma symptoms, a significant decrease in β-agonist use, and a significantly lower percentage of patients who required treatment with corticosteroids (6% vs. 16%). Furthermore, six months of treatment with zileuton reduced peripheral eosinophil counts by more than 20% (108). Although most of the improvement in airway function occurs within two to four weeks after the initiation of drug therapy, the improvement in FEV_1 was maintained over the course of the trial, extending previous findings that patients do not become tolerant of the effects of 5-LO inhibition or blockade.

The effect on FEV_1 also appears to be greater in patients with more severe airway obstruction. Zafirlukast improved FEV_1 by only 40 mL in patients whose baseline FEV_1 was more than 80% predicted, compared with an increase of 800 mL in those whose FEV_1 was less than 45% predicted (128). Among patients using inhaled corticosteroids, pranlukast allowed a 50% reduction in the dose of inhaled corticosteroid compared with placebo, without loss of asthma control (130). In general these agents have been shown to improve asthma control and can reduce days lost from school or work, unscheduled medical care episodes, and days with asthma symptoms (131–133).

Treatment once daily with montelukast appears to confer the same benefit as more frequent treatment with other agents (134). Furthermore, the leukotriene receptor antagonists have been systemically studied in children and are approved for use in children as young as two years of age (135–137). In children with moderate persistent asthma, treatment with montelukast (one 5-mg tablet at bedtime) was associated with improved lung function at baseline, decreased asthma symptoms, and decreased need for asthma rescue medication use. Asthma-specific quality of life improved a "clinically significant" amount in children receiving active treatment, while such an effect was not observed in children treated with placebo. These effects were present in patients also receiving inhaled corticosteroids as an asthma treatment. Montelukast, given as a single 5-mg tablet daily, inhibited the bronchospasm induced by exercise by an average of 50%; these effects were observed up to 24 hours after the last medication dose, indicating a prolonged effect. In children with exercise-induced asthma, zafirlukast, 40 mg/day, was effective in preventing exercise-induced bronchospasm (138).

How do leukotriene modifiers fare as monotherapy in comparison to other controller therapies? Several studies have compared the effectiveness of leukotriene modifiers and inhaled corticosteroids (124,139,140). In a study comparing montelukast and beclomethasone as monotherapy in patients with moderate asthma, there were greater peak expiratory flow rate and quality of life, fewer nocturnal awakenings and asthma attacks, more asthma-control days, and fewer days with asthma exacerbations following treatment with either active agent than with placebo (141). Both classes of therapy caused similar decreases in peripheral blood eosinophil counts. Although beclomethasone in general had a greater mean effect on FEV_1 than montelukast (percentage change from baseline in FEV_1 was 13.1% with beclomethasone, 7.4% with montelukast), montelukast had a faster onset of action and a greater initial effect. While other studies corroborate the findings that inhaled corticosteroids show greater improvement in FEV_1 and peak flow than leukotriene modifiers, they demonstrate no significant difference in exacerbation rates or days of asthma control (140,142–145). While inhaled corticosteroids often demonstrated greater effects on inflammatory indicators, several investigators found that both of these agents were effective at reducing airway inflammation and airway hyperresponsiveness (146); inhaled steroid use resulted in greater adrenal suppression and a rise in osteocalcin levels, an important marker of bone turnover (115).

Studies by Edelman et al. (95) and Villaran et al. (147) showed montelukast to be more effective than the long-acting β-agonist salmeterol in the acute and chronic treatment of exercise-induced asthma. In a four-week study comparing zafirlukast and salmeterol in patients with persistent asthma with established β-adrenergic responsiveness, both salmeterol and montelukast improved pulmonary function, asthma symptoms, and supplemental albuterol use (148). While salmeterol treatment resulted in significantly greater improvements from baseline than zafirlukast for morning peak flow (29.6 vs. 13.0 L/min), percentage of symptom-free days (22.4% vs. 8.8), and percentage of days and nights with no supplemental albuterol use (30.5% vs. 11.3), there was no significant difference in the improvement in FEV_1. In another study comparing salmeterol with zafirlukast over four weeks in 301 patients with persistent asthma, salmeterol was more effective than zafirlukast in improving pulmonary function and symptom control. However, asthma exacerbation rates and adverse event profiles were similar between the two drugs (149).

When zileuton was compared with twice-daily theophylline in a three-month trial, the two drugs resulted in similar increases in FEV_1 and had similar safety profiles. Theophylline gave somewhat greater symptomatic relief in the first two months of the trial, but there was no significant difference in maximal effect (150). When zafirlukast and cromolyn were compared to each other and to placebo in the treatment of patients with mild asthma, the medications were found to be superior to placebo but comparable to each other in terms of symptom scores and β-agonist usage (151,152).

Leukotriene Modifiers as Add-On Therapy

Several investigators have demonstrated that leukotriene modifiers decrease
the need for oral corticosteroid rescue therapy and permit the safe reduc-

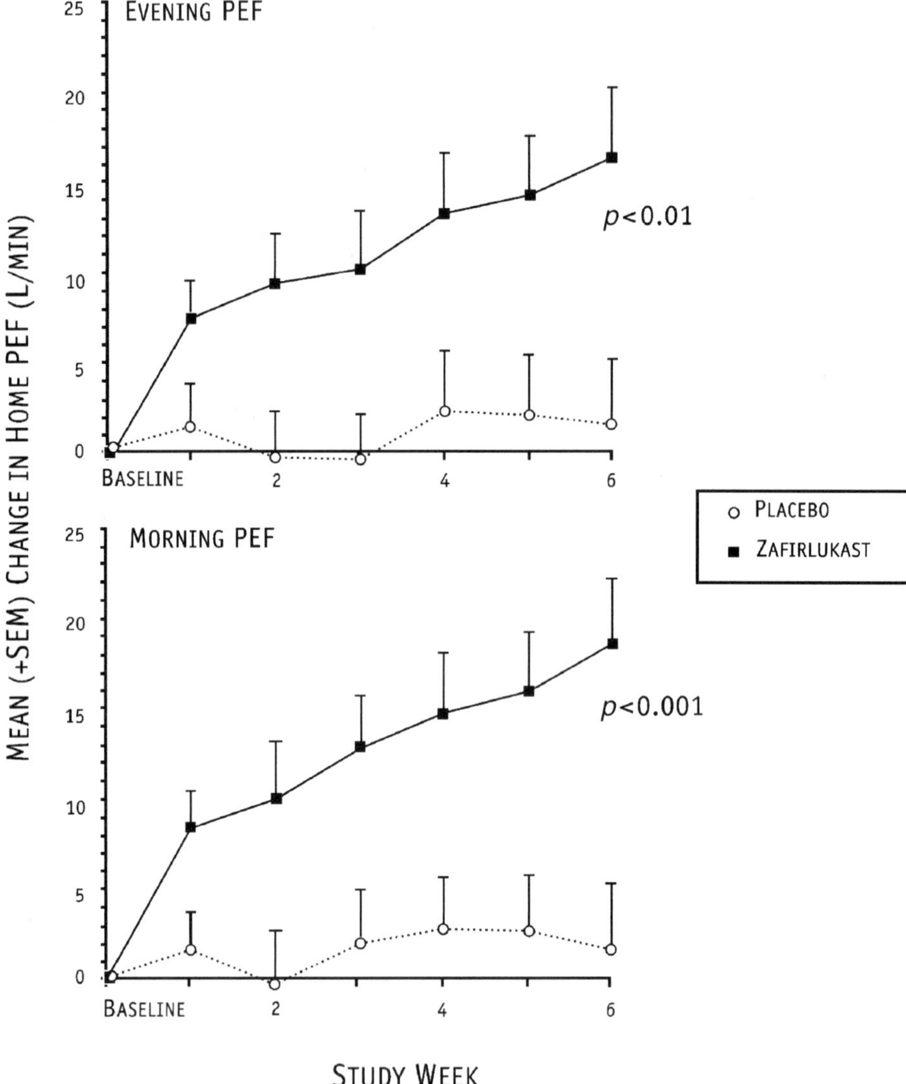

Figure 2   Effect of zafirlukast compared with placebo on A.M. and P.M. peak expiratory flow in 368 adults who had persistent asthma symptoms despite >1200 μg of
inhaled corticosteroids. Zafirlukast significantly improved A.M. and P.M. peak flows.
Source: From Ref. 155.

tion of inhaled glucocorticoid doses (153,154). Virchow and colleagues (155) showed that zafirlukast improves both pulmonary function and asthma symptoms in patients taking high-dose inhaled corticosteroids, and also resulted in a reduction in asthma exacerbations (Fig. 2). Laviolette et al. (156) demonstrated that the addition of montelukast to inhaled beclomethasone in patients marginally controlled with beclomethasone alone led to a significant improvement in FEV_1, daytime asthma symptom scores, and nocturnal awakenings (Fig. 3). For patients with asthma and persistent symptoms despite budesonide treatment, concomitant therapy with montelukast significantly improves asthma control with fewer nighttime awakenings, and results in greater improvements in rescue β-agonist use (157). Another double-blind, 16-week study compared the clinical benefits of adding montelukast to budesonide with doubling the budesonide dose in adults with asthma (158). The addition of montelukast was an effective and well-tolerated alternative to doubling budesonide dose with respect to peak flow, symptoms, exacerbations, and asthma-specific quality of life.

How does the combination of a leukotriene modifier and an inhaled corticosteroid compare with combination therapy of a long-acting β-agonist and an inhaled corticosteroid? While the LABA/ICS combination generally results in greater improvements in FEV_1 and peak flow, there were no

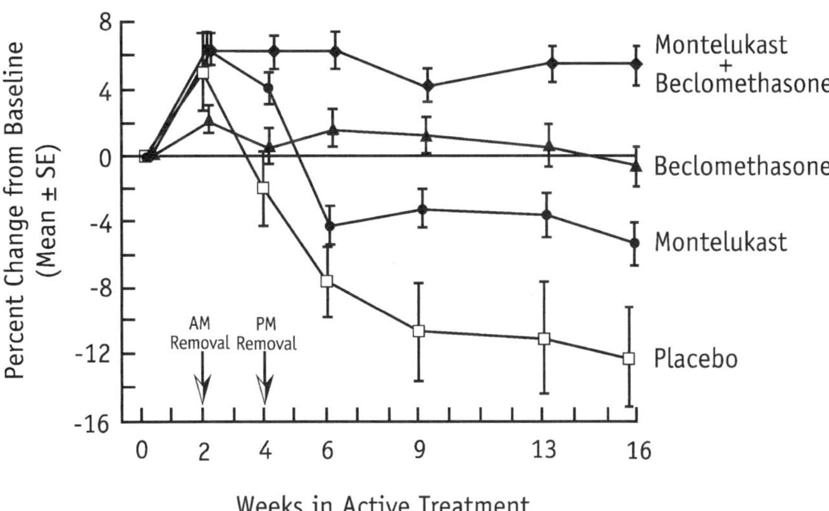

Figure 3 Mean FEV_1 percent change from baseline in subjects receiving montelukast + beclomethasone (*closed diamonds*), beclomethasone alone (*closed triangles*), montelukast alone (*closed circles*), or placebo (*open squares*). Both montelukast and beclomethasone resulted in greater improvement in FEV_1 than placebo. The addition of montelukast to beclomethasone yielded greater results than the use of either agent alone. *Source*: From Ref. 156.

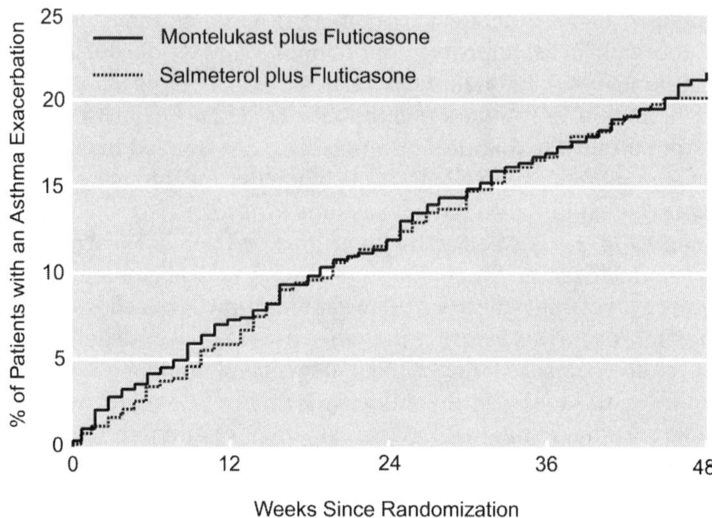

Figure 4 Percentage of patients experiencing an asthma exacerbation during treatment with either montelukast plus fluticasone versus salmeterol plus fluticasone. There was no significant difference in exacerbation rates between the two groups. *Source*: From Ref. 159.

differences between groups with respect to asthma exacerbations (159,160) (Fig. 4). Wilson et al. (161) also compared the efficacy of salmeterol and montelukast as second-line therapy in patients with asthma not controlled by inhaled steroids. While both montelukast and salmeterol produced significant improvements in asthma control when given with inhaled corticosteroid therapy, montelukast also produced significant effects on adenosine monophosphate bronchial challenge and blood eosinophil count, suggesting additive anti-inflammatory activity. This benefit was even observed when montelukast was added to the combination of long-acting β-agonist and inhaled corticosteroid (120).

IV. Leukotriene Modifiers: Safety Considerations

Standard asthma treatments may be complicated by several adverse effects. For instance, β-agonists may cause tachycardia, palpitations, and headaches. Theophylline has a very narrow toxic-therapeutic window, interacts with many medications, and may cause tremors, nausea, and several other ill effects. While systemic corticosteroids have a myriad of adverse effects, including hyperglycemia, growth retardation, hypertension, insomnia, and edema, even inhaled corticosteroids pose risks, including cataracts, thrush, adrenal suppression, and bone loss (162,163). In contrast, the leukotriene modifiers continue to have an excellent safety profile and offer the opportunity to minimize dosage and potential risks of many of the aforementioned medications. In the clinical trials leading to the approval of zileuton, zafirlukast, montelukast, and pranlukast, these drugs were very well tolerated and had side-effect profiles similar to those of placebo. The most common adverse effects included headache, dyspepsia, nausea, diarrhea, nonspecific pain, and myalgia (164). Nevertheless, as the number of patients taking these medications has increased, systemic adverse effects have been reported with these medications. For instance, in long-term safety studies of zileuton, approximately 5% of patients receiving the drug had clinically significant increases in transaminases within the first few months of therapy, while only 2% of patients in the usual-care group had an increase. These effects reversed with drug withdrawal, but it is generally felt that patients receiving the drug require monitoring of liver function at the onset of treatment and periodically thereafter (165). This complication does not occur with zafirlukast at the recommended dose of 20 mg twice daily, but it does occur at an appreciable frequency with higher doses. There has been no report of elevated liver function tests with montelukast therapy.

There have been single-case reports of drug-induced lupus (166) and of tubulointerstitial nephritis (167) with some of these drugs, but of most concern is the potential association with the Churg–Strauss syndrome (CSS). Within six months after the release of zafirlukast, eight patients who received the drug for moderate to severe asthma developed eosinophilia, pulmonary infiltrates, cardiomyopathy, and other signs of vasculitis, which are characteristic of CSS (168). All of the patients had discontinued high-dose corticosteroid use within three months of presentation, and all developed the syndrome within four months of zafirlukast initiation; the syndrome dramatically improved in each patient upon reinitiation of corticosteroid therapy. Since that report, there have been several similar cases in other patients receiving zafirlukast (169–171), as well as with montelukast (172–175) and pranlukast (176). While many potential mechanisms for this association have been postulated, including increased syndrome reporting due to bias, potential for allergic reaction, and leukotriene imbalance resulting from leukotriene receptor blockade, careful analysis of all reported cases suggests that the CSS developed only in those patients taking leukotriene modifiers who had an underlying eosinophilic disorder that was being masked by corticosteroid treatment and unmasked by leukotriene receptor antagonist-mediated steroid withdrawal, similar to the "forme fruste" of CSS (177). Since that time there have been numerous reports of CSS in asthma patients not receiving leukotriene modifiers (178), and overall it appears that there has been no increase in the incidence of CSS and that none of these drugs are directly causative of this rare syndrome. Although physicians must be alert for the signs and symptoms of CSS, particularly in patients with moderate-to-severe asthma in whom corticosteroids are tapered, the leukotriene modifiers remain safe and effective for the treatment of asthma.

V. Conclusions: The Role of Leukotriene Modifiers in the Treatment of Asthma and Future Directions

A. What Is the Role of Leukotriene Modifiers in the Treatment of Asthma?

On the basis of their relative effectiveness in mediating asthma symptoms and maintaining lung function, their comparative efficacy with respect to other asthma treatment modalities, their excellent safety profile, and most important their ease of administration, each of the leukotriene modifiers has earned an important place in the treatment of asthma. But where do these medications fit in the complex treatment paradigms that physicians use in treating this disease? In addition to their clear benefits in patients with aspirin-sensitive asthma, exercise-induced asthma, and cold-sensitive asthma, and their synergistic benefits in allergen-associated asthma, these drugs may be used as first-line therapy for mild persistent asthma and as add-on treatment for those patients whose asthma is not controlled by inhaled corticosteroids.

First-Line Asthma Treatment

First-line asthma treatment is medication given to a patient whose asthma is no longer controlled by rescue use of inhaled β-agonists, i.e., when the use of rescue treatment exceeds 120 puffs/mo or 8 inhalers/yr. The goals of first-line asthma therapy have been defined by the National Asthma Education and Prevention Program: asthma control with near normal airway function, absence of asthma symptoms, maintenance of activity without limitation, prevention of exacerbations, and an acceptable tolerability profile (179). However, a study demonstrated that the outpatient management of most asthma patients did not comply with the consensus guidelines and that asthma knowledge was quite poor (180). Furthermore, many patients with persistent asthma cannot attain these treatment goals with a single controller medication even at high doses (181), and the use of multiple therapies often complicates treatment regimens (182). For instance, despite the fact that inhaled corticosteroids have been advocated as the principal maintenance treatment for all degrees of asthma, one report indicated that multiple daily administration contributed to poor patient compliance and that compliance with inhaled medications (30–60%) was less than that with oral medications (70–80%) (182). One important therapeutic advantage of the leukotriene modifiers is that all marketed forms of these drugs are taken orally. Not only are these medications easier to take and less fraught with potential technical and coordination problems that may arise with inhalers, the limited compliance that patients have demonstrated with inhaled medications makes any pill form of asthma treatment a more desirable one. In the same vein, the availability of a once-daily medication (montelukast) enhances patient compliance even further. While inhaled steroids have been demonstrated to be more potent than leukotriene modifiers, the leukotriene modifiers may have greater overall effectiveness in real-world use due to enhanced patient compliance and simpler medication administration in the pill form. Furthermore, leukotriene modifiers more than adequately meet the requirements for efficacy and patient expectations as outlined by the NAEP. In addition to reducing symptoms and β-agonist use, agents active on the leukotriene pathway reduce exacerbations by 60% to 80% (183) and nearly double symptom-free days and days without asthma, while halving absence from school and work (131). Now that these medications are approved for children as young as age two, physicians have a safe alternative to inhaled corticosteroids. Given their effectiveness, safety record, and convenience of administration with expected superior compliance, the leukotriene modifiers have emerged as an excellent choice for first-line therapy in patients with mild persistent asthma.

Add-On Treatment to Inhaled Corticosteroids or ICS/LABA Combinations

Before the availability of leukotriene modifiers, one of the challenges of physicians who treat patients with moderate to severe asthma was minimizing corticosteroid dose and adverse effects while maintaining control of symptoms. Several investigators have demonstrated that leukotriene modifiers decrease the need for oral corticosteroid rescue therapy and permit the safe reduction of inhaled glucocorticoid doses (153,184,185). In Lofdahl's study (184), 226 subjects receiving high doses of inhaled corticosteroids were randomized to receive montelukast or placebo. Compared with placebo, montelukast allowed significant reduction in the inhaled corticosteroid dose (montelukast 47% vs. placebo 30%), and fewer patients on montelukast [18 (16%) vs. 34 (30%) placebo] required discontinuation because of failed rescue. For severe asthmatics who receive oral corticosteroid therapy, leukotriene modifiers may help minimize corticosteroid risks by allowing for reduction of dose or conversion to inhaled formulations. In severely asthmatic patients in whom steroids are being tapered, it is important to be alert for signs of potential underlying Churg–Strauss vasculitis that was being masked by corticosteroid use.

B. Future Directions: Pharmacogenetics and Novel Therapies

Leukotriene Modifiers and Pharmacogenetics

For any given disease, including asthma, there is variability of a given individual's response to a given pharmacotherapy (interindividual variability) and there is variability of a given individual's response to a given therapy on repeated occasions (intraindividual repeatability). Pharmacogenetics is the term applied to the study of the contribution of genetic differences among individuals to the variability in the responses to pharmacotherapy among individuals (186–188). As the response to leukotriene modifiers is not uniform across all asthmatics, and not every asthmatic responds to these medications to the same degree (189), it is hypothesized that an important determinant of responsiveness to these therapies is genetic. Several of the genes involved in the regulation of leukotriene synthesis and degradation have been studied and assessed for functional polymorphic variants that could account for differences in therapeutic responses to these agents. Polymorphisms of the 5-LO promoter gene and the LTC4 synthase gene have been studied and have been determined to play important roles in the response to leukotriene modifier therapy.

For example, Drazen and colleagues (190) postulated that since asthma patients harboring mutant forms of the 5-LO core promoter might have diminished 5-LO gene transcription, their asthma may be less dependent on leukotriene formation, and therefore they may be less sensitive to the antiasthma effects of 5-LO inhibition. To test this hypothesis, they stratified, by genotype at the 5-LO promoter, a cohort of 221 mild-to-moderate asthmatics who had completed a double-blind, randomized, placebo-controlled trial with a 5-LO inhibitor, ABT-761, which is clinically similar to zileuton (190). After 84 days of treatment, the 64 patients with wild-type genotype at the 5-LO core promoter locus who had received treatment with the 5-LO inhibitor had a substantially greater improvement in FEV_1 than that in the 10 patients with no wild-type allele at the 5-LO core promoter receiving the same dose of medication (18.8% improvement vs. 1.1% decline $p < 0.0001$) (Fig. 5). They also had a significantly greater improvement than the 69 patients with the same genotype who received placebo (only 5.1% improvement, $p = 0.0037$). This was the first demonstration in which genotype at a locus in a gene was of value in prospectively identifying a group of patients with an altered response to treatment and provided a rationale for the pharmacogenetic tailoring of medication regimens to the genetic makeup of the patient receiving treatment. In addition to studies of the 5-LO promoter, polymorphisms of other enzymes in the leukotriene pathway have been examined, including polymorphisms of the LTC4 synthase gene (191). Sampson and colleagues demonstrated that in a small group of asthmatic subjects with variant LTC4 synthase genotypes, administration of the leukotriene receptor antagonist zafirlukast for two weeks resulted in an increase in FEV_1 by 9%, while patients with wild-type genotype had a 12% decrease in FEV_1 (192). While these results failed to have statistical significance (likely due to the small sample size), the trend in differential response based on LTC4 synthase polymorphisms suggests that this locus, too, may have a role in determining response to asthma therapy. These findings are important as they highlight the fact that in the future, one may be able to

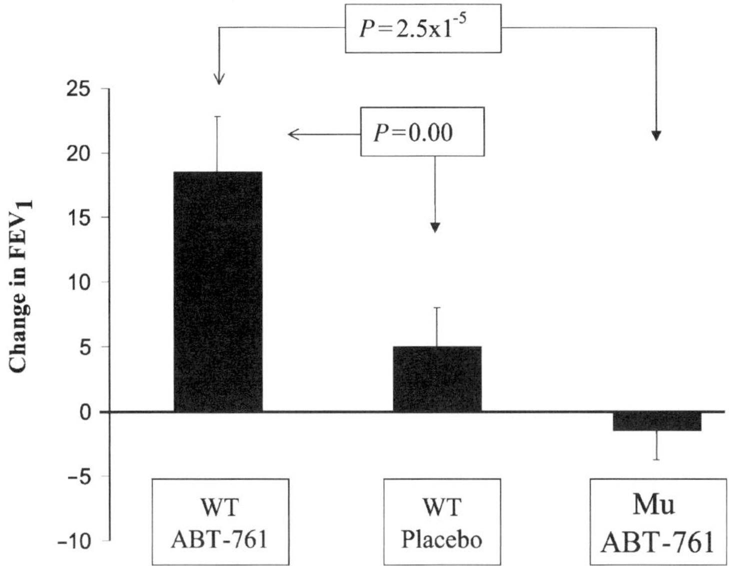

Figure 5 Percent change in FEV$_1$ from baseline in subjects with wild-type genotype at the 5-LO core promoter locus treated with the 5-LO inhibitor ABT-761 or placebo and for patients with no wild-type alleles treated with ABT-761. *Source*: From Ref. 190.

utilize pharmacogenetics to determine which patients may be responders to these therapies and, perhaps, which individuals may develop particular side effects from these therapies.

Novel Therapies and Indications

Future directions of research regarding leukotriene modifiers will revolve around novel therapies and new indications. An active area of investigation is the search for new medications that target specific areas of the 5-LO cascade. Current research involves the development and clinical evaluation of new 5-LO inhibitors and cysteinyl leukotriene receptor antagonists, as well as PLA2 inhibitors, FLAP inhibitors, and LTB4 receptor antagonists. For instance, the FLAP inhibitor MK-0591 was given to patients with moderately severe asthma who required treatment with inhaled corticosteroids, and those who received 125 mg of the drug twice daily had a significantly greater rise in mean FEV$_1$ and peak flow rates compared to those receiving placebo and also had fewer asthma symptoms and no adverse events (193). Similarly, when another FLAP inhibitor, BAYx1005, was given to 67 patients with moderate chronic asthma receiving corticosteroids, there were small but significant increases in FEV$_1$ after four weeks of treatment (194).

These classes of promising drugs may contribute significantly to asthma therapy in the future. While the potential role of these agents is very exciting, so is the potential use of current leukotriene modifiers, which have been shown to cause rapid benefit in the setting of acute asthma in the emergency department (195).

Leukotriene modifiers are currently being prescribed to patients with COPD, rhinosinusitis, and RSV infection. While there might be some theoretical and anecdotal basis for their use in these conditions, there have been no clinical trials to date documenting definitive efficacy or safety in these populations, and no drugs involved in the 5-LO pathway are currently approved for these or other inflammatory conditions. As we learn more about leukotrienes and their functions through further investigation, we will undoubtedly uncover much about the pathobiology of asthma and other inflammatory entities.

VI. Summary

Leukotrienes play an important role in asthmatic bronchoconstriction. Cysteinyl leukotriene receptor antagonists and 5-LO inhibitors are important medications that have been developed to specifically target this pathologic pathway. While these medications are particularly useful in the treatment of aspirin-sensitive asthma, exercise-induced asthma, and allergen-mediated asthma, their safety profile, efficacy, and ease of administration make leukotriene modifiers an excellent choice for first-line therapy in patients with mild persistent asthma. In more severe asthma, these medications allow for tapering of systemic and high-dose inhaled corticosteroids and minimize adverse effects while maintaining good lung function. As new, more potent leukotriene modifiers are developed, and as the burgeoning field of pharmacogenetics develops, the role of these important compounds in combating asthma will undoubtedly further evolve.

References

1. Danzig M, Cuss F. Inhibition of interleukin-5 with a monoclonal antibody attenuates allergic inflammation. Allergy 1997; 52(8):787–794.
2. Kellaway CH, Trethewie ER. The liberation of a slow-reacting smooth muscle stimulating substance in anaphylaxis. Q J Exp Physiol 1940; 30:121–145.
3. Brocklehurst WE. The release of histamine and the formation of a slow-reacting substance (SRS-A) during anaphylactic shock. J Physiol (Lond) 1960; 151:416–435.
4. Drazen JM, Austen KF. Effects of intravenous administration of slow-reacting substance of anaphylaxis, histamine, bradykinin, and prostaglandin F2alpha on pulmonary mechanics in the guinea pig. J Clin Invest 1974; 53: 1679–1685.

5. Samuelsson B, Dahlen SE, Lindgren JA, Rouzer CA, Serhan CN. Leukotrienes and lipoxins: structures, biosynthesis, and biological effects. Science 1987; 237:1171–1176.

6. Samuelsson B. Leukotrienes: mediators of immediate hypersensitivity reactions and inflammation. Science 1983; 220:568–575.

7. Schleimer RP, MacGlashan DW Jr, Peters SP, Pinckard RN, Adkinson NF Jr, Lichtenstein LM. Characterization of inflammatory mediator release from purified human lung mast cells. Am Rev Respir Dis 1986; 133:614–617.

8. Weller PF, Lee CW, Foster DW, Corey EJ, Austen KF, Lewis RA. Generation and metabolism of 5-lipoxygenase pathway leukotrienes by human eosinophils: predominant production of leukotriene C4. Proc Natl Acad Sci USA 1983; 80:7626–7630.

9. Schonfeld W, Schluter B, Hilger R, Konig W. Leukotriene generation and metabolism in isolated human lung macrophages. Immunology 1988; 65:529–536.

10. Holtzman MJ. Arachidonic acid metabolism in airway epithelial cells. Annu Rev Physiol 1992; 54:303–329.

11. Eling TE, Danilowicz RM, Henke DC, Sivarajah K, Yankaskas JR, Boucher RC. Arachidonic acid metabolism by canine tracheal epithelial cells. Product formation and relationship to chloride secretion. J Biol Chem 1986; 261:12841–12849.

12. Feinmark SJ, Cannon PJ. Endothelial cell leukotriene C4 synthesis results from intercellular transfer of leukotriene A4 synthesized by polymorphonuclear leukocytes. J Biol Chem 1986; 261:16466–16472.

13. Jackson RM, Chandler DB, Fulmer JD. Production of arachidonic acid metabolites by endothelial cells in hyperoxia. J Appl Physiol 1986; 61:584–591.

14. Piper PJ, Galton SA. Generation of leukotriene B4 and leukotriene E4 from porcine pulmonary artery. Prostaglandins 1984; 28:905–914.

15. Bjorck T, Dahlen SE. Evidence indicating that leukotrienes C4, D4 and E4 are major mediators of contraction induced by anti-IgE in human bronchi. Agents Actions 1989; 26:87–89.

16. Orning L, Hammarstrom S. Inhibition of leukotriene C and leukotriene D biosynthesis. J Biol Chem 1980; 255:8023–8026.

17. Togias AG, Naclerio RM, Peters SP, Nimmagadda I, Proud D, Kagey-Sobotka A, Adkinson NF Jr, Norman PS, Lichtenstein LM. Local generation of sulfidopeptide leukotrienes upon nasal provocation with cold, dry air. Am Rev Respir Dis 1986; 133:1133–1137.

18. Knapp HR, Sladek K, Fitzgerald GA. Increased excretion of leukotriene-E4 during aspirin-induced asthma. J Lab Clin Med 1992; 119:48–51.

19. Israel E, Fischer AR, Rosenberg MA, Lilly CM, Callery JC, Shapiro J, et al. The pivotal role of 5-lipoxygenase products in the reaction of aspirin-sensitive asthmatics to aspirin. Am Rev Respir Dis 1993; 148:1447–1451.

20. Dahlen B, Margolskee DJ, Zetterstrom O, Dahlen SE. Effect of the leukotriene receptor antagonist MK-0679 on baseline pulmonary function in aspirin sensitive asthmatic subjects. Thorax 1993; 48:1205–1210.

21. Morganroth ML, Stenmark KR, Zirrolli JA, Mauldin R, Mathias M, Reeves JT, et al. Leukotriene C4 production during hypoxic pulmonary vasoconstriction in isolated rat lungs. Prostaglandins 1984; 28:867–875.

22. Taniguchi H, Taki F, Takagi K, Satake T, Sugiyama S, Ozawa T. The role of leukotriene B4 in the genesis of oxygen toxicity in the lung. Am Rev Respir Dis 1986; 133:805–808.

23. Taylor IK, Ward PS, Taylor GW, Dollery CT, Fuller RW. Inhaled PAF Stimulates Leukotriene and Thromboxane-A2 Production in Humans. J Appl Physiol 1991; 71:1396–1402.

24. Woods JW, Evans JF, Ethier D, Scott S, Vickers PJ, Hearn L, et al. 5-Lipoxygenase and 5-lipoxygenase activating protein are localized in the nuclear envelope of activated human leukocytes. J Exp Med 1993; 178:1935–1946.

25. Goldman DW, Gifford LA, Young RN, Marotti T, Cheung MK, Goetzl EJ. Affinity labeling of the membrane protein-binding component of human polymorphonuclear leukocyte receptors for leukotriene B4. J Immunol 1991; 146: 2671–2677.

26. Slipetz DM, Scoggan KA, Nicholson DW, Metters KM. Photoaffinity labelling and radiation inactivation of the leukotriene B4 receptor in human myeloid cells. Eur J Pharmacol 1993; 244:161–173.

27. Ford-Hutchinson AW. Leukotriene B4 in inflammation. Crit Rev Immunol 1990; 10:1–12.

28. Rola-Pleszczynski M, Thivierge M, Gagnon N, Lacasse C, Stankova J. Differential regulation of cytokine and cytokine receptor genes by PAF, LTB4 and PGE2. J Lipid Mediat 1993; 6:175–181.

29. Mong S, Wu HL, Miller J, Hall RF, Gleason JG, Crooke ST. SKF 104353, a high affinity antagonist for human and guinea pig lung leukotriene D4 receptor, blocked phosphatidylinositol metabolism and thromboxane synthesis induced by leukotriene D4. Mol Pharmacol 1987; 32:223–229.

30. Mong S, Hoffman K, Wu HL, Crooke ST. Leukotriene-induced hydrolysis of inositol lipids in guinea pig lung: mechanism of signal transduction for leukotriene-D4 receptors. Mol Pharmacol 1987; 31:35–41.

31. Crooke ST, Mattern M, Sarau HM, Winkler JD, Balcarek J, Wong A, et al. The signal transduction system of the leukotriene D4 receptor. Trends Pharmacol Sci 1989; 10:103–107.

32. Crooke ST, Sarau H, Saussy D, Winkler J, Foley J. Signal transduction processes for the LTD4 receptor. Adv Prost Thromb Leukot Res 1990; 20: 127–137.

33. Buckner CK, Krell RD, Laravuso RB, Coursin DB, Bernstein PR, Will JA. Pharmacological evidence that human intralobar airways do not contain different receptors that mediate contractions to leukotriene C4 and leukotriene D4. J Pharmacol Exp Ther 1986; 237:558–562.

34. Jones TR, Davis C, Daniel EE. Pharmacological study of the contractile activity of leukotriene C4 and D4 on isolated human airway smooth muscle. Can J Physiol Pharmacol 1982; 60:638–643.

35. Davis C, Kannan MS, Jones TR, Daniel EE. Control of human airway smooth muscle: in vitro studies. J Appl Physiol 1982; 53:1080–1087.

36. Muccitelli RM, Tucker SS, Hay DW, Torphy TJ, Wasserman MA. Is the guinea pig trachea a good in vitro model of human large and central airways? Comparison on leukotriene-, methacholine-, histamine- and antigen-induced contractions. J Pharmacol Exp Ther 1987; 243:467–473.

37. Dewar JC, Wilkinson J, Wheatley A, Thomas NS, Doull I, Morton N, et al. The glutamine 27 beta(2)-adrenoceptor polymorphism is associated with elevated IgE levels in asthmatic families. J Allerg Clin Immunol 1997; 100(2): 261–265.

38. Porreca E, Difebbo C, Disciullo A, Angelucci D, Nasuti M, Vitullo P, et al. Cysteinyl leukotriene D_4 induced vascular smooth muscle cell proliferation: a possible role in myointimal hyperplasia. Thromb Haemost 1996; 76(1): 99–104.

39. Cohen P, Noveral JP, Bhala A, Nunn SE, Herrick DJ, Grunstein MM. Leukotriene D_4 facilitates airway smooth muscle cell proliferation via modulation of the IGF axis. Am J Physiol 1995; 13:L151–L157.

40. Drazen JM. Inhalation challenge with sulfidopeptide leukotrienes in human subjects. Chest 1986; 89:414–419.

41. Bisgaard H, Groth S, Madsen F. Bronchial hyperreactivity to leucotriene D4 and histamine in exogenous asthma. Br Med J (Clin Res Ed) 1985; 290: 1468–1471.

42. Hui KP, Lotvall J, Chung KF, Barnes PJ. Attenuation of Inhaled Allergen-Induced Airway Microvascular Leakage and Airflow Obstruction in Guinea Pigs by a 5-Lipoxygenase Inhibitor (A-63162). Am Rev Respir Dis 1991; 143: 1015–1019.

43. Wasserman MA, Welton AF, Renzetti LM. Synergism exhibited by LTD_4 and PAF receptor antagonists in decreasing antigen-induced airway microvascular leakage. Prostaglandins Relat Compounds 1995; 23:273.

44. Pasquale D, Chikkappa G. Lipoxygenase products regulate proliferation of granulocyte-macrophage progenitors. Exp Hematol 1993; 21(10):1361–1365.

45. Porreca E, Difebbo C, Disciullo A, Angelucci D, Nasuti M, Vitullo P, et al. Cysteinyl leukotriene D_4 induced vascular smooth muscle cell proliferation: a possible role in myointimal hyperplasia. Thromb Haemost 1996; 76(1): 99–104.

46. Cohen P, Noveral JP, Bhala A, Nunn SE, Herrick DJ, Grunstein MM. Leukotriene D_4 facilitates airway smooth muscle cell proliferation via modulation of the IGF axis. Am J Physiol 1995; 13:L151–L157.

47. Laitinen LA, Laitinen A, Haahtela T, Vilkka V, Spur BW, Lee TH. Leukotriene-E(4) and granulocytic infiltration into asthmatic airways. Lancet 1993; 341:989–990.

48. Munoz NM, Leff AR. Blockade of eosinophil migration by 5-lipoxygenase and cyclooxygenase inhibition in explanted guinea pig trachealis. Am J Physiol 1995; 12:L446–L454.

49. Laitinen LA, Laitinen A, Haahtela T, Vilkka V, Spur BW, Lee TH. Leukotriene-E(4) and granulocytic infiltration into asthmatic airways. Lancet 1993; 341:989–990.

50. Munoz NM, Leff AR. Blockade of eosinophil migration by 5-lipoxygenase and cyclooxygenase inhibition in explanted guinea pig trachealis. Am J Physiol 1995; 12:L446–L454.

51. Lewis RA, Austen KF, Soberman RJ. Leukotrienes and other products of the 5-lipoxygenase pathway. Biochemistry and relation to pathobiology in human diseases. N Engl J Med 1990; 323:645–655.

52. Bjorck T, Dahlen SE. Evidence indicating that leukotrienes C4, D4 and E4 are major mediators of contraction induced by anti-IgE in human bronchi. Agents Actions 1989; 26:87–89.

53. Togias AG, Naclerio RM, Peters SP, Nimmagadda I, Proud D, Kagey-Sobotka A, et al. Local generation of sulfidopeptide leukotrienes upon nasal provocation with cold, dry air. Am Rev Respir Dis 1986; 133:1133–1137.

54. Knapp HR, Sladek K, Fitzgerald GA. Increased excretion of leukotriene-E4 during aspirin-induced asthma. J Lab Clin Med 1992; 119:48–51.

55. Schleimer RP, MacGlashan DW Jr, Peters SP, Pinckard RN, Adkinson NF Jr, Lichtenstein LM. Characterization of inflammatory mediator release from purified human lung mast cells. Am Rev Respir Dis 1986; 133:614–617.

56. Weller PF, Lee CW, Foster DW, Corey EJ, Austen KF, Lewis RA. Generation and metabolism of 5-lipoxygenase pathway leukotrienes by human eosinophils: predominant production of leukotriene C4. Proc Natl Acad Sci USA 1983; 80:7626–7630.

57. Rankin JA, Hitchcock M, Merrill W, Bach MK, Brashler JR, Askenase PW. IgE-dependent release of leukotriene C4 from alveolar macrophages. Nature 1982; 297:329–331.

58. Schonfeld W, Schluter B, Hilger R, Konig W. Leukotriene generation and metabolism in isolated human lung macrophages. Immunology 1988; 65: 529–536.

59. Okubo T, Takahashi H, Sumitomo M, Shindoh K, Suzuki S. Plasma levels of leukotrienes C4 and D4 during wheezing attack in asthmatic patients. Int Arch Allergy Appl Immunol 1987; 84:149–155.

60. Lam S, Chan H, LeRiche JC, Chan-Yeung M, Salari H. Release of leukotrienes in patients with bronchial asthma. J Allergy Clin Immunol 1988; 81:711–717.

61. Wenzel SE, Larsen GL, Johnston K, Voelkel NF, Westcott JY. Elevated levels of leukotriene C4 in bronchoalveolar lavage fluid from atopic asthmatics after endobronchial allergen challenge. Am Rev Respir Dis 1990; 142:112–119.

62. Wenzel SE, Trudeau JB, Kaminsky DA, Cohn J, Martin RJ, Westcott JY. Effect of 5-lipoxygenase inhibition on bronchoconstriction and airway inflammation in nocturnal asthma. Am J Respir Crit Care Med 1995; 152: 897–905.

63. Sladek K, Dworski R, Fitzgerald GA, Buitkus KL, Block FJ, Marney SR Jr, et al. Allergen-stimulated release of thromboxane A2 and leukotriene E4 in humans. Effect of indomethacin. Am Rev Respir Dis 1990; 141:1441–1445.

64. Drazen JM, Obrien J, Sparrow D, Weiss ST, Martins MA, Israel E, et al. Recovery of leukotriene-E4 from the urine of patients with airway obstruction. Am Rev Respir Dis 1992; 146:104–108.

65. Bellia V, Bonanno A, Cibella F, Cuttitta G, Mirabella A, Profita M, et al. Urinary leukotriene E_4 in the assessment of nocturnal asthma. J Allerg Clin Immunol 1996; 97(3):735–741.

66. Kumlin M, Dahlen B, Bjorck T, Zetterstrom O, Granstrom E, Dahlen SE. Urinary excretion of leukotriene-E4 and 11-dehydro-thromboxane-B2 in response to bronchial provocations with allergen, aspirin, leukotriene-D4, and histamine in asthmatics. Am Rev Respir Dis 1992; 146:96–103.

67. Jones AT, Evans TW. NO: COPD and beyond. Thorax 1997; 52(suppl 3): S16–S21.
68. Ferreri NR, Howland WC, Stevenson DD, Spiegelberg HL. Release of leukotrienes, prostaglandins, and histamine into nasal secretions of aspirin-sensitive asthmatics during reaction to aspirin. Am Rev Respir Dis 1988; 137(4): 847–854.
69. Christie PE, Tagari P, Fordhutchinson AW, Charlesson S, Chee P, Arm JP, et al. Urinary leukotriene-E4 concentrations increase after aspirin challenge in aspirin-sensitive asthmatic subjects. Am Rev Respir Dis 1991; 143: 1025–1029.
70. Drazen JM, Obrien J, Sparrow D, Weiss ST, Martins MA, Israel E, et al. Recovery of Leukotriene-E4 from the Urine of Patients with Airway Obstruction. Am Rev Respir Dis 1992; 146:104–108.
71. Antczak A, Montuschi P, Kharitonov S, Gorski P, Barnes PJ. Increased Exhaled Cysteinyl-Leukotrienes and 8-Isoprostane in Aspirin-induced Asthma. Am J Respir Crit Care Med 2002; 166(3):301–306.
72. Lam S, Chan H, LeRiche JC, Chan-Yeung M, Salari H. Release of leukotrienes in patients with bronchial asthma. J Allergy Clin Immunol 1988; 81:711–717.
73. Wenzel SE, Larsen GL, Johnston K, Voelkel NF, Westcott JY. Elevated levels of leukotriene C4 in bronchoalveolar lavage fluid from atopic asthmatics after endobronchial allergen challenge. Am Rev Respir Dis 1990; 142:112–119.
74. Israel E, Dermarkarian R, Rosenberg M, Sperling R, Taylor G, Rubin P, et al. The effects of a 5-lipoxygenase inhibitor on asthma induced by cold, dry air. N Engl J Med 1990; 323:1740–1744.
75. Smith LJ, Geller S, Ebright L, Glass M, Thyrum PT. Inhibition of leukotriene D4-induced bronchoconstriction in normal subjects by the oral LTD4 receptor antagonist ICI 204,219. Am Rev Respir Dis 1990; 141:988–992.
76. Spector SL, Smith LJ, Glass M. Effects of 6 weeks of therapy with oral doses of ICI 204,219, a leukotriene D4 receptor antagonist, in subjects with bronchial asthma. ACCOLATE Asthma Trialists Group. Am J Respir Crit Care Med 1994; 150(3):618–623.
77. Nakagawa T, Mizushima Y, Ishii A. Effect of a leukotriene antagonist on experimental and clinical bronchial asthma. Adv Prost Thromb Leukot Res 1990; 21:465–468.
78. Delepeleire I, Reiss TF, Rochette F, Botto A, Zhang J, Kundu S, et al. Montelukast causes prolonged, potent leukotriene D4-receptor antagonism in the airways of patients with asthma. Clin Pharmacol Ther 1997; 61(1): 83–92.
79. Oshaughnessy TC, Georgiou P, Howland K, Dennis M, Compton CH, Barnes NC. Effect of pranlukast, an oral leukotriene receptor antagonist, on leukotriene D4 (LTD4) challenge in normal volunteers. Thorax 1997; 52(6): 519–522.
80. Calhoun WJ, Lavins BJ, Minkwitz MC, Evans R, Gleich GJ, Cohn J. Effect of zafirlukast (Accolate) on cellular mediators of inflammation: bronchoalveolar lavage fluid findings after segmental antigen challenge. Am J Respir Crit Care Med 1998; 157(5):1381–1389.

81. Israel E, Dermarkarian R, Rosenberg M, Sperling R, Taylor G, Rubin P, et al. The effects of a 5-lipoxygenase inhibitor on asthma induced by cold, dry air. N Engl J Med 1990; 323:1740–1744.

82. Fischer AR, Mcfadden CA, Frantz R, Awni WM, Cohn J, Drazen JM, et al. Effect of chronic 5-lipoxygenase inhibition on airway hyperresponsiveness in asthmatic subjects. Am J Respir Crit Care Med 1995; 152:1203–1207.

83. Taylor IK, Wellings R, Taylor GW, Fuller RW. Urinary leukotriene-E4 excretion in exercise-induced asthma. J Appl Physiol 1992; 73:743–748.

84. Anderson SD. Is there a unifying hypothesis for exercise-induced asthma? J Allergy Clin Immunol 1984; 73(5 pt 2):660–665.

85. Kikawa Y, Miyanomae T, Inoue Y, Saito M, Nakai A, Shigematsu Y, et al. Urinary leukotriene E4 after exercise challenge in children with asthma. J Allergy Clin Immunol 1992; 89:1111–1119.

86. Reiss TF, Hill JB, Harman E, Zhang J, Tanaka WK, Bronsky E, et al. Increased urinary excretion of LTE_4 after exercise and attenuation of exercise-induced bronchospasm by montelukast, a cysteinyl leukotriene receptor antagonist. Thorax 1997; 52(12):1030–1035.

87. Finnerty JP, Wood-Baker R, Thomson H, Holgate ST. Role of leukotrienes in exercise-induced asthma: inhibitory effect of ICI-204, 219, a potent LTD4 receptor antagonist. Am Rev Respir Dis 1992; 145:746–749.

88. Bronsky EA, Kemp JP, Zhang J, Guerreiro D, Reiss TF. Dose-related protection of exercise bronchoconstriction by montelukast, a cysteinyl leukotriene-receptor antagonist, at the end of a once-daily dosing interval. Clin Pharmacol Ther 1997; 62(5):556–561.

89. Leff JA, Busse WW, Pearlman D, Bronsky EA, Kemp J, Hendeles L, et al. Montelukast, a leukotriene-receptor antagonist, for the treatment of mild asthma and exercise-induced bronchoconstriction [see comments]. N Engl J Med 1998; 339(3):147–152.

90. Adelroth E, Inman MD, Summers E, Pace D, Modi M, Obyrne PM. Prolonged protection against exercise-induced bronchoconstriction by the leukotriene D_4-receptor antagonist cinalukast. J Allerg Clin Immunol 1997; 99(2):210–215.

91. Makker HK, Lau LC, Thomson HW, Binks SM, Holgate ST. The protective effect of inhaled leukotriene-D_4 receptor antagonist ICI-204, 219 against exercise-induced asthma. Am Rev Respir Dis 1993; 147:1413–1418.

92. Meltzer SS, Hasday JD, Cohn J, Bleecker ER. Inhibition of exercise-induced bronchospasm by zileuton: a 5-lipoxygenase inhibitor. Am J Respir Crit Care Med 1996; 153:931–935.

93. Inman MD, O'Byrne PM. The effect of regular inhaled albuterol on exercise-induced bronchoconstriction. Am J Respir Crit Care Med 1996; 153:65–69.

94. Reiss TF, Chervinsky P, Dockhorn RJ, Shingo S, Seidenberg B, Edwards TB, et al. Montelukast a once daily leukotriene receptor antagonist in the treatment of chronic asthma. Arch Int Med 1998; 158:1213–1220.

95. Edelman JM, Turpin JA, Bronsky EA, Grossman J, Kemp JP, Ghannam AF, et al. Oral montelukast compared with salmeterol to prevent exercise-induced bronchoconstriction. Ann Int Med 2000; 132(2):97–104.

96. Cowburn AS, Sladek K, Soja J, Adamek L, Nizankowska E, Szczeklik A, et al. Overexpression of leukotrine C4 synthase in bronchial biopsies from patients with aspirin-intolerant asthma. J Clin Invest 1998; 101:834–846.

97. Dahlen B, Kumlin M, Margolskee DJ, Larsson C, Blomqvist H, Williams VC, et al. The leukotriene-receptor antagonist MK-0679 blocks airway obstruction induced by inhaled lysine-aspirin in aspirin-sensitive asthmatics. Eur Respir J 1993; 6:1018–1026.

98. Menendez R, Venzor J, Ortiz G. Failure of zafirlukast to prevent ibuprofen-induced anaphylaxis. Ann Allergy Asthma Immunol 1998; 80(3):225–226.

99. Enrique E, GarciaOrtega P, Gaig P, SanMiguel MM. Failure of montelukast to prevent anaphylaxis to diclofenac. Allergy 1999; 54(5):529–530.

100. Fuller RW, Black PN, Dollery CT. Effect of the oral leukotriene D4 antagonist LY171883 on inhaled and intradermal challenge with antigen and leukotriene D4 in atopic subjects. J Allergy Clin Immunol 1989; 83: 939–944.

101. Rasmussen JB, Margolskee DJ, Eriksson LO, Williams VC, Andersson KE. Leukotriene (LT) D4 is involved in antigen-induced asthma: a study with the LTD4 receptor antagonist, MK-571. Ann NY Acad Sci 1991; 629:436.

102. Taylor IK, O'Shaughnessy KM, Fuller RW, Dollery CT. Effect of cysteinyl-leukotriene receptor antagonist ICI-204, 219 on allergen-induced broncho-constriction and airway hyperreactivity in atopic subjects. Lancet 1991; 337: 690–694.

103. Dahlen SE, Dahlen B, Eliasson E, Johansson H, Bjorck T, Kumlin M, et al. Inhibition of allergic bronchoconstriction in asthmatics by the leukotriene-antagonist ICI-204, 219. Adv Prost Thromb Leukot Res 1991; 21A:461–464.

104. Hamilton A, Faiferman I, Stober P, Watson RM, O'Byrne PM. Pranlukast, a cysteinyl leukotriene receptor antagonist, attenuates allergen-induced early and late phase bronchoconstriction and airway hyperresponsiveness in asthmatic subjects [see comments]. J Allergy Clin Immunol 1998; 102(2): 177–183.

105. Hamilton AL, Watson RM, Wyile G, O'Byrne PM. Attenuation of early and late phase allergen-induced bronchoconstriction in asthmatic subjects by a 5-lipoxygenase activating protein antagonist, BAYx1005. Thorax 1997; 52(4): 348–354.

106. Roquet A, Dahlen B, Kumlin M, Ihre E, Anstren G, Binks S, et al. Combined antagonism of leukotrienes and histamine produces predominant inhibition of allergen-induced early and late phase airway obstruction in asthmatics. Am J Respir Crit Care Med 1997; 155(6):1856–1863.

107. Hui KP, Barnes NC. Lung function improvement in asthma with a cysteinyl-leukotriene receptor antagonist. Lancet 1991; 337:1062–1063.

108. Liu MC, Dube LM, Lancaster J. Acute and chronic effects of a 5-lipoxygen-ase inhibitor in asthma: a 6-month randomized multicenter trial. J Allerg Clin Immunol 1996; 98(5 part 1):859–871.

109. Gaddy JN, Margolskee DJ, Bush RK, Williams VC, Busse WW. Bronchodila-tion with a potent and selective leukotriene D4 (LTD4) antagonist (MK-571) in patients with asthma. Am Rev Respir Dis 1992; 146:358–363.

110. Impens N, Reiss TF, Teahan JA, Desmet M, Rossing TH, Shingo S, et al. Acute bronchodilation with an intravenously administered leukotriene-D(4) antagonist, MK-679. Am Rev Respir Dis 1993; 147:1442–1446.

111. Reiss TF, Altman LC, Chervinsky P, Bewtra A, Stricker WE, Noonan GP, et al. Effects of montelukast (MK-0476), a new potent cysteinyl leukotriene (LDT(4)) receptor antagonist, in patients with chronic asthma. J Allerg Clin Immunol 1996; 98(3):528–534.

112. Israel E, Rubin P, Kemp JP, Grossman J, Pierson WE, Siegel SC, et al. The effect of inhibition of 5-lipoxygenase by zileuton in mild to moderate asthma. Ann Intern Med 1993; 119:1059–1066.

113. Salvi SS, Krishna MT, Sampson AP, Holgate ST. The anti-inflammatory effects of leukotriene-modifying drugs and their use in asthma. Chest 2001; 119(5):1533–1546.

114. Fujimura M, Sakamoto S, Kamio Y, Matsuda T. Effect of a leukotriene antagonist, ONO-1078, on bronchial hyperresponsiveness in patients with asthma. Respir Med 1993; 87:133–138.

115. Dempsey OJ, Kennedy G, Lipworth BJ. Comparative efficacy and anti-inflammatory profile of once-daily therapy with leukotriene antagonist or low-dose inhaled corticosteroid in patients with mild persistent asthma. J Allergy Clin Immunol 2002; 109(1):68–74.

116. Parameswaran K, Watson R, Gauvreau GM, Sehmi R, O'Byrne PM. The effect of pranlukast on allergen-induced bone marrow eosinophilopoiesis in subjects with asthma. Am J Respir Crit Care Med 2004; 169(8):915–920.

117. Reiss TF, Chervinsky P, Dockhorn RJ, Shingo S, Seidenberg B, Edwards TB, et al. Montelukast a once daily leukotriene receptor antagonist in the treatment of chronic asthma. Arch Int Med 1998; 158:1213–1220.

118. Strauch E, Moske O, Thoma S, Storm vGK, Ihorst G, Brandis M, et al. A Randomized Controlled Trial on the Effect of Montelukast on Sputum Eosinophil Cationic Protein in Children with Corticosteroid-Dependent Asthma. Pediatr Res 2003; 54(2):198–203.

119. Bratton DL, Lanz MJ, Miyazawa N, White CW, Silkoff PE. Exhaled nitric oxide before and after montelukast sodium therapy in school-age children with chronic asthma: a preliminary study. Pediatr Pulmonol 1999; 28(6):402–407.

120. Currie GP, Lee DKC, Haggart K, Bates CE, Lipworth BJ. Effects of montelukast on surrogate inflammatory markers in corticosteroid-treated patients with asthma. Am J Respir Crit Care Med 2003; 167(9):1232–1238.

121. Sandrini A, Ferreira IM, Gutierrez C, Jardim JR, Zamel N, Chapman KR. Effect of montelukast on exhaled nitric oxide and nonvolatile markers of inflammation in mild asthma. Chest 2003; 124(4):1334–1340.

122. Straub DA, Moeller A, Minocchieri S, Hamacher J, Sennhauser FH, Hall GL, et al. The effect of montelukast on lung function and exhaled nitric oxide in infants with early childhood asthma. Eur Respir J 2005; 25(2):289–294.

123. Straub DA, Minocchieri S, Moeller A, Hamacher J, Wildhaber JH. The Effect of montelukast on exhaled nitric oxide and lung function in asthmatic children 2 to 5 years old. Chest 2005; 127(2):509–514.

124. Malmstrom K, Rodriguez-Gomez G, Guerra J, Villaran C, Pineiro A, Wei LX, et al. Oral montelukast, inhaled beclomethasone, and placebo for chronic asthma. A randomized controlled trial. Ann Int Med 1999; 130:487–495.

125. Minoguchi K, Kohno Y, Minoguchi H, Kihara N, Sano Y, Yasuhara H, et al. Reduction of eosinophilic inflammation in the airways of patients with asthma using montelukast. Chest 2002; 121(3):732–738.

126. Henderson WR, Lewis DB, Albert RK, Zhang Y, Lamm WJE, Chiang GKS, et al. The importance of leukotrienes in airway inflammation in a mouse model of asthma. J Exp Med 1996; 184(4):1483–1494.

127. Henderson WR Jr, Tang LO, Chu SJ, Tsao SM, Chiang GKS, Jones F, et al. A role for cysteinyl leukotrienes in airway remodeling in a mouse asthma model. Am J Respir Crit Care Med 2002; 165(1):108–116.

128. Spector SL, Smith LJ, Glass M. Effects of 6 weeks of therapy with oral doses of ICI-204, 219, a leukotriene D4 receptor antagonist, in subjects with bronchial asthma. ACCOLATE Asthma Trialists Group. Am J Respir Crit Care Med 1994; 150(3):618–623.

129. Barnes NC, Pujet JC. Pranlukast, a novel leukotriene receptor antagonist: results of the first european, placebo controlled, multicentre clinical study in asthma. Thorax 1997; 52(6):523–527.

130. Tamaoki J, Kondo M, Sakai N, Nakata J, Takemura H, Nagai A, et al. Leukotriene antagonist prevents exacerbation of asthma during reduction of high-dose inhaled corticosteroid. The Tokyo Joshi-Idai Asthma Research Group. Am J Respir Crit Care Med 1997; 155(4):1235–1240.

131. Suissa S, Dennis R, Ernst P, Sheehy O, Wooddauphinee S. Effectiveness of the leukotriene receptor antagonist zafirlukast for mild-to-moderate asthma—a randomized, double-blind, placebo-controlled trial. Ann Intern Med 1997; 126(3):177.

132. Fish JE, Kemp JP, Lockey RF, Glass M, Hanby LA, Bonuccelli CM. Zafirlukast for symptomatic mild-to-moderate asthma: a 13-week multicenter study. The Zafirlukast Trialists Group. Clin Ther 1997; 19(4):675–690.

133. Barnes N, Thomas M, Price D, Tate H. The national montelukast survey. J Allergy Clin Immunol 2005; 115(1):47–54.

134. Reiss TF, Chervinsky P, Dockhorn RJ, Shingo S, Seidenberg B, Edwards TB. Montelukast, a once-daily leukotriene receptor antagonist, in the treatment of chronic asthma: a multicenter, randomized, double-blind trial. Montelukast Clinical Research Study Group. Arch Intern Med 1998; 158(11):1213–1220.

135. Knorr B, Franchi LM, Bisgaard H, Vermeulen JH, LeSouef P, Santanello N, et al. Montelukast, a leukotriene receptor antagonist, for the treatment of persistent asthma in children aged 2 to 5 years. Pediatrics 2001; 108(3):e48.

136. Knorr B, Matz J, Bernstein JA, Nguyen H, Seidenberg BC, Reiss TF, et al. Montelukast for chronic asthma in 6- to 14-year-old children: a randomized, double-blind trial. Pediatric Montelukast Study Group. JAMA 1998; 279(15): 1181–1186.

137. Pearlman DS, Ostrom NK, Bronsky EA, Bonuccelli CM, Hanby LA. The leukotriene D4-receptor antagonist zafirlukast attenuates exercise-induced bronchoconstriction in children. J Pediatr 1999; 134:273–279.

138. Knorr B, Matz J, Bernstein JA, Nguyen H, Seidenberg BC, Reiss TF, et al. Montelukast for chronic asthma in 6- to 14-year-old children: a randomized, double-blind trial. Pediatric Montelukast Study Group. JAMA 1998; 279(15): 1181–1186.

139. Bleecker ER, Welch MJ, Weinstein SF, Kalberg C, Johnson M, Edwards L, et al. Low-dose inhaled fluticasone propionate versus oral zafirlukast in the treatment of persistent asthma. J Allergy Clin Immunol The 2000; 105: 1123–1129.

140. Busse W, Raphael GD, Galant S, Kalberg C, Goode-Sellers S, Srebro S, et al. Low-dose fluticasone propionate compared with montelukast for first-line treatment of persistent asthma: a randomized clinical trial. J Allergy Clin Immunol 2001; 107(3):461–468.

141. Malmstrom K, Rodriguez-Gomez G, Guerra J, Villaran C, Pineiro A, Wei LX, et al. Oral montelukast, inhaled beclomethasone, and placebo for chronic asthma. A randomized controlled trial. Ann Int Med 1999; 130:487–495.

142. Israel E, Chervinsky PS, Friedman B, van Bavel J, Skalky CS, Ghannam AF, et al. Effects of montelukast and beclomethasone on airway function and asthma control. J Allergy Clin Immunol 2002; 110(6):847–854.

143. Baumgartner RA, Martinez G, Edelman JM, Rodriguez GGG, Bernstein M, Bird S, et al. Distribution of therapeutic response in asthma control between oral montelukast and inhaled beclomethasone. Eur Respir J 2003; 21(1): 123–128.

144. Wenzel S, Chervinsky P, Kerwin E, Silvers W, Faiferman I, Dubb J, et al. Oral pranlukast (Ultair) versus inhaled beclomethasone: results of a 12 week trial in patients with asthma (abstr). Am J Respir Crit Care Med 1997; 155:A203.

145. Laitinen LA, Naya IP, Binks S, Harris A. Comparative efficacy of zafirlukast and low dose steroids in asthmatics on prnbeta-agonists. Eur Resp J 1997; 10:419S.

146. Leigh R, Vethanayagam D, Yoshida M, Watson RM, Rerecich T, Inman MD, et al. Effects of montelukast and budesonide on airway responses and airway inflammation in asthma. Am J Respir Crit Care Med 2002; 166(9):1212–1217.

147. Villaran C, O'Neill SJ, Helbling A, van Noord JA, Lee TH, Chuchalin AG, et al. Montelukast versus salmeterol in patients with asthma and exercise-induced bronchoconstriction. J Allergy Clin Immunol 1999; 104(3):547–553.

148. Busse W, Nelson H, Wolfe J, Kalberg C, Yancey SW, Rickard KA. Comparison of inhaled salmeterol and oral zafirlukast in patients with asthma. J Allerg Clin Immunol 1999; 103(6):1075–1080.

149. Rickard KA, Wolfe JD, LaForce CF, Anderson WH, Kalberg CJ. A comparison of salmeterol and zafirlukast in patients with persistent asthma (abstr). Chest 1998; 114:297S.

150. Schwartz HJ, Petty T, Dube LM, Swanson LJ, Lancaster JF. A randomized controlled trial comparing zileuton with theophylline in moderate asthma. Arch Intern Med 1998; 158(2):141–148.

151. Nathan RA, Glass M, Snader L. Effects of 13 weeksof treatmet with ICI-204, 219 (Accolate) or cromolyn sodium (Intal) in patients with mild to moderate asthma (abstr). J Allergy Clin Immunol 1995; 95:388.

152. Holgate ST, Anderson KD, Rodgers EM. Comparison of Accolate (zafirlukast) with sodium cromoglycate in mild to moderate asthmatic patients (abstr). Allergy 1995; 50:319–320.

153. Tamaoki J, Kondo M, Sakai N, Nakata J, Takemura H, Nagai A, et al. Leukotriene antagonist prevents exacerbation of asthma during reduction of high-dose inhaled corticosteroid. Am J Respir Crit Care Med 1997; 155: 1235–1240.

154. Kanniess F, Richter K, Janicki S, Schleiss MB, Jorres RA, Magnussen H. Dose reduction of inhaled corticosteroids under concomitant medication with montelukast in patients with asthma. Eur Respir J 2002; 20(5):1080–1087.

155. Virchow JC Jr, Prasse A, Naya I, Summerton L, Harris A, and the Zafirlukast Study Group. Zafirlukast improves asthma control in patients receiving high-dose inhaled corticosteroids. Am J Respir Crit Care Med 2000; 162: 578–585.

156. Laviolette M, Malmstrom K, Lu S, Chervinsky P, Pujet JC, Peszek I, et al. Montelukast added to inhaled beclomethasone in treatment of asthma. Am J Respir Crit Care Med 1999; 160:1862–1868.

157. Vaquerizo MJ, Casan P, Castillo J, Perpina M, Sanchis J, Sobradillo V, et al. Effect of montelukast added to inhaled budesonide on control of mild to moderate asthma. Thorax 2003; 58(3):204–210.

158. Price DB, Hernandez D, Magyar P, Fiterman J, Beeh KM, James IG, et al. Randomised controlled trial of montelukast plus inhaled budesonide versus double dose inhaled budesonide in adult patients with asthma. Thorax 2003; 58(3):211–216.

159. Bjermer L, Bisgaard H, Bousquet J, Fabbri LM, Greening AP, Haahtela T, et al. Montelukast and fluticasone compared with salmeterol and fluticasone in protecting against asthma exacerbation in adults: one year, double blind, randomised, comparative trial. BMJ 2003; 327(7420):891–896.

160. Nelson H, Busse WW, Kerwin E, Church N, Emmett A, Rickard K, et al. Fluticasone propionate/salmeterol combination provides more effective asthma control than low-dose inhaled corticosteroid plus montelukast. J Allergy Clin Immunol 2000; 106(6):1088–1095.

161. Wilson AM, Dempsey OJ, Sims EJ, Lipworth BJ. A comparison of salmeterol and montelukast as second-line therapy in asthmatic patients not controlled on inhaled corticosteroids. Thorax 1999; 54:A66.

162. Kamada AK, Szefler SJ, Martin RJ, Boushey HA, Chinchilli VM, Drazen JM, et al. Issues in the use of inhaled glucocorticoids. The Asthma Clinical Research Network. Am J Respir Crit Care Med 1996; 153(6 pt 1):1739–1748.

163. Simons FER. Benefits and risks of inhaled glucocorticoids in children with persistent asthma. J Allerg Clin Immunol 1998; 102(5):S77–S84.

164. Anonymous. Physicians Desk Reference. 54th. 2000. Montvale, NJ, Medical Economics. Ref Type: Serial (Book,Monograph).

165. Lazarus SC, Lee T, Kemp JP, Wenzel S, Dube LM, Ochs RF, et al. Safety and clinical efficacy of zileuton in patients with chronic asthma. Am J Manag Care 1998; 4(6):841–848.

166. Finkel TH, Hunter DJ, Paisley JE, Finkel RS, Larsen GL. Drug-induced lupus in a child after treatment with zafirlukast (Accolate). J Allergy Clin Immunol 1999; 103:533–534.

167. Schurman SJ, Alderman JM, Massanari M, Lacson AG, Perlman SA. Tubulointerstitial nephritis induced by the leukotriene receptor antagonist pranlukast. Chest 1998; 114(4):1220–1223.

168. Wechsler ME, Garpestad E, Flier SR, Kocher O, Weiland DA, Polito AJ, et al. Pulmonary infiltrates, eosinophilia, and cardiomyopathy following corticosteroid withdrawal in patients with asthma receiving zafirlukast. JAMA 1998; 279(6):455–457.

169. Katz RS, Papernik M. Zafirlukast and Churg-Strauss syndrome [letter; comment]. JAMA 1998; 279(24):1949.

170. Green RL, Vayonis AG. Churg-Strauss syndrome after zafirlukast in two patients not receiving steroid treatment. Lancet 1999; 353:725–726.

171. Knoell DL, Lucas J, Allen JN. Churg-Strauss syndrome associated with zafirlukast. Chest 1998; 114(1):332–334.

172. Franco J, Artes MJ. Pulmonary eosinophilia associated with montelukast. Thorax 1999; 54(6):558–560.

173. Wechsler ME, Finn D, Gunawardena D, Westlake R, Barker A, Haranath SP, et al. Churg-strauss syndrome in patients receiving montelukast as treatment for asthma. Chest 2000; 117:708–713.

174. Haranath SP, Freston C, Fucci M, Lee E, Anwar MS. Montelukast-associated Churg-Strauss syndrome. Am J Respir Crit Care Med 1999; 159(3):A646.

175. Wechsler ME, Finn D, Jordan M, Gunawardena D, Drazen JM. Montelukast and the Churg-Strauss syndrome. Am J Respir Crit Care Med 1999; 159(3): A646.

176. Kinoshita M, Shiraishi T, Koga T, Ayabe M, Rikimaru T, Oizumi K. Churg-Strauss syndrome after corticosteroid withdrawal in an asthmatic patient treated with pranlukast. J Allerg Clin Immunol 1999; 103:534–535.

177. Churg A, Brallas M, Cronin SR, Churg J. Formes frustes of Churg-Strauss syndrome. Chest 1995; 108:320–323.

178. Bili A, Condemi JJ, Bottone SM, Ryan C. Seven cases of complete and incomplete forms of Churg-Strauss syndrome not related to leukotriene receptor antagonists. J Allerg Clin Immunol 1999; 104(5):1060–1065.

179. National Asthma Education Program. Guidelines for the diagnosis and treatment of asthma II. Bethesda, MD: National Institutes of Health, 1997.

180. Taylor D, Auble TE, Calhoun WJ, Mosesso VN. Current outpatient management of asthma shows poor compliance with international consensus guidelines. Chest 1999; 116(6):1638–1645.

181. Woolcock A, Lundback B, Ringdal N, Jacques LA. Comparison of addition of salmeterol to inhaled steroids with doubling of the dose of inhaled steroids. Am J Respir Crit Care Med 1996; 153:1481–1488.

182. Kelloway JS, Wyatt RA, Adlis SA. Comparison of patient's compliance with prescribed oral and inhaled asthma medications. Arch Int Med 1994; 154: 1349–1352.

183. Horwitz RJ, Mcgill KA, Busse WW. The role of leukotriene modifiers in the treatment of asthma. Am J Respir Crit Care Med 1998; 157(5):1363–1371.

184. Lofdahl CG, Reiss TF, Leff JA, Israel E, Noonan MJ, Finn AF, et al. Randomised, placebo controlled trial of effect of a leukotriene receptor antagonist, montelukast, on tapering inhaled corticosteroids in asthmatic patients. Brit Med J 1999; 319(7202):87–90.

185. Israel E, Cohn J, Dube L, Drazen JM. Effect of treatment with zileuton, a 5-lipoxygenase inhibitor, in patients with asthma: a randomized controlled trial. JAMA 1996; 275(12):931–936.

186. Roses AD. Pharmacogenetics and the practice of medicine. Nature 2000; 405(6788):857–865.

187. Lai E, Riley J, Purvis I, Roses A. A 4-Mb high-density single nucleotide polymorphism-based map around human APOE. Genomics 1998; 54(1):31–38.

188. Palmer LJ, Silverman ES, Weiss ST, Drazen JM. Pharmacogenetics of asthma. Am J Respir Crit Care Med 2002; 165(7):861–866.

189. Malmstrom K, Rodriguez-Gomez G, Guerra J, Villaran C, Pineiro A, Wei LX, et al. Oral montelukast, inhaled beclomethasone, and placebo for chronic asthma. A randomized controlled trial. Ann Int Med 1999; 130:487–495.

190. Drazen JM, Yandava C, Dube L, Szczerback N, Hippensteel R, Pillari A, et al. Pharmacogenetic association between ALOX5 promoter genotype and the response to anti-asthma treatment. Nature Genetics 1999; 22:170–172.

191. Asano K, Shiomi T, Hasgawa N, Nakamura H, Kudo H, Matsuzaki T, et al. Leukotriene C4 synthase gene A(-444)C polymorphism and clinical response to a CYS-LT(1) antagonist, pranlukast, in Japanese patients with moderate asthma. Pharmacogenetics 2002; 12(7):565–570.

192. Sampson AP, Siddiqui S, Buchanan D, Howarth PH, Holgate ST, Holloway JW, et al. Variant LTC(4) synthase allele modifies cysteinyl leukotriene synthesis in eosinophils and predicts clinical response to zafirlukast. Thorax 2000; 55(suppl 2):S28–S31.

193. Diamant Z, Timmers MC, Vanderveen H, Friedman BS, DeSmet M, Depre M, et al. The effect of MK-0591, a novel 5-lipoxygenase activating protein inhibitor, on leukotriene biosynthesis and allergen-induced airway responses in asthmatic subjects in vivo. J Allergy Clin Immunol 1995; 95:42–51.

194. Fischer AR, Rosenberg MA, Roth M, Loper M, Jungerwirth S, Israel E. Effect of a novel 5-lipoxygenase activating protein inhibitor, BAYx1005, on asthma induced by cold dry air. Thorax 1997; 52:1074–1077.

195. Camargo CA, Smithline HA, Malice MP, Green SA, Reiss TF. A randomized controlled trial of intravenous montelukast in acute asthma. Am J Respir Crit Care Med 2003; 167(4):528–533.

196. Deykin A, Israel E. Newer therapeutic agents for asthma. Dis Month 1999; 45:117–144.

6

Theophylline and Phosphodiesterase Inhibitors

MILES WEINBERGER

Department of Pediatrics, Allergy and Pulmonary Division, University of Iowa College
  of Medicine
Iowa City, Iowa, U.S.A.

I. History

For decades theophylline was used as a bronchodilator for the relief of acute asthmatic symptoms, initially in patients unresponsive to injected epinephrine (1), and subsequently as an oral agent in fixed dose combination with a weak sympathomimetic bronchodilator, ephedrine (2). It had also been used as a respiratory stimulant for Cheyne-Stokes respirations (3), as a diuretic in the treatment of acute pulmonary edema (4,5), to prevent episodes of apnea and bradycardia in premature newborns (6,7), as an aid in weaning very low birth weight infants from mechanical ventilation (8), and extensively in the treatment of chronic obstructive pulmonary disease (COPD) (9,10). It's most important use eventually became as maintenance therapy for controlling the symptoms of chronic asthma (11). Studies of the pharmacodynamic and pharmacokinetic characteristics of theophylline, the development of reliably absorbed slow-release formulations, and the availability of rapid, specific serum assays improved both the efficacy and safety of this drug (12). Identification of anti-inflammatory effects for theophylline has increased current interest in this venerable medication (13).

II. Pharmacological Activities Potentially Relevant for Asthma

Although traditionally classified as a bronchodilator and initially used primarily for acute bronchodilatation, the ability of theophylline as maintenance therapy to control chronic asthma has always appeared disproportionately greater than was explainable by its modest degree of bronchodilator activity alone (14–22). In addition to bronchodilatation, theophylline has bronchoprotective (23–26), anti-inflammatory (27–30), and immunomodulatory (22) effects that potentially contribute to its efficacy as a maintenance medication for controlling chronic asthma.

Theophylline attenuates airway responsiveness to histamine (23), methacholine (23), allergen (27), sulfur dioxide (24), distilled water (25), toluene diisocyanate (31), and adenosine (32). While the degree of attenuation is modest for most of these bronchoconstrictors, theophylline can completely inhibit airway responsiveness to exercise at serum concentration of $\geq 15\,\mu g/mL$ (26), the upper half of the $10–20\,\mu g/mL$ range shown to provide optimal control of chronic asthma (14,33–35). None of these bronchoprotective effects correlate well with the degree of bronchodilatation produced by theophylline before the challenge. For substances such as methacholine and histamine that directly stimulate bronchial smooth muscle contraction, the bronchoprotection may be effected by direct inhibition of smooth muscle contraction, i.e., functional antagonism. In contrast, attenuation of the early response to allergen by theophylline may involve inhibition of synthesis or release of leukotrienes from the mast cells (36), attenuation of the effects of cysteinyl leukotrienes at the Cyst LT_1 receptor (37), or blocking of adenosine enhancement of mediator release from mast cells (38).

Theophylline down-regulates inflammatory and immune cell function in vitro and in vivo in animals with airway inflammation (39,40). In patients with allergic asthma, it attenuates the late phase increase in airway obstruction and airway responsiveness to histamine (27) and decreases allergen-induced migration of activated eosinophils into the bronchial mucosa (30). Moreover, withdrawal of theophylline from 27 adults with severe chronic asthma receiving high doses of inhaled corticosteroid therapy resulted in increased symptoms of asthma, especially at night, accompanied by an increase in the number of activated cytotoxic T lymphocytes in the bronchial mucosa and an increase in helper T lymphocytes in the airway epithelium (22). The decrease in lung function that occurs at night in many patients with asthma is reduced by theophylline, and this reduction has been associated with both a decrease in the percentage of neutrophils and a decrease in stimulated leukotriene B_4 from macrophages in early morning bronchoalveolar lavage fluid (41). These anti-inflammatory effects have been identified at serum concentrations over $5\,\mu g/mL$ (22,30), but it is not known if the anti-inflammatory effect is greater at serum concentrations over 10 µg/mL, where optimal clinical effect has been demonstrated in other studies (14,33–35).

These findings suggest that theophylline has anti-inflammatory, immunomodulatory, and bronchoprotective effects that contribute to its efficacy as maintenance prophylactic therapy for chronic asthma. Theophylline also decreases fatigue of diaphragmatic muscles (42), increases mucociliary clearance (43), acts centrally to block the decrease in ventilation that occurs with sustained hypoxia (44), and decreases microvascular leakage of plasma into the airways (45). While unlikely to be important in chronic asthma, some of these actions may provide a rationale for the addition of theophylline in the treatment of acute asthma unresponsive to vigorous use of inhaled β_2-adrenergic agonist drugs and systemically administered corticosteroids. These latter actions may also be relevant to the use of theophylline in other clinical situations where clinical efficacy has been reported, such as chronic obstructive pulmonary disease, apnea of prematurity, or ventilator weaning in premature infants.

III. Molecular Mechanisms

Although several molecular mechanisms have been proposed to explain the actions of theophylline, nonspecific inhibition of phosphodiesterase (PDE) isozymes and non-selective antagonism of specific cell-surface receptors for adenosine are the only ones known to occur at clinically relevant drug concentrations. Theophylline increases the intracellular concentration of cyclic nucleotides in airway smooth muscle and inflammatory cells by inhibiting PDE-mediated hydrolysis. Several distinct isoenzyme families have now been distinguished, based on substrate specificity and the development of selective inhibitors (46). Theophylline is a nonspecific PDE inhibitor that inhibits activation of inflammatory cell types, including T lymphocytes, eosinophils, mast cells, and macrophages, in vitro (47). Inhibition of PDE types 3 and 4 have been reported to relax smooth muscles in pulmonary arteries and in airways (48), while anti-inflammatory and immunomodulatory actions appear to result largely from inhibition of the type IV isoenzymes (40,49).

In vitro studies have demonstrated effects on mononuclear cells and lymphocytes that may be relevant to its anti-inflammatory effect. Inhibition of the L-arginine-dependent production of nitric oxide (50) and suppression of interleukin-4 production (51) has been demonstrated in peripheral blood mononuclear cells of asthmatics. Dust mite–induced lymphocyte proliferation and production of proinflammatory Th2 cytokines, interleukins 5 and 13, were suppressed by theophylline in another report (52).

Theophylline's bronchoprotective effects against the early response to antigen- and leukotriene D_4–induced bronchoconstriction appear to be mediated by a common, but unknown, molecular mechanism that does not involve PDE inhibition or adenosine receptor antagonism (37). In contrast, centrally mediated stimulation of respiration (53), nausea and vomiting (54), and ventricular arrhythmias that result from toxic serum concentrations are probably mediated by PDE inhibition, but it is unknown which isozymes are involved.

While theophylline inhibits adenosine receptors that act as a bronchoconstrictor (32), it is unlikely that adenosine receptor antagonism is involved in the bronchodilator action of theophylline. Enprofylline, a methylxanthine that does not antagonize adenosine receptors, is a more potent inhibitor of PDE and a more potent bronchodilator than theophylline, while 8-phenyltheophylline, a potent adenosine receptor antagonist that does not inhibit PDE, does not relax bronchial smooth muscle in vivo (37). However, nonspecific adenosine receptor antagonism appears to be the mechanism by which theophylline increases ventilation during hypoxia, decreases fatigue of diaphragmatic muscles, and decreases adenosine enhancement of mediator release from mast cells (37). Some adverse effects of theophylline, such as increased psychomotor activity, sinus tachycardia, gastric acid secretion, diuresis, and antagonism of gamma aminobutyric acid-benzodiazepine receptors in the brain, probably also result from adenosine receptor antagonism (37). Adenosine antagonism also may be responsible for the modest decrease in cerebral blood flow observed after a single dose of theophylline (55), although no evidence indicates that this effect is clinically important, especially after multiple doses when adenosine A_1 receptors are upregulated.

Theophylline activates histone deacetylase, the activity of which is reduced in asthmatic airways. This suppresses the expression of inflammatory genes (56). The mechanism by which theophylline at low doses activates histone deacetylase has not been identified, but it is not mediated by either PDE inhibition or adenosine receptor antagonism. This activity of theophylline appears to require activated glucocorticoid receptors. Low concentrations of theophylline markedly potentiate the anti-inflammatory effects of corticosteroids in vitro, with 100- to 1000-fold potentiation, and this may be the explanation for the benefit of low-dose theophylline added to inhaled corticosteroids seen in clinical studies of patients with asthma. Furthermore, theophylline, through direct activation of histone deacetylase, has been shown to reverse the effect of oxidative stress and cigarette smoke with the consequent restoration of corticosteroid responsiveness (13).

IV. Pharmacodynamics

A. Efficacy for Treating Acute Symptoms from Asthma

The traditional role of theophylline as an acute intervention measure has changed with more aggressive use of inhaled β_2-agonists and systemic corticosteroids. A controlled clinical trial of 44 adults seen for acute asthma in an emergency department showed no greater benefit from theophylline (as intravenous aminophylline) than placebo when added to vigorous use of inhaled β_2-adrenergic agonist drugs and systemic corticosteroids (57). In patients with severe exacerbations requiring hospitalization, data on the value of adding theophylline are conflicting (58–61). In one study of 39 hospitalized adults, the addition of theophylline to inhaled albuterol (salbutamol) and oral prednisone was not beneficial (58). In contrast, another study of 21 adults treated with inhaled albuterol, intravenous methylprednisolone, and theophylline or placebo found that the theophylline-treated patients had greater improvement in FEV_1 at 3 and 48 hours and needed rescue therapy with inhaled albuterol less often; there was no accompanying increase in the frequency of adverse effects (59). Using the same protocol, theophylline was not beneficial in children treated at the same institution (60). The author common to these two reports speculated that the difference in results was the more vigorous use of inhaled β_2-agonists on the pediatric service.

Theophylline thus appears superfluous for routine use during acute exacerbations of asthma when inhaled β_2-adrenergic agonists and corticosteroids are used optimally. However, patients with respiratory failure were excluded from these studies, a precaution that was necessary for ethical reasons, and addition of theophylline may yet be justified for patients with severe acute symptoms not rapidly responding to these measures. In this situation, a single loading dose can be given; a continuous infusion can then be instituted if benefit is observed.

B. Efficacy as Maintenance Therapy for Chronic Asthma

Theophylline has been repeatedly demonstrated to be effective as a single maintenance medication in the management of chronic asthma. The first studies of this in the early 1970s demonstrated that symptoms were markedly diminished, and need for intervention with measures to treat acute symptoms were virtually eliminated for most patients (14,15). Subsequent studies compared theophylline with alternative medications. Theophylline was associated with more asymptomatic days than cromolyn sodium (disodium cromoglycate) when both were used as monotherapy in patients with severe chronic asthma (16), although efficacy appeared similar in patients with milder asthma (62–64).

Comparison with oral β_2-agonists have shown clinical advantage for theophylline, especially for nocturnal symptoms (65,66). Although inhaled albuterol is far more potent for acute bronchodilatation than theophylline, a controlled clinical trial demonstrated that theophylline nonetheless provided more stable clinical effect (19). In contrast, longer acting β_2-agonists, salmeterol and formoterol, are used as twice-daily maintenance medications for chronic asthma. In a two-week comparison study with theophylline (67), salmeterol was more effective than theophylline, but only 98 of 141 patients (median age 51) completed the trial, and over half the patients had serum theophylline concentrations below the 10–20 µg/mL range despite initially determined dosage that attained serum concentrations of 10–20 µg/mL, where maximal efficacy is most likely (14,34,35). Other large-scale multicenter trials have suffered from the same problem with most patients having serum concentrations consistently below 10 µg/mL during the trial (68,69). A study of 15 patients reported little difference between salmeterol and theophylline on nocturnal asthma during a two-week study with a range of serum theophylline concentrations from less than 8 to greater than 15 µg/mL (median 11 µg/mL) (70). Although several large trials have reported sustained bronchodilatation and clinical efficacy with long-term use of salmeterol (71), there is concern regarding loss of bronchoprotective effect against challenge with methacholine (72), exercise (73,74), and allergen inhalation (75) after as little as two weeks. The effect from continuous use of β_2-agonists may be particularly important for certain genetic polymorphisms of the β_2-receptor (76). In contrast, attenuation of airway responsiveness to exercise is sustained with theophylline (77).

Theophylline has substantial additive effect with inhaled (17,20,22) or alternate morning oral corticosteroids (17), reducing symptoms (Fig. 1), improving exercise tolerance, and decreasing requirements for inhaled bronchodilator and the need for short courses of corticosteroids because of bronchodilator subresponsiveness (17). Moreover, abrupt discontinuation of theophylline in patients with severe asthma results in precipitous deterioration even though other drugs such as cromolyn, inhaled steroids, and β_2-agonists are continued (20). This has been observed even among patients receiving a mean of 1500 µg/day of beclomethasone (22). In contrast, cromolyn sodium (disodium cromoglycate) has not shown additive effect with either theophylline (16) or inhaled corticosteroids in three placebo-controlled studies (78–80). Trials of nedocromil in adults at doses of 4 mg (81) and 8 mg (82) four times daily showed only a small additive effect with inhaled corticosteroids. A small additive effect with inhaled corticosteroids has been observed for a leukotriene antagonist, montelukast (83), but this appears to be less than is seen from adding salmeterol (84). Of currently marketed non-steroidal medications, only salmeterol has had additive benefit of a magnitude similar to theophylline for patients already receiving an inhaled corticosteroid (85,86).

The degree of clinical effect from theophylline described above is most readily apparent when serum concentrations are maintained between 10 and 20 µg/mL (14,33–35), and the magnitude of effect can be demonstrated to relate to serum concentration (26,35,87,88). Measures of effect on airway hyper-responsiveness to histamine (23), methacholine (23,89), or exercise (26) relate closely to serum concentration. Inhibition of exercise-induced bronchospasm relates to serum concentration, with clinically important

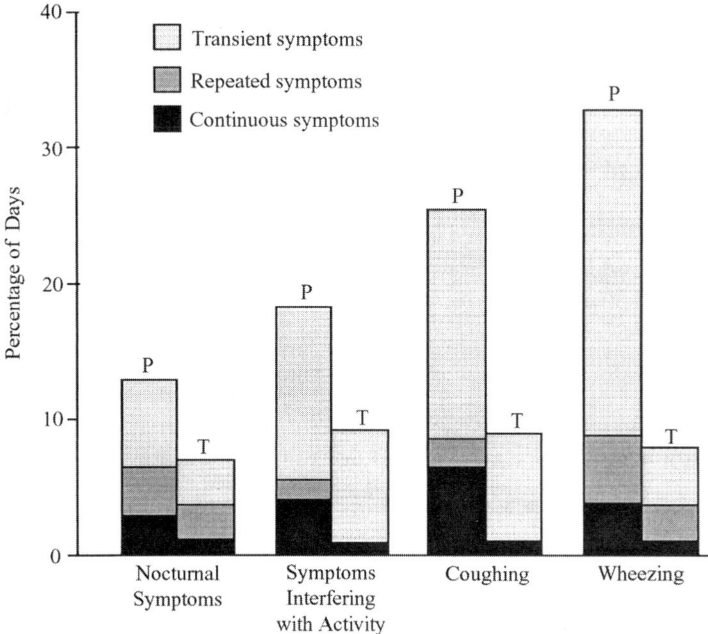

Figure 1 Mean frequency of symptoms in 21 children with asthma receiving a constant dose of beclomethasone dipropionate (mean of 550 µg/day, 11 puffs per day) and treated in randomized sequence for four weeks with each of placebo (*P*) or theophylline at dosage previously individualized to achieve a peak serum concentration of 10–20 µg/mL (*T*). Nocturnal symptoms of cough, wheeze, or dyspnea that disturbed sleep were recorded each morning, and interference with activity, cough, and wheeze during the day were recorded each evening as absent, transient, repeated, or continuous. In addition to significantly fewer symptoms, theophylline was also associated with significantly less airway responsiveness to exercise and significantly fewer interventions with both inhaled β_2-adrenergic agonists and short courses of oral corticosteroids. *Source*: From Ref. 17.

effects most apparent above 10 µg/mL and even greater effects above 15 µg/ mL (26). At these concentrations theophylline is more effective than cromolyn in attenuating exercise-induced bronchospasm (26), although it generally does not match the acute benefits from an inhaled β_2-receptor agonist.

C. Toxicity

The therapeutic benefit from theophylline has required consideration for its use in a manner that minimizes its potential for adverse effects (90). Drug interactions or alterations in clearance for other reasons have the potential to cause toxicity. However, toxicity has occurred most commonly from errors in dosage (91,92). Fortunately, most cases of toxicity are mild and readily reversible without residual effects. In virtually every case where there has been serious toxicity such as seizures with neurological damage, serious errors in dosage occurred, often compounded by other factors such as drug interactions or failing to be alert for early signs of toxicity such as nausea, vomiting, central nervous stimulation, or tachycardia.

Some adverse effects from theophylline have been overplayed, particularly in the lay news media where headlines have proclaimed "Asthma Drug Hard on Kids" (*USA Today*, December 2, 1986, 1), and an advertisement for an ABC Television news show, Prime Time Live, ominously described "An Asthma Drug that Can Take Your Breath Away, *Permanently!*" (*TV Guide* advertisement for Prime Time Live, American Broadcasting Company) aired February 7, 1991. In actuality, severe toxic effects from theophylline are quite rare in clinical practice. In a study as part of the Boston Collaborative Drug Surveillance Program, the frequency of toxicity was assessed among 36,000 patients who filled 225,000 prescriptions for theophylline over nine years. Severe toxicity occurred in only one patient per 1000 patient years of exposure, and seizures occurred in only two patients (one child and one adult) with serum concentrations of about 50 µg/mL. Nonetheless, the prescribing clinician needs to be aware that theophylline has the greatest potential for serious acute toxicity of any medication used for asthma. Extensive reviews of the world's English language literature of reported cases of theophylline toxicity are recorded elsewhere (93–95).

Initiation of treatment is commonly associated with caffeine-like side effects, including a minor degree of central nervous system (CNS), stimulation and/or nausea. These occur frequently after a loading dose and appear to have little direct relationship to serum concentration (96). Although few complaints are elicited from the acutely ill patient in need of a rapid bronchodilator effect, these minor side effects can be troublesome in many ambulatory patients with chronic asthma. They can generally be avoided by beginning with low doses and slowly attaining full therapeutic doses over a period of 7 to 10 days. When this procedure is followed and serum concentrations do not exceed 20 µg/mL, adverse effects are rare and minor (Table 1) (97). Even subclinical effects are difficult to detect. Sleep, for example appears to be unaffected during chronic therapy (70,98,99), despite the common complaint of insomnia during initiation of therapy. On the other hand, subclinical tremor, without patient awareness, is detectable in association with theophylline use (100), and potentiation of tremor is seen when theophylline is used concomitantly with oral β_2-agonists (101).

Behavioral and learning problems have been attributed to theophylline, but with more concern than reason (102). In point of fact, a controlled evaluation of various behavior and psychologic variables showed a pattern of small but statistically significant effects similar to those associated with dietary caffeine ingestion. These effects were not clinically apparent to the patients, and not all of them were "adverse" effects (e.g., patients

Table 1 Frequency of Apparent Adverse Effects from Theophylline Among 404 Patients Under Care of the University of Iowa Pediatric Allergy and Pulmonary Clinic

Serum concentration (μg/mL)	Frequency of adverse effects [no. subjects affected/no. subjects studied (%)]	
	Children	Adults
< 10	0/29	0/12
10–19.9	5/258 (2)	3/38 (8)
$\geq$ 20	17/61 (28)	4/6 (67)

Data obtained by questioning patients at time initial blood sample was collected in sequentially treated ambulatory patients whose dose had been titrated over nine days, according to previously prescribed published guidelines. *Source*: From Ref. 97.

demonstrated significantly improved ability to memorize number sequences during theophylline therapy). Several well-controlled studies have failed to confirm earlier suggestions or even parents' impressions of effects on behavior and learning (103–106). The performance on standardized achievement tests of asthmatic children in Iowa receiving theophylline has been compared with non-asthmatic sibling controls, demonstrating that mean scores of the children with asthma were well above the national average and no different, on average, from their siblings (106). In that study, 85% of children with chronic symptoms of asthma requiring maintenance medication seen over a one-year period at two clinical settings were receiving theophylline for greater than three months, most for greater than one year. Nevertheless, there may be a small subpopulation of children in whom theophylline therapy may cause unacceptable persistent central nervous system side effects at therapeutic serum concentrations. Alternative therapy should be used in such patients.

The risk of actual toxicity from theophylline increases in likelihood and severity as concentrations exceed 20 μg/mL and include nausea, vomiting, headache, diarrhea, irritability, and insomnia (107–109). In one report adverse effects were documented retrospectively among 75% of patients with serum concentrations over 25 μg/mL, but were uncommon at concentrations between 15 and 20 μg/mL and absent below 15 μg/mL (109). At higher serum levels, there is a progressively increasing risk of toxic encephalopathy with hyperthermia, seizures, brain damage, and death; hyperglycemia, hypokalemia, hypotension, and cardiac arrhythmias may also be observed at these higher levels (107–113). However, there is considerable variability in the toxic response to theophylline.

Severe toxicity and death most often have been the result of therapeutic misadventure in which multiple excessive doses were administered; in early reports, this was commonly associated with the use of suppositories in infants and small children (114–116). Irritability, vomiting of material resembling coffee grounds, and seizures from which the patient never regained consciousness characterized the clinical course in many such cases. Age over 60 appears to be associated with increased risk for theophylline-induced seizures when serum concentrations are excessive during repeated dosing (117). Serious theophylline intoxication has frequently been reported with cardiac decompensation or hepatic dysfunction (107,118,119). In these individuals clearance of the drug was impaired and excessive serum concentrations accumulated (107,108,119). Administration of a 0.9 mg/kg/hr constant intravenous infusion of aminophylline (equivalent to 0.7 mg/kg/hr anhydrous theophylline) was common among these and other reports of toxicity associated with theophylline in adults during the 1970s and early 1980s (107–109,118–120). A report from a major inner-city hospital identified greater than 10-hour delays in house officers responding to excessive serum concentrations as the most common cause of theophylline toxicity (92). Other common causes of toxicity include failure to recognize the need for reduced dosage in patients with physiologic conditions or concomitant drug therapy that slows theophylline elimination, failure to recognize obvious early signs of toxicity, failure to recognize previous toxicity at the administered dose, and inappropriate increases in dosage.

Theophylline-induced seizures can occur in patients without a previous history of neurologic disease when serum concentrations are excessive (107,108,112,121,122). Zwillich et al. (108) reported a mean serum concentration of 54 µg/mL among eight patients with seizures, compared with 35 µg/mL for those with minor adverse effects, and a mean concentration of 19 µg/mL in patients in a medical intensive care unit for severe respiratory symptoms without symptoms of toxicity. Four of the eight patients with seizures died without regaining consciousness. Most noteworthy was the failure to recognize minor adverse effects in seven of these eight severely ill patients in an intensive care unit prior to the seizure. Although typically present when looked for, minor symptoms of toxicity such as nausea and vomiting cannot be relied upon as a dosing end point; *only serum theophylline measurements can reliably forewarn the physician of impending life-threatening toxicity.*

Two distinct clinical patterns of theophylline-induced seizures have been reported. In patients with an underlying neurologic disorder, transient focal seizures, with or without generalization and without neurologic sequelae, have been reported at serum concentrations as low as 15–25 µg/mL (123). This is rare in patients without a history of neurologic disease (124). In contrast, at higher serum concentrations theophylline-induced seizures appear to be a manifestation of a toxic encephalopathy. They are then typically generalized, persistent, resistant to anticonvulsant therapy, and followed by a comatose period with cerebral edema that frequently produces permanent brain damage or death. An electroencephalogram (EEG) obtained at the time of the seizure often demonstrates a pattern of periodic epileptiform discharges. Neurologic sequelae from theophylline toxicity appear not to occur in the absence of seizures (125,126).

Interestingly, one report indicated asymptomatic abnormal paroxysmal EEG activity at serum concentrations at or somewhat above the upper end of the therapeutic range in a greater proportion of asthmatic patients than would be expected to occur in a group of individuals of similar age (127). This suggests that theophylline lowers the seizure threshold. Brain injury or disease has also been suggested as a risk factor for prolonged seizures and death from theophylline at serum concentrations not usually associated with such severe outcomes (128).

The duration of an excessive serum concentration appears to play a major role in the severity of CNS toxicity from theophylline. There is a progressive risk of seizures in association with serum concentrations greater than 30–40 µg/mL when the intoxication occurred after multiple doses. However, seizures are uncommon from a single overdose in an ingestion such as a suicide attempt, unless concentrations are greater than 100 µg/ mL (117,122,129). These findings suggest that the amount of theophylline accumulating in brain tissue may be a more important determinant of seizure activity than serum concentration. The mechanism of this toxic effect has not been defined, but findings consistent with brain anoxia and neuronal loss have been found at necropsy in patients who died of theophylline-induced seizures (111).

Another difference between acute and chronic overdoses is the electrolyte abnormalities, particularly hypokalemia, associated commonly with acute but much less frequently with chronic overdoses (130). Other metabolic and electrolyte abnormalities that commonly accompany hypokalemia include hypophosphatemia, hypomagnesemia, hyperglycemia, and acidosis (113,131). Some of these effects may be, in part, due to elevated levels of norepinephrine and epinephrine transiently released by very high levels of theophylline (132). Potentiation of hypokalemia and hyperglycemia have been described from combined systemic administration of a β_2-agonist and theophylline (133,134) but not from combined use of theophylline and an inhaled β_2-agonist (135). The hypokalemia induced by theophylline overdose appears to be transient and is considerably less in patients presenting to an emergency room more than six hours after ingestion than those presenting earlier, even at similar serum theophylline concentrations (136). Since the hypokalemia occurs early in the course of theophylline prior to sufficient vomiting to account for gastrointestinal loss, intracellular sequestration is the most likely mechanism. Aggressive potassium administration is therefore not indicated and may, in fact, lead to subsequent hyperkalemia with associated electrocardiographic changes (137).

Arrhythmias from theophylline have been most evident in adults (117, 122,129). Although tachycardia commonly occurs in premature newborns at concentrations above 10 µg/mL, most other patients experience this effect only at concentrations greater than 20 µg/mL (107,110,117,122). In patients with COPD, however, theophylline serum concentrations in the range of 15–20 µg/mL may increase the frequency of ventricular arrhythmias (138) or multifocal atrial tachycardia (139). At higher concentrations, ventricular tachycardia or runs of premature ventricular contractions may occur in patients with no prior history of cardiac arrhythmias (107,110,117,122). Hypotension and sudden cardiac arrest have been associated with rapid administration of intravenous theophylline, particularly when injected directly into a central venous catheter (140). Adverse effects on the electric stability of the heart are probably an accentuation of the positive chronotropic action of theophylline, which is mediated by a direct effect on the myocardium, a release of local norepinephrine, and, to a lesser extent, a transient diminution of peripheral vagal control (141).

Other adverse reactions from theophylline are uncommon. Dehydration in children has resulted from a combination of a loss of fluids caused by vomiting, decreased fluid intake, and the transient diuretic action of the drug. In fact, when diabetic ketoacidosis has been excluded, the combination of persistent vomiting and diuresis may be pathognomonic of theophylline intoxication, since oliguria would be expected to result from dehydration (142). In patients with ulcer disease, theophylline may stimulate gastric acid secretion (143) and increase epigastric pain. It has been suggested that xanthines, including theophylline, may increase the risk of fibrocystic breast disease (144–146), but case–controlled studies supported neither this (147,148) nor a hypothesized effect on breast epithelial cells (145). There have been isolated reports of theophylline causing urinary retention in elderly men with benign prostatic hypertrophy (149), hypercalcemia (150), rhabdomyolysis after an overdose (151), and esophageal ulcerations from incomplete swallowing of a slow-release tablet (152).

We have observed, in an uncontrolled manner, the suggestion that patients with migraine may have an increased frequency of acute migraine symptoms in association with therapeutic use of theophylline. A possible mechanism for this may relate to the evidence that theophylline can inhibit adenine-related vasodilatation of cerebrovasculature (153). Although there have been no published reports, let alone controlled studies, of this association, alternative therapy to theophylline should be used if an increased frequency of headaches occurs in the absence of excessive serum concentrations.

Allergic reactions to theophylline have been reported only in association with the administration of aminophylline, presumably to the ethylenediamine component, and have included urticaria and exfoliative dermatitis (154,155). Asthmatic symptoms in these patients can be safely treated with an oral or intravenous theophylline formulation that does not contain ethylenediamine.

V. Biopharmaceutics and Pharmacokinetics

A. Absorption

Theophylline is rapidly, consistently, and completely absorbed from oral liquids and plain uncoated tablets (96,156). Absorption of theophylline may be somewhat slowed by concurrent ingestion of food (157,158), antacids (aluminum or magnesium hydroxide) (159,160), the recumbent position (161,162), or when the dose is increased (156,163). However, the extent of absorption is unchanged and these alterations are unimportant clinically with preparations that undergo rapid dissolution. The rate of disintegration and dissolution in the stomach is the major determinant of the rate and completeness of absorption from rapid-release formulations. Absorption of theophylline lags at night during sleep with more rapid absorption in the early morning hours resulting in higher morning trough concentrations (164–166).

Since maximal solubility of theophylline in water is about 8 mg/mL at physiologic pH and temperature, intramuscular administration results in precipitation of the drug at the injection site and slow absorption (167). Moreover, this route is painful and irritating, since these solutions have a pH of about nine. The rate and extent of absorption of theophylline from rectal solutions (168) approaches that of oral solutions, but commercially available rectal suppositories made from a cocoa butter base have repeatedly been associated with slow and erratic absorption (167,169,170). While rectal solutions were frequently used in the past for acute care, there is currently little indication for these formulations.

Slow release preparations became the formulations of choice for theophylline as maintenance therapy for chronic asthma. The extent and rate of absorption differed among the various slow-release formulations (171–175) and occasionally between lots (172) or different strengths (171) of the same brand. Even among completely absorbed products, differences in rates of absorption were sufficient to be of clinical importance since effect from theophylline related directly to the blood level at any given point in time (175). Absorption of some formulations were shown to differ markedly in rate and/or completeness of absorption when taken fasting or following food (176–185). This issue was of particular importance for some products marketed for once-daily dosing.

B. Distribution

Once theophylline enters the systemic circulation, about 40% becomes bound to plasma protein (186), while the remaining free drug distributes throughout body water. Although earlier studies had reported 60% protein binding (187,188), this was an artifact of failing to recognize the pH and temperature dependency of protein binding and the consequent need to simulate in vivo conditions (186).

Distribution is sufficiently rapid that serum concentrations are in equilibrium with tissue concentrations of the drug within one hour after an intravenous injection (87). The apparent volume of distribution, the space into which theophylline distributes, ranges from 0.3 to 0.7 L/kg (30–70% of ideal body weight) (189,190) and averages about 0.45 L/kg in both children (191,192) and adults (96,191,193). The mean volume of distribution for premature newborns (194), adults with hepatic cirrhosis (195,196), uncorrected acidemia (197), the elderly (198), acutely ill patients with COPD (199), and in women during the third trimester of pregnancy (200) is slightly larger, since protein binding is reduced in these patients. In most other circumstances, even when theophylline clearance is altered, volume of distribution remains relatively unaffected.

Theophylline freely crosses the placenta (201,202) and passes into breast milk (203,204), although only minor adverse effects have been reported for infants indirectly receiving the drug in this manner (201,202). Theophylline crosses the blood–brain barrier more slowly than caffeine, but cerebrospinal fluid concentrations were reported to be 90% of serum concentrations in premature infants after distribution (205). In contrast, cerebrospinal fluid theophylline concentrations in older children are approximately 50% of the serum concentration (206). Concentrations in saliva average about 60% of serum levels (187,207,208), corresponding to the amount of unbound drug in the blood.

C. Metabolism

Theophylline is eliminated from the body by hepatic biotransformation into relatively inactive metabolites that are rapidly excreted in the urine (209). About 85% to 90% of a dose is metabolized (210) primarily by cytochrome P450 1A2 and to a lesser extent by 3A3 and 2E1 (211). This occurs over multiple parallel pathways by both first-order and capacity-limited kinetic processes (163,210,212). The major metabolite, 1,3-dimethyluric acid, is formed by hydroxylation in the C-8 position, whereas 3-methylxanthine and the intermediate metabolite, 1-methylxanthine, result from N-demethylation (210). The intermediate metabolite, 1-methylxanthine, is rapidly converted by xanthine oxidase to 1-methyluric acid (213). Since the rate of formation of 1-methylxanthine is slower than the conversion to 1-methyluric acid, highly sensitive assays are able to detect only small amounts of 1-methylxanthine in blood and urine (210). About 6% of a dose of theophylline is N-methylated to caffeine in adults, which in turn is converted to paraxanthine (214).

Since the hepatic extraction ratio for theophylline is only about 10% (215), there is little loss of available drug from first-pass metabolism; serum concentration–time curves are similar after both oral and intravenous administration (96). Renal clearance of theophylline is dependent upon urine flow rate (216), but less than 15% of a dose is excreted in the urine unchanged beyond the neonatal period (210,216). Therefore, dosage adjustments are not generally required because of renal dysfunction (217) except in neonates during the first few months of life when renal clearance plays a larger role because of hepatic immaturity (218). In patients with normal renal function, the renal clearance of theophylline metabolites far exceeds the normal glomerular filtration rate, suggesting that tubular secretion plays a role in their elimination (210). This relationship explains why 3-methylxanthine, the only active metabolite, does not exert pharmacologic effects.

In the premature infant, about 50% of the dose is excreted in the urine unchanged, and the remainder undergoes N-methylation to caffeine and C-8 hydroxylation to 1,3-demethyluric acid (211,219). As only small amounts of 3-methylxanthine and 1-methyluric acid have been recovered in urine from premature newborns, cytochrome P450 2A2 activity, which mediates the N-demethylation pathway (211), seems to be relatively deficient in this patient population (219,220). The conversion of theophylline to caffeine is not unique to neonates, but it is clinically more important because of the extremely long half-life of caffeine in this population, which results in accumulation. Caffeine serum concentrations average 30% of the theophylline concentration but may be substantially higher in some neonates (221,222). However, measurement of caffeine serum levels in a neonate receiving theophylline is necessary only when adverse effects appear and the theophylline concentration is within the 5–10 µg/mL therapeutic range. Theophylline is only a minor metabolite of caffeine in the neonate (221).

The various metabolic pathways of theophylline undergo capacity-limited kinetics, i.e., clearance is more rapid at lower serum concentrations than at higher, as a consequence of saturation of enzyme systems (210). Since values for the Michalis–Menten constants that describe enzyme kinetics, K_m and V_{max}, for 1,3-dimethyluric acid, the major metabolite, are high relative to the other metabolites, this pathway saturates enzyme systems at higher serum concentrations, and thus elimination appears more linear at usually attained serum concentrations than other major pathways for theophylline metabolism.

D. Elimination

In 1972, Jenne et al. (33) first described the interpatient variation in theophylline elimination rate, dosage requirements, and serum concentration. A fixed dose of oral medication administered continuously to a group of asthmatic adults resulted in a wide range of serum concentrations. When dosage was adjusted to maintain serum concentrations within the 10–20 µg/mL range, defined as providing maximum likelihood of effectiveness without risk of toxicity, requirements varied from 400 to 2000 mg/day.

A similar variability in rate of elimination was demonstrated for children (223). However, since children, on average, metabolize theophylline at a faster rate than do adults, weight-adjusted dosage requirements to achieve a therapeutic serum concentration are higher in children (Fig. 2) (224). Interestingly, dose requirements to attain peak serum concentrations of 10–20 µg/mL examined during the period from 1990 to 1995 averaged about 25% lower than when dose requirements were examined from 1978 to 1983 (97) (Fig. 3).

While theophylline elimination was initially described as first order, i.e., the rate of elimination appeared proportional to the concentration (191–193), dose dependency of elimination rate has been repeatedly demonstrated (225–228). This tendency is clinically relevant in that changes in dosage can result in disproportionate changes in serum concentration (Fig. 4).

E. Physiologic Factors Associated with Alteration in Theophylline Disposition

Total body clearance, the product of volume of distribution and elimination rate constant, quantifies theophylline removal from the body. While intrapatient variability in clearance is small (223,229), interpatient variability is large and appears to be from differences in the rate of hepatic biotransformation, which changes with age, concurrent illness, smoking, pregnancy, aberrations in diet, and intake of other drugs. The volume of distribution is a somewhat larger fraction of body weight in infancy and varies inversely with body fat. However, the major variable of the two components of clearance is the elimination rate, often expressed as a half-life of elimination. Because of immature hepatic enzymes, metabolic clearance of theophylline is very slow in the neonate, and even more so in the premature, with elimination half-lives averaging greater than 24 hours. Consequently, dosage requirements are markedly reduced in neonates (194,255) and increase during the first year of life (230). Maturation occurs over the course of the first year of life, so that elimination half-lives average the same from age one to nine and then slowly decrease until mean elimination half-lives in adults average twice that seen in children from one to nine years. Girls begin to have decreased weight-adjusted dosage requirements at a somewhat earlier age than males (97); this decrease in clearance appears to be related to sexual maturation that begins earlier in girls (231).

Conflicting reports have been published on the influence of obesity (189,190,232–235), old age (198,236,237), and gender (238–240) on theophylline clearance. Available evidence suggests that there is no clinically important difference in theophylline clearance between males and females of comparable age and/or development (97,238). Free-drug clearance appears to be lower in elderly patients than in younger adults, because of decreased protein binding (198). The decrease in theophylline clearance

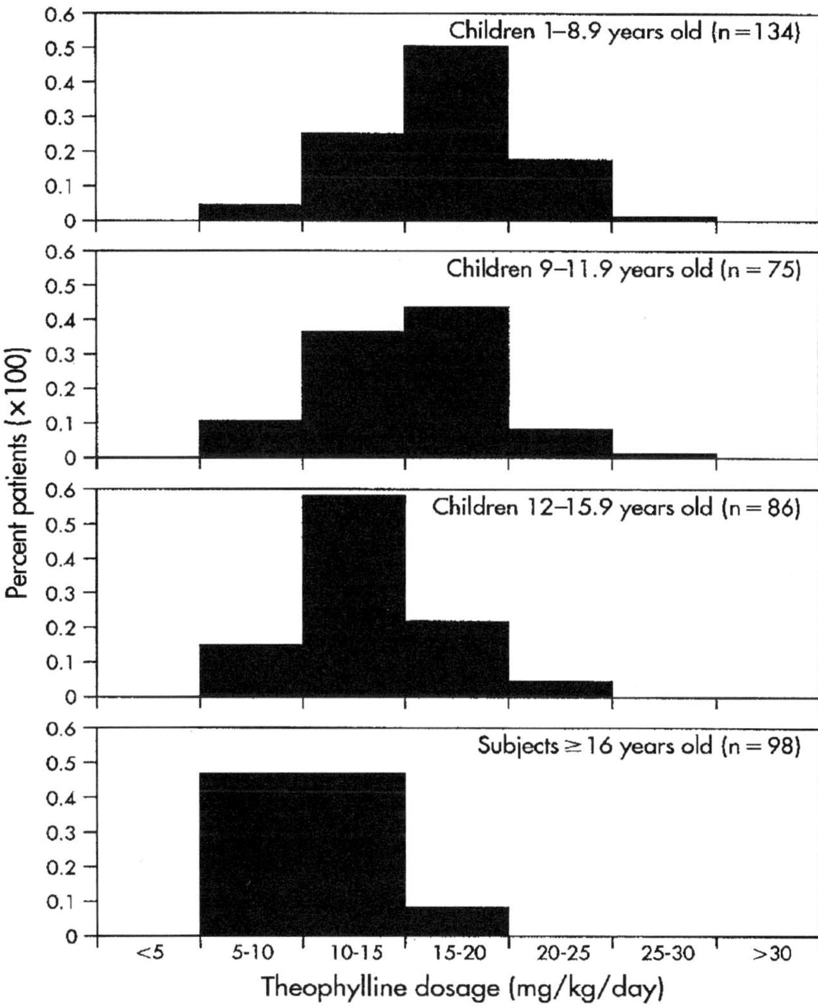

Figure 2 Distribution of dosage requirements needed to attain serum theophylline concentrations at various ages. *Source*: From Ref. 224.

associated with hepatic cirrhosis (195,196), acute hepatitis (241), cholestasis (241), cardiac decompensation (242–244), cor pulmonale (245), hypothyroidism (246), and sepsis with multiorgan failure (247) can be large and of major clinical importance.

Clearance is also reduced during febrile illnesses of various etiology (223,248–251). Fever experimentally induced with etiocholanolone has been shown to reduce the clearance of antipyrine, another drug N-demethylated by cytochrome P450 1A2 (252). Increased theophylline serum concentrations

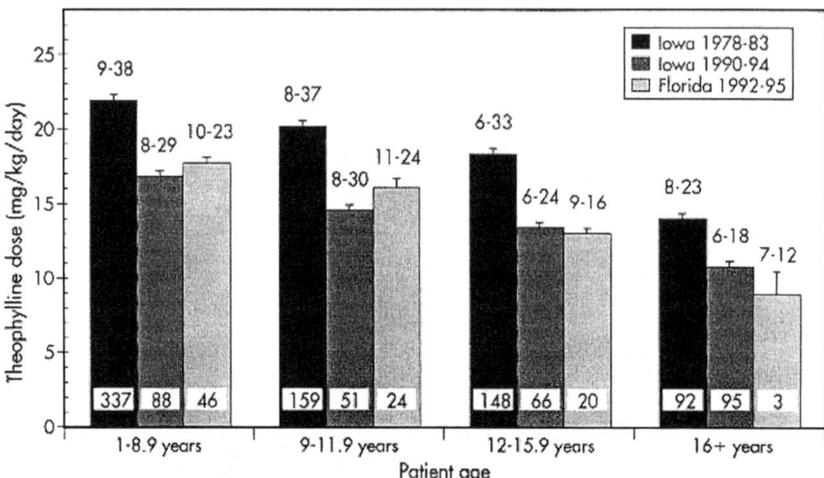

Figure 3 Comparison of mean dosage requirements needed to attain serum theophylline concentrations between 10 and 20 µg/mL (mean 14 µg/mL) in Iowa during the period from 1978 to 1983 and from 1990 to 1995 at two clinics. The shift to lower doses among all groups indicates decreased population clearance of theophylline, presumably from some difference in environmental stimulus of theophylline metabolism; the difference in exposure to active and passive cigarette smoke during these two time periods is postulated to be in the cause of this. *Source*: From Ref. 224.

have also been associated with herpes simplex viral infection (253). While there has been speculation that viral respiratory infections can reduce theophylline elimination in the absence of fever, extensive clinical experience in young children who got multiple viral respiratory infections while on maintenance therapy with theophylline and controlled studies in adults (254) and children with respiratory syncytial virus infection (255) have not supported any clinically important role for viral infections in the absence of sustained high fever, e.g., $\geq 102°$F for > 24 hours.

In studies of non-asthmatic volunteers, increased clearance rates have been reported for cigarette and marijuana smokers (239,256). Compared with adolescents of similar age, patients with cystic fibrosis have a greater clearance and shorter elimination half-life of theophylline (261). This could be because of some aspect of their diet or delayed maturation compared with age-matched controls rather than inherently faster metabolism. A high protein, low-carbohydrate diet increases the rate of theophylline elimination, whereas a low protein, high-carbohydrate diet decreases theophylline clearance compared with a normal diet (257,258). Ingestion of charcoal-broiled beef also can increase clearance (259). However, the changes in clearance caused by diet are, on average, not large and are unlikely to require changes in dosage requirements except when radical and persistent

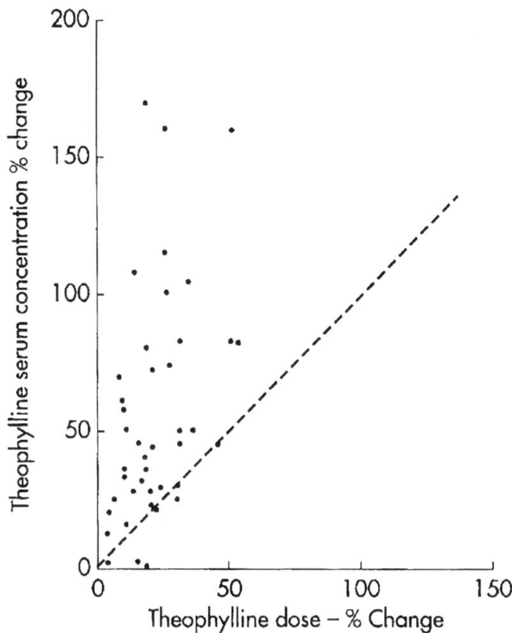

Figure 4 Relationship between changes in steady-state concentration and change in dose among 42 patients who had at least two serum concentration measurements at different doses of the same product (from 200 charts reviewed). In 30 of these children, percent change in serum concentration was at least 50% greater than percent change in dose (% change in concentration divided by % change in dose > 1.5). Thus, dose-dependent kinetics of a sufficient magnitude to be of potential clinical importance occurred in at least 15% of 200 children. *Source*: From Ref. 226.

alterations in diet occur (e.g., a heavy meat eater adopting a high-carbohydrate vegetarian diet or a low protein, hypocaloric diet) (260).

Chronic hypoxia in patients with severe COPD requiring supplemental oxygen was associated with a significantly lower theophylline clearance among patients with a PaO_2 of less than 45 mmHg while breathing room air for 48 hours (261). However, administration of supplemental oxygen did not result in an increase in theophylline clearance in those patients, suggesting that the decreased clearance is a function of the disease for which the oxygen is being used rather than the oxygen itself.

F. Drugs That Alter Theophylline Disposition

Most commonly used drugs do not interact adversely with theophylline. Amoxicillin (262,263), ampicillin with (264) or without sulbactam (265), cefaclor (266,267), metronidazole (268), co-trimoxazole (269), tetracycline

(270), azithromycin (271), terfenadine (272), and montelukast (data on file, Merck Pharmaceuticals) have been specifically studied and have no effect on theophylline clearance, nor is there evidence that other related medications have drug interactions with theophylline. On the other hand, while the quinolone antibiotics ofloxacin (273,274), norfloxacin (275,276), lomefloxacin (277–281), and flosequinan (282) have little or no effect on theophylline clearance, ciprofloxacin, enoxacin, and perfloxacin do slow theophylline elimination. Similarly, the H_2 blockers famotidine (283), ranitidine (284), and nizatidine (285) have no effect on theophylline clearance, while cimetidine, uniquely in that class, can substantially slow theophylline clearance. Controlled clinical studies have demonstrated little or no effect of corticosteroids on theophylline elimination (286,287). Several drugs that do have some effect on theophylline clearance (288,289) cause sufficiently small effect to be of little clinical relevance. However, there is a growing list of medications that have sufficient effect on the hepatic P450 1A2 enzyme responsible for theophylline metabolism to cause at least a 20% change in the rate of elimination for theophylline (Table 2) (290). In contrast, therapeutic serum concentrations of theophylline lower drug levels of erythromycin (291), zafirlukast (data on file, Zeneca Pharmaceuticals), and lithium (292). There are also drug interactions with theophylline that involve alteration of pharmacologic effects without affecting serum concentrations of either drug. Theophylline is likely to antagonize the cardiac antiarrhythmic effect of adenosine (Adenogard product information, Fujisawa USA Inc.), decrease the CNS depressant effect of benzodiazepines (293), and antagonize the neuromuscular blocking effects of pancuronium (294). Ephedrine (15) and, to a lesser extent, more selective oral β_2-agonsists (295) increase the adverse effects of theophylline. There is an increased risk of ventricular arrhythmias when halothane and theophylline are used concurrently (296), and ketamine may lower the seizure threshold to theophylline (297).

Influenza vaccine, once suggested to slow theophylline elimination and thus potentially cause toxicity (298), has subsequently been shown to have little (299) or no effect (300–305). Kramer and McClain (306) reported that hepatic metabolism of aminopyrine, a sensitive indirect measurement of N-demethylation, was reduced in 12 afebrile volunteers two to seven days after immunization with trivalent influenza vaccine; the effect lasted as long as 21 days in many subjects. They proposed that vaccination stimulated the production of interferon, which decreased cytochrome P_{450} activity, as the mechanism for this interaction. Trivalent influenza vaccine has been reported to slow theophylline elimination (298,307,308), but in subsequent studies the interaction could not be demonstrated (309–312). The discrepancies in these reports probably relate to the timing of the theophylline clearance measurement and the pre-vaccination clearance value in the subjects. Meredith et al. (301) demonstrated a small but transient decrease in clearance after vaccination in subjects with a higher prevaccination

Table 2 Pharmacokinetic Drug Interactions with Theophylline Likely to Cause at Least a 20% Change in Serum Concentration (Using Usual Dose Unless Otherwise Specified)

Interacting drug	Mean % increase in clearance	Mean % decrease in concentration[a]
Drugs that increase theophylline clearance		
Aminoglutethimide	32	24
Carbamazepine	50	34
Moricizine	32	25
Phenobarbital	34	25
Phenytoin	60	40
Rifampin	80	40
Sulfinpyrazone	22	20

Interacting drug	Mean % decrease in clearance	Mean % increase in concentration[a]
Drugs that decrease theophylline clearance		
Alcohol	25	34
Allopurinol (high dose)	21	26
Cimetidine	40	70
Ciprofloxacin	30	40
Clarithromycin	20	25
Disulfiram	32	50
Enoxacin	75	300
Erythromycin	26	35
Estrogen-containing oral contraceptives	25	34
Fluvoxamine	30	40
Interferon	50	100
Methotrexate	19	20
Mexiletine	45	80
Pentoxifylline	Not measured	30
Propafenone	31	40
Propranolol	50	100
Tacrine	48	90
Thiabendazole	66	190
Ticlopidine	37	60
Troleandomycin	25–50 depending on dose	33–100 depending on dose
Verapamil	18	20
Zileuton	50	100

[a]New C_{ss} = (original C_{ss}) [1 ÷ (1 − fractional change in clearance)].
Source: From Ref. 290.

clearance. The effect was present 24 hours after vaccination in association with elevated serum concentrations but was gone seven days later. Thus, there does not appear to be a need to reduce theophylline dosage routinely after influenza vaccination.

VI. Clinical Usage

A. Dosage for Acute Bronchodilatation

When theophylline is used as an acute bronchodilator, the goal of obtaining a therapeutic serum concentration is best accomplished with an intravenous loading dose (118,313). Because of rapid distribution into body fluids, the serum concentration obtained from an initial loading dose is related primarily to the volume of distribution, the apparent space into which the drug diffuses. If a mean volume of distribution of about 0.5 L/kg is assumed (actual range is 0.3–0.7 L/kg), each mg/kg (ideal body weight) of theophylline administered in a rapidly absorbed form results in an average 2 µg/mL increase in serum concentration. Thus a 15- to 30-minute infusion of 7.5 mg/kg results in a mean peak serum theophylline concentration increase of approximately 15 µg/mL with a range of 11–25 µg/mL (96).

B. Dosage for Maintenance Therapy of Chronic Asthma

The interpatient variability in clearance, combined with the narrow therapeutic index of theophylline, results in an overlap of therapeutic and potentially toxic doses, i.e., doses optimal for some patients may be excessive for patients with slower clearance. Furthermore, initiation of therapy with theophylline may be associated with mild, transient caffeine-like side effects such as nausea, headache, nervousness, and insomnia even at low serum concentrations (96). These symptoms can generally be avoided or minimized by beginning with low doses, no more than about two-thirds of average dosage for age and size, and increasing only slowly as tolerated at intervals no more frequent than three-days, approaching but not exceeding average doses for age (Table 3).

VII. Indications for Theophylline

Medications for asthma include those used for intervention to relieve acute symptoms of asthma when they occur, and those used for maintenance to prevent symptoms of chronic asthma. The use of theophylline as intervention for acute bronchodilatation has largely been supplanted by the current generation of inhaled bronchodilators, such as albuterol, which are specific for β_2-adrenergic agonist receptors and can safely be given in higher doses

Table 3 Theophylline Dosage Guidelines for Children Beyond Early Infancy[a] and Adults Who Have No Risk Factors for Decreased Theophylline Clearance[b]

	Weight-adjusted dose and maximum dose	Comments
Initial dose	~10 mg/kg/day maximum of 300 mg/day	If initial dose is tolerated, increase dose no sooner than three days to the first increment
First increment	~13 mg/kg/day maximum of 450 mg/day	If the first incremental increase is tolerated, increase dose no sooner than three days to the second increment
Second increment	~16 mg/kg/day maximum of 600 mg/day	If the second incremental increase is tolerated, measure an estimate of the peak serum concentration[c] after at least three days

Serum theophylline concentration	Dose adjustment
<10 μg/mL	Increase dose ~25%
10 to 15.9 μg/mL	Maintain dose if tolerated
16 to 19.9 μg/mL	Consider ~10% dose reduction[d]
20–25 μg/mL	Hold next dose, then resume first incremental dose
>25 μg/mL	Hold next two doses, then resume initial dose

These are based on the principle of beginning with about two-thirds of average doses and increasing slowly, only as tolerated, approaching but not exceeding average doses for age.

[a] For infants 6–26 weeks of age, the initial daily dosage is expressed by the regression equation: dose (in milligrams per kilogram per day) = (0.2) (age in weeks) + 5.0; this is 2/3 of the median dose. Subsequent dosage increases in this age group should be based on a peak serum concentration measurement no sooner than three days after the start of therapy.

[b] This schedule uses dosage that is lower than previous (97) and current FDA approved dosing guidelines, to account for the most recent assessment of population dosage requirements, and to further minimize risk of even minor adverse effects. Using these guidelines, one to two measurements of serum theophylline concentration are usually sufficient to determine dose requirement; annual recheck is than adequate unless clinically indicated sooner.

[c] The time to peak serum concentration depends on the rate of absorption, rate of elimination, and dosing interval.

[d] This decreases the likelihood of side effects from fluctuations in absorption or elimination rate that may result in serum concentrations >20 μg/mL and is especially important for patients who require doses higher than the second increment.

than older adrenergic bronchodilators. However, a therapeutic trial of theophylline may be justified in selected patients inadequately responsive to an inhaled β_2-adrenergic agonist and systemic corticosteroid.

The low cost of theophylline has resulted in some continued enthusiasm for its use as maintenance therapy in third-world countries. However, the relative value of that without the ready ability to monitor serum theophylline concentrations is likely to limit its efficacy or safety, depending on the choice of dosage. The primary indication for theophylline currently is then as additive therapy to low-dose inhaled corticosteroids as an occasional alternative to a long-acting β_2-agonist such as salmeterol or formoterol (76).

VIII. Post-theophylline Phosphodiesterase Inhibitors

More selective PDE inhibitors have been under investigation for their antiasthmatic potential. Rolipram is a specific inhibitor of PDE 4 that did not match theophylline in anti-inflammatory effects, whereas a dual selective inhibitor of PDEs 3 and 4, zardaverine, exhibited greater effect in vitro (314). Another specific inhibitor of PDEs 3 and 4, identified as Org 20241, both relaxes airways smooth muscle and inhibits eosinophil activation in various in vitro systems to a greater degree than rolipram (315). However, a report examining theophylline and rolipram on antigen-induced airway responses in neonatally immunized rabbits demonstrated prevention of airway hyper-responsiveness following allergen aerosol from rolipram but not theophylline, although both inhibited eosinophil recruitment (316). Another agent, identified as CDP840, is a specific inhibitor of PDE 4 that was more active than rolipram in reducing antigen-induced bronchoconstriction and pulmonary eosinophilic inflammation (317).

An inhaled PDE 3 inhibitor, olprinone, was reported to have bronchodilator effect in asthmatic patients of a magnitude similar to albuterol (318). A later report indicated that olprinone given intravenously produced more bronchodilatation then theophylline at doses that produced a mean concentration of about $10\,\mu g/mL$ (319). Identified as a second generation PDE4 inhibitor, cilomilast is an oral agent that has demonstrated some improved lung function in asthmatics (320). Roflumilast, another PDE 4 inhibitor, demonstrated a reduction in exercise-induced asthma in association with a reduction of tumor necrosis factor alpha, a surrogate marker for the inhibition of inflammatory cell activation (321). Despite the efforts to investigate these more specific PDE inhibitors in an attempt to find an alternative to theophylline without the potential for adverse effects, the more specific agents have thus far not been free from the nausea and emetic potential that characterizes higher serum concentrations of theophylline (322). Investigations are therefore continuing.

IX. Summary

Theophylline is an old drug that is demonstrably efficacious for asthma. Originally classified as a bronchodilator, considerable data has demonstrated anti-inflammatory effect that appears to contribute to its role as maintenance therapy in the management of chronic asthma. A narrow therapeutic index and the development of alternatives have greatly decreased its use and indications. Its primary indication currently is as an alternative to long-acting β_2-agonists added to an inhaled corticosteroid. Optimal safety and efficacy requires therapeutic drug monitoring. Theophylline is a nonspecific PDE inhibitor. Because its mechanism of anti-inflammatory effect appears to be mediated through inhibition of PDE 4, more specific PDE 4 inhibitors have been developed and investigated in an attempt to find an agent with improved efficacy and safety over theophylline. While investigations are ongoing, no such product has yet been identified with distinct advantage over theophylline.

References

1. Herrmann G, Aynesworth MB. Successful treatment of persistent extreme dyspnea "status asthmaticus." J Lab Clin Med 1937; 23:135–148
2. Brown EA. New type of medication to be used in bronchial asthma and other allergic conditions. N Engl J Med 1940; 223:843–846.
3. Dowell AR, Heyman A, Sieker HO, Tripathy K. Effect of aminophylline on respiratory center sensitivity in Cheyne-Stokes respirations and in pulmonary emphysema. N Engl J Med 1965; 273:1447–1453.
4. May CD. History of the introduction of theophylline into the treatment of asthma. Clin Allergy 1974; 4:211–217.
5. Schultze-Werninghaus G, Meier-Sydow J. The clinical and pharmacological history of theophylline: first report on the bronchospasmolytic action in man by SR Hirsch in Frankfurt (Main) 1922. Clin Allergy 1982; 12:211–215.
6. Shannon DC, Gotay F, Stein IM, Rogers MC, Todres ID, Moylan FM. Prevention of apnea and bradycardia in low-birthweight infants. Pediatrics 1975; 55:589–594.
7. Uauy R, Shapiro DL, Smith B, Warshaw JP. Treatment of severe apnea in prematures with orally administered theophylline. Pediatrics 1975; 55:595–598.
8. Barr PA. Weaning very low birthweight infants from mechanical ventilation using intermittent mandatory ventilation and theophylline. Arch Dis Child 1978; 53:598–600.
9. Murciano D, Auclair MH, Pariente R, Aubier M. A randomized controlled trial of theophylline in patients with severe chronic obstructive pulmonary disease. N Engl J Med 1989; 320:1521–1525.
10. Chrystyn H, Mulley BA, Peake MD. Dose response relation to oral theophylline in severe chronic obstructive airways disease. BMJ 1988; 297:1506–1510.

11. Weinberger M, Hendeles L. Theophylline in asthma. N Eng J Med 1996; 334:1384–1388.

12. Hendeles L, Weinberger M. Theophylline. A State-of-the-Art review. Pharmacotherapy 1983; 3:2–44.

13. Barnes PJ. Theophylline: New perspectives for an old drug. Am J Respir Crit Care Med 2003; 167:813–818.

14. Weinberger MM, Bronsky EA. Evaluation of oral bronchodilator therapy in asthmatic children. J Pediatr 1974; 84:421–427.

15. Weinberger MM, Bronsky EA. Interaction of ephedrine and theophylline. Clin Pharmacol Ther 1975; 17:585–592.

16. Hambleton G, Weinberger M, Taylor J, Cavanaugh M, Ginchansky E, Godfrey S, Tooly M, Bell T, Greenberg S. Comparison of cromoglycate (cromolyn) and theophylline in controlling symptoms of chronic asthma. Lancet 1977; 1:381–385.

17. Nassif EG, Weinberger MM, Thompson R, Huntley W. The value of maintenance theophylline for steroid dependent asthma. N Engl J Med 1981; 304: 71–75.

18. Dusdieker L, Green M, Smith GD, Ekwo EE, Weinberger M. Comparison of orally administered metaproterenol and theophylline in the control of chronic asthma. J Pediatr 1982; 101:281–287.

19. Joad J, Ahrens RC, Lindgren SD, Weinberger MM. Relative efficacy of maintenance therapy with theophylline, inhaled albuterol, and the combination for chronic asthma. J Allergy Clin Immunol 1987; 79:78–85.

20. Brenner M, Berkowitz R, Marshall N, Strunk RC. Need for theophylline in severe steroid-requiring asthmatics. Clin Allergy 1988; 18:143–150.

21. Rivington RN, Boulet LP, Cote J, Kreisman H, Small DI, Alexander M, Day A, Harsanyi Z, Darke AC. Efficacy of Uniphyl, salbutamol, and their combination in asthmatic patients on high-dose inhaled steroids. Am J Respir Crit Care Med 1995; 151:325–332.

22. Kidney J, Dominguez M, Taylor PM, Rose M, Chung KF, Barnes PJ. Immunomodulation by theophylline in asthma. Demonstration by withdrawal therapy. Am J Respir Crit Care Med 1995; 151:1907–1914.

23. Magnussen H, Reuss G, Jorres R. Theophylline has a dose-related effect on the airway response to inhaled histamine and methacholine in asthmatics. Am Rev Respir Dis 1987; 136:1163–1167.

24. Koenig JQ, Dumler K, Rebolledo V, Williams PV, Pierson WE. Theophylline mitigates the bronchoconstrictor effects of sulfur dioxide in subjects with asthma. J Allergy Clin Immunol 1992; 89:789–794.

25. Fabbri LM, Alessandri MV, De Marzo N, Zocca E, Paleari D, Pozzan M, Mapp CE. Long-lasting protective effect of slow-release theophylline on asthma induced by ultrasonically nebulized distilled water. Ann Allergy 1986; 56:171–176.

26. Pollock J, Kiechel F, Cooper D, Weinberger MM. Relationship of serum theophylline concentration to inhibition of exercise-induced bronchospasm and comparison with cromolyn. Pediatrics 1977; 60:840–844.

27. Hendeles L, Harman E, Huang D, O'Brien R, Blake K, Delafuente J. Theophylline attenuation of airway responses to allergen: comparison with cromolyn metered-dose inhaler. J Allergy Clin Immunol 1995; 95:505–514.

28. Sullivan P, Bekir S, Jaffar Z, Page C, Jeffery P, Costello J. Anti-inflammatory effects of low-dose oral theophylline in atopic asthma. Lancet 1994; 343: 1006–1008.

29. Jaffar ZH, Sullivan P, Page C, Costello J. Low-dose theophylline modulates T-lymphocyte activation in allergen-challenged asthmatics. Eur Respir J 1996; 9:456–462.

30. Kraft M, Torvik JA, Trudeau JB, Wenzel SE, Martin RJ. Theophylline: potential anti-inflammatory effects in nocturnal asthma. J Allergy Clin Immunol 1996; 97:1242–1246.

31. Crescioli S, De Marzo N, Boschetto P, Spinazzi A, Plebani M, Mapp CE, Fabbri LM, Ciaccia A. Theophylline inhibits late asthmatic reactions induced by toluene diisocyanate in sensitized subjects. Eur J Pharmacol 1992; 228: 45–50.

32. Holgate ST, Mann JS, Cushley MJ. Adenosine as a bonchoconstrictor mediator in asthma and its antagonism by methylxanthines. J Allergy Clin Immunol 1984; 74:302–306.

33. Jenne JW, Wyze MS, Rood FS, MacDonald FM. Pharmacokinetics of theophylline: Application to adjustment of the clinical dose of aminophylline. Clin Pharmacol Ther 1972; 13:349–360.

34. Simons FE, Lucuik GH, Simons KJ. Sustained-release theophylline for treatment of asthma in preschool children. Am J Dis Child 1982; 136:790–793.

35. Neijens HJ, Duiverman EJ, Graatsma BH, Kerrebijn KF. Clinical and bronchodilating efficacy of controlled-release theophylline as a function of its serum concentrations in preschool children. J Pediatr 1985; 107:811–815.

36. Rabe KF, Morton BE, Dent G, Coleman RA, Magnussen. Methylxanthine phosphodiesterase inhibitors block allergen-induced bronchoconstriction of human airways in-vitro. Am J Resp Crit Care Med 1995; 151:A388 (abstract).

37. Howell RE. Multiple mechanisms of xanthine actions on airway reactivity. J Pharmacol Exp Ther 1990; 255:1008–1014.

38. Welton AF, Simko BA. Regulatory role of adenosine in antigen-induced histamine release from the lung tissue of actively sensitized guinea-pigs. Biochem Pharmacol 1980; 29:1085–1092.

39. Scordamaglia A, Ciprandi G, Ruffoni S, Caria M, Paolieri F, Venuti D, Canconica GW. Theophylline and the immune response: In vitro and in vivo effects. Clin Immunol Immunopathol 1988; 48:238–246.

40. Lagente V, Pruniaux M, Junien J, Moodley I. Modulation of cytokine-induced eosinophil infiltration by phosphodiesterase inhibitors. Am J Respir Crit Care Med 1995; 151:1720–1724.

41. Kraft M, Pak J, Borish L, Martin RJ. Theophylline's effect on neutrophil function and the late asthmatic response. J Allergy Clin Immunol 1996; 98:251–257.

42. Murciano D, Aubier M, Lecocguic Y, Pariente R. Effects of theophylline on diaphragmatic strength and fatigue in patients with chronic obstructive pulmonary disease. N Engl J Med 1984; 311:349–353.

43. Cotromanes E, Gerrity TR, Garrard CS, Harshbarger RD, Yeates DB, Kendzierski DL, Lourenco RV. Aerosol penetration and mucociliary transport in the healthy human lung. Effect of low serum theophylline levels. Chest 1985; 88:194–200.

44. Easton PA, Anthonisen NR. Ventilatory response to sustained hypoxia after pretreatment with aminophylline. J Appl Physiol 1988; 64:1445–1450.

45. Erjefalt I, Persson CG. Anti-asthma drugs attenuate inflammatory leakage of plasma into airway lumen. Acta Physiol Scand 1986; 128:653–654.

46. Barnes PJ. Cyclic nucleotides and phosphodiesterases and airway function. Eur Respir J 1995; 8:457–462.

47. Banner KH, Page CP. Theophylline and selective phosphodiesterase inhibitors as anti-inflammatory drugs in the treatment of bronchial asthma. Eur Respir J 1995; 8:996–1000.

48. Rabe KF, Tenor H, Dent G, Nakashima M, Schudt C, Magnussen H. Theophylline relaxes human airways and pulmonary arteries in-vitro through phosphodiesterase inhibition. Am Rev Respir Dis 1993; 147:A184.

49. Banner KH, Marchini F, Buschi A, Moriggi E, Semeraro C, Page CP. The effect of selective phosphodiesterase inhibitors in comparison with other anti-asthma drugs on allergen-induced eosinophilia in guinea-pig airways. Pulm Pharmacol 1995; 8:37–42.

50. Sansone GR, Matin A, Wang SF, Bouboulis D, Frieri M. Theophylline inhibits the production of nitric oxide by peripheral blood mononuclear cells from patients with asthma. Ann Allergy Asthma Immunol 1998; 81:90–95.

51. Tohda Y, Nakahara H, Kubo H, Muraki M, Fukuoka M, Nakajima S. Theophylline suppresses the release of interleukin-4 by peripheral blood mononuclear cells. Int Arch Allergy Immunol 1998; 115:42–46.

52. Kimura M, Okafuji I, Yoshida T. Theophylline suppresses IL-5 and IL-13 production, and lymphocyte proliferation upon stimulation with house dust mite in asthmatic children. Int Arch Allergy Immunol 2003; 131:189–194.

53. Howell LL, Morse WH, Spealman RD. Respiratory effects of xanthines and adenosine analogs in rhesus monkeys. J Pharmacol Exp Ther 1990; 254: 786–791.

54. Howell RE, Muehsam WT, Kinnier WJ. Mechanism for the emetic side effect of xanthine bronchodilators. Life Sci 1990; 46:563–568.

55. Bowton DL, Haddon WS, Prough DS, Adair N, Alford PT, Stump DA. Theophylline effect on the cerebral blood flow response to hypoxemia. Chest 1988; 94:371–375.

56. Ito K, Lim S, Caramori G, Cosio B, Chung KF, Adcock IM, Barnes PJ. A molecular mechanism of action of theophylline: induction of histone deacetylase activity to decrease inflammatory gene expression. Proc Natl Acad Sci USA 2002; 99:8921–8926.

57. Murphy DG, McDermott MF, Rydman RJ, Sloan EP, Zalenski RJ. Aminophylline in the treatment of acute asthma when β_2-adrenergics and steroids are provided. Arch Intern Med 1993; 153:1784–1788.

58. Self TH, Abou-Shala N, Burns R, Stewart CF, Ellis RF, Tsiu SJ, Kellermann AL. Inhaled albuterol and oral prednisone in hospitalized adult asthmatics. Does aminophylline add any benefit? Chest 1990; 98:1317–1321.

59. Huang D, O'Brien RG, Harman E, Aull L, Reents S, Visser J, Shieh G, Hendeles L. Does aminophylline benefit adults admitted to the hospital for an acute exacerbation of asthma? Ann Intern Med 1993; 119:1155–1160.

60. Carter E, Cruz M, Chesrown S, Shieh G, Reilly K, Hendeles L. Efficacy of intravenous theophylline in children hospitalized with severe asthma. J Pediatr 1993; 122:470–476.

61. DiGiulio GA, Kercsmar CM, Krug SE, Alpert SE, Marx CM. Hospital treatment of asthma: lack of benefit from theophylline given in addition to nebulized albuterol and intravenously administered corticosteroid. J Pediatr 1993; 122:464–469.

62. Glass J, Archer LN, Adams W, Simpson H. Nebulized cromoglycate, theophylline, and placebo in preschool asthmatic children. Arch Dis Child 1981; 56:648–651.

63. Furukawa CT, Shapiro GG, Bierman CW, Kraemer MJ, Ward DJ, Pierson WE. A double-blind study comparing the effectiveness of cromolyn sodium and sustained-release theophylline in childhood asthma. Pediatrics 1984; 74:453–459.

64. Newth CJ, Newth CV, Turner JA. Comparison of nebulised sodium cromoglycate and oral theophylline in controlling symptoms of chronic asthma in preschool children: A double-blind study. Aust N Z J Med 1982; 12:232–238.

65. Dusdieker L, Green M, Smith GD, Ekwo EE, Weinberger M. Comparison of orally administered metaproterenol and theophylline in the control of chronic asthma. J Pediatr 1982; 101:281–287.

66. Heins M, Kurtin L, Oellerich M, Maes R, Sybrecht GW. Nocturnal asthma: slow-release terbutaline versus slow-release theophylline therapy. Eur Respir J 1988; 1:306–310.

67. Fjellbirkeland L, Gulsvik A, Palmer JB. The efficacy and tolerability of inhaled salmeterol and individually dose-titrated, sustained-release theophylline in patients with reversible airways disease. Respir Med 1994; 88:599–607.

68. Pollard SJ, Spector SL, Yancey SW, Cox FM, Emmett A. Salmeterol versus theophylline in the treatment of asthma. Ann Allergy Asthma Immunol 1997; 78:457–464.

69. Paggiaro PL, Giannini D, Di Franco A, Testi R. Comparison of inhaled salmeterol and individually dose-titrated slow-release theophylline in patients with reversible airway obstruction. Eur Respir J 1996; 9:1689–1695.

70. Selby C, Engleman HM, Fitzpatrick MF, Sime PM, Mackay TW, Douglas NJ. Inhaled salmeterol or oral theophylline in nocturnal asthma? Am J Respir Crit Care Med 1997; 155:104–108.

71. Weinberger M. Salmeterol for the treatment of asthma (Guest editorial). Ann Allergy 1995; 75:209–211.

72. Cheung D, Timmers MC, Zwinderman AH, Bel EH, Dijkman JH, Sterk PJ. Long-term effects of a long-acting β_2-adrenoreceptor agonist, salmeterol, on airway hyperresponsiveness in patients with mild asthma. N Engl J Med 1992; 327:1198–1203.

73. Ramage L, Lipworth BJ, Ingram CG, Cree IA, Dhillon DP. Reduced protection against exercise induced bronchoconstriction after chronic dosing with salmeterol. Respir Med 1994; 88:363–368.

74. Simons FER, Gerstner TV, Cheang MS. Tolerance to the bronchoprotective effect of salmeterol in adolescents with exercise-induced asthma using concurrent inhaled glucocorticoid treatment. Pediatrics 1997; 99:655–659.

75. Giannini D, Carletti A, Dente FL, Bacci E, Bancalari L, DiFranco A, Vagaggini B, Paggiaro PL. Tolerance to salmeterol in allergen induced bronchoconstriction. Am J Resp Crit Care Med 1995; 151(part 2):A39.

76. Weinberger M. What are the clinical implications of β_2-adrenoreceptor polymorphisms for the treatment of asthma? J Pediatr Pharmacol Ther 2003; 8:6–9.

77. Bierman CW, Shapiro GG, Pierson WE, Dorsett CS. Acute and chronic theophylline therapy in exercise-induced bronchospasm. Pediatrics 1977; 60: 845–849.

78. Toogood JH, Jennings B, Lefcoe NM. A clinical trial of combined cromolyn/ beclomethasone treatment for chronic asthma. J Allergy Clin Immunol 1981; 67:317–324.

79. Hiller EJ, Milner AD. Betamethasone 17 valerate aerosol and disodium cromoglycate in severe childhood asthma. Br J Dis Chest 1975; 69:103–106.

80. Dawood AG, Hendry AT, Walker SR. The combined use of betamethasone valerate and sodium cromoglycate in the treatment of asthma. Clin Allergy 1977; 7:161–165.

81. Svendsen UG, Jorgensen H. Inhaled nedocromil sodium as additional treatment to high dose inhaled corticosteroids in the management of bronchial asthma. Eur Respir J 1991; 4:992–999.

82. O'Hickey SP, Rees PJ. High-dose nedocromil sodium as an addition to inhaled corticosteroids in the treatment of athma. Respir Med 1994; 88:499–502.

83. Phipatanakul W, Greene C, Downes SJ, Cronin B, Eller TJ, Schneider LC, Irani AM. Montelukast improves asthma control in asthmatic children maintained on inhaled corticosteroids. Ann Allergy Asthma Immunol 2003; 91: 49–54.

84. Fish JE, Israel E, Murray JJ, Emmett A, Boone R, Yancey SW, Rickard KA. Salmeterol powder provides significantly better benefit than montelukast in asthmatic patients receiving concomitant inhaled corticosteroid therapy. Chest 2001; 120:423–430.

85. Greening AP, Ind P, Northfield M, Shaw G. Added salmeterol versus higher-dose corticosteroid in asthma patients with symptoms on existing inhaled corticosteroid (Allen & Hanburys Limited UK Study Group). Lancet 1994; 344:219–224.

86. Woolcock A, Lundback B, Ringdal N, Jacques LA. Comparison of addition of salmeterol to inhaled steroids with doubling of the dose of inhaled steroid. Am J Respir Crit Care Med 1996; 153:1481–1488.

87. Levy G, Koysooko R. Pharmacokinetic analysis of the effect of theophylline on pulmonary function in asthmatic children. J Pediatr 1975; 86:789–793.

88. Richer C, Mathieu M, Bah H, Thuillez C, Duroux P, Giudicelli JF. Theophylline kinetics and ventilatory flow in bronchial asthma and chronic airflow obstruction: Influence of erythromycin. Clin Pharmacol Ther 1982; 31: 579–586.

89. Magnussen H, Reuss G, Jörres R. Theophylline has a dose-related effect on the airway response to inhaled histamine and methacholine in asthmatics. Am Rev Respir Dis 1987; 136:1163–1167.

90. Hendeles L, Weinberger M, Szefler S, Ellis E. Safety and efficacy of theophylline in children with asthma. J Pediatr 1992; 120:177–183.

91. Sessler CN. Theophylline toxicity: clinical features of 116 consecutive cases. Am J Med 1990; 88:567–576.

92. Schiff GD, Hegde HK, LaCloche L, Hryhorczuk DO. Inpatient theophylline toxicity: preventable factors. Ann Int Med 1991; 114:748–753.

93. Hendeles L, Weinberger M. Theophylline. In: Ellis E, et al. ed. Allergy: Principles and Practice. 2nd ed. St. Louis: C.V. Mosby, 1983:535–574.

94. Tsiu SJ, Self TH, Burns R. Theophylline toxicity: update. Ann Allergy 1990; 64:241–257.

95. Paloucek FP, Rodvold KA. Evaluation of theophylline overdose and toxicities. Ann Emerg Med 1988; 17:135–144.

96. Hendeles L, Weinberger M, Bighley L. Disposition of theophylline after a single intravenous infusion of aminophylline. Am Rev Respir Dis 1978; 118: 97–103.

97. Milavetz G, Vaughan L, Weinberger M, Hendeles L. Evaluation of a scheme for establishing and maintaining dosage of theophylline in ambulatory patients with chronic asthma. J Pediatr 1986; 109:351–354.

98. Avital A, Steljes DG, Pasterkamp H, Kryger M, Sanchez I, Chernick V. Sleep quality in children with asthma treated with theophylline or cromolyn sodium. J Pediatr 1991; 119:979–984.

99. Martin RJ, Pak J. Overnight theophylline concentrations and effects on sleep and lung function in chronic obstructive pulmonary disease. Am Rev Respir Dis 1992; 145:540–544.

100. Joad J, Ahrens RC, Lindgren SD, Weinberger M. Extrapulmonary effects of maintenance therapy with theophylline and inhaled albuterol in patients with chronic asthma. J Allergy Clin Immunol 1986; 78:1147–1153.

101. Ahrens RC. Skeletal muscle tremor and the influence of adrenergic drugs. J Asthma 1990; 27:11–20.

102. Weinberger M, Lindgren S, Bender B, Lerner JA, Szefler S. Effects of theophylline on learning and behavior: reason for concern or concern without reason? J Pediatr 1987; 111:471–474

103. Rappaport L, Coffman H, Guare R, Fenton T, DeGraw C, Twarog F. Effects of theophylline on behavior and learning in children with asthma. Am J Dis Child 1989; 143:368–372.

104. Schlieper A, Alcock D, Beaudry P, Feldman W, Leikin L. Effect of therapeutic plasma concentrations of theophylline on behavior, cognitive processing, and affect in children with asthma. J Pediatr 1991; 118:449–455.

105. Bender B, Milgrom H. Theophylline-induced behavior change in children. An objective evaluation of parents' perceptions. JAMA 1992; 267:2621–2624.

106. Lindgren S, Lokshin B, Stromquist A, Weinberger M, Nassif E, McCubbin M, Frasher R. Does asthma or treatment with theophylline limit academic performance in children? N Eng J Med 1992; 237:926–930.

107. Hendeles L, Bighley L, Richardson RH, Hepler CD, Carmichael J. Frequent toxicity from IV aminophylline infusions in critically ill patients. Drug Intel Clin Pharm 1977; 11:12–18.

108. Zwillich CW, Sutton FD, Neff TA, Cohn WM, Matthay RA, Weinberger MM. Theophylline-induced seizures in adults; correlation with serum concentrations. Ann Intern Med 1975; 82:784–787.

109. Jacobs MH, Senior RM, Kessler G. Clinical experience with theophylline: relationships between dosage, serum concentration and toxicity. JAMA 1976; 235:1983–1986.

110. Helliwell M, Berry D. Theophylline poisoning in adults. Br Med J 1979; 2:1114.

111. Culberson CG, Langston JW, Herrick M. Aminophylline encephalopathy: A clinical electroencephalographic and neuropathological analysis. Tran Am Neurol Assoc 1979; 104:224–226.

112. Mountain RD, Neff TA. Oral theophylline intoxication. A serious error of patient and physician understanding. Arch Intern Med 1984; 144:724–727.

113. Hall KW, Dobson KE, Dalton JG, Ghignone MC, Penner SB. Metabolic abnormalities associated with intentional theophylline overdose. Ann Intern Med 1984; 101:457–462.

114. White BH, Daeschner CW. Aminophylline (theophylline ethylenediamine) poisoning in children. J Pediatr 1956; 49:262–271.

115. Nolke AC. Severe toxic effects from aminophylline and theophylline suppositories in children. JAMA 1956; 161:693–697.

116. Veum J, Schwartz AB. Toxic effects of half-strength aminophylline suppositories in asthmatic children. J Pediatr 1956; 49:703–707.

117. Shannon M. Predictors of major toxicity after theophylline overdose. Ann Intern Med 1993; 119:1161–1167.

118. Weinberger MM, Matthay R, Ginchansky E, Chidsey C, Petty T. Intravenous aminophylline dosage: use of serum theophylline measurement for guidance. JAMA 1976; 235:2110–2113.

119. Jacobs MH, Senior RM. Theophylline toxicity due to impaired theophylline degradation. Am Rev Respir Dis 1974; 110:342–345.

120. Kordash TR, Van Dellen RG, McCall JT. Theophylline concentrations in asthmatic patients after administration of aminophylline. JAMA 1977; 238: 139–141.

121. Yarnell PR, Chu NS. Focal seizures and aminophylline. Neurology 1975; 25:819–822.

122. Olson KR, Benowitz NL, Woo OF, Pond SM. Theophylline overdose: acute single ingestion versus chronic repeated overmedication. Am J Emer Med 1985; 3:386–394.

123. Nakada T, Kwee IL, Lerner AM, Remler MP. Theophylline-induced seizures: clinical and pathophysiologic aspects. West J Med 1983; 138:371–374.

124. Richards W, Church JA, Brent DK. Theophylline associated seizures in children. Ann Allergy 1985; 54:276–279.

125. Gal P, Roop C, Robinson H, Erkan NV. Theophylline-induced seizures in accidentally overdosed neonates. Pediatrics 1980; 65:547–549.
126. Simons FE, Friesen FR, Simons KJ. Theophylline toxicity in term infants. Am J Dis Child 1980; 134:39–41.
127. Schucard DW, Spector SL, Euwer RL, Cummins KR, Shucard JL, Friedman A. Central nervous system effects of antiasthma medication-an EEG study. Ann Allergy 1985; 54:177–184.
128. Bahls FH, Ma KK, Bird TD. Theophylline-associated seizures with "therapeutic" or low toxic serum concentrations: risk factors for serious outcome in adults. Neurology 1991; 41:1309–1312.
129. Gaudreault P, Wason S, Lovejoy FJ. Acute pediatric theophylline overdose: a summary of 28 cases. J Pediatr 1983; 102:474–476.
130. Shannon M, Lovejoy FH Jr. Hypokalemia after theophylline intoxication. The effects of acute vs chronic poisoning. Arch Intern Med 1989; 149:2725–2729.
131. Sawyer WT, Caravati EM, Ellison MJ, Krueger KA. Hypokalemia, hyperglycemia, and acidosis after intentional theophylline overdose. Am J Emerg Med 1985; 3:408–411.
132. Kearney TE, Manoguerra AS, Curtis GP, Ziegler MG. Theophylline toxicity and the beta-adrenergic system. Ann Intern Med 1985; 102:766–769.
133. Smith SR, Kendall MJ. Potentiation of the adverse effects of intravenous terbutaline by oral theophylline. Br J Clin Pharmacol 1986; 21:451–453.
134. Whyte KF, Reid C, Addis GJ, Whitesmith R, Reid JL. Salbutamol induced hypokalaemia: the effect of theophylline alone and in combination with adrenaline. Br J Clin Pharmacol 1988; 25:571–578.
135. Deenstra M, Haalboom JR, Struyvenberg A. Decrease of plasma potassium due to inhalation of beta-2-agonists: absence of an additional effect of intravenous theophylline. Eur J Clin Invest 1988; 18:162–165.
136. Amitai Y, Lovejoy FH Jr. Hypokalemia in acute theophylline poisoning. Am J Emerg Med 1988; 6:214–218.
137. D'Angio R, Sabatelli F. Management considerations in treating metabolic abnormalities associated with theophylline overdose. Arch Intern Med 1987; 147:1837–1838.
138. Patel AK, Skatrud JB, Thomsen JH. Cardiac arrhythmias due to oral aminophylline in patients with chronic obstructive pulmonary disease. Chest 1981; 80:661–665.
139. Levine JH, Michael JR, Guarnieri T. Multifocal atrial tachycardia: a toxic effect of theophylline. Lancet 1985; 1:12–14.
140. Camarata SJ, Weil MH, Hanashiro PK, Shubin H. Cardiac arrest in the critically ill. I. A study of predisposing causes in 132 patients. Circulation 1971; 44:688–695.
141. Urthaler F, James TN. Both direct and neurally mediated components of the chronotropic actions of aminophylline. Chest 1976; 70:24–32.
142. Ellis EF. Theophylline and derivatives. In: Middleton E, Reed CE, Ellis EF, eds. Allergy Principles and Practice 2nd ed. St. Louis: The C.V. Mosby Co., 1978:434.
143. Foster LJ, Trudeau WL, Goldman AL. Bronchodilator effects on gastric acid secretion. JAMA 1979; 241:2613–2615.

144. Hindi-Alexander MC, Zielezny MA, Montes N, Bullough B, Middleton E, Rosner DH, London WM, Middleton E Jr. Theophylline and fibrocystic breast disease. J Allergy Clin Immunol 1985; 75:709–715.

145. Minton JP, Abou-Issa H, Reiches N, Roseman JM. Clinical and biochemical studies on methylxanthine-related fibrocystic breast disease. Surgery 1981; 90:299–304.

146. La Vecchia C, Franceschi S, Parazzini F, Regallo M, Decarli A, Gallus G, Di Pietro S, Tognoni G. Benign breast disease and consumption of beverages containing methylxanthines. JNCI 1985; 74:995–1000.

147. Lubin F, Ron E, Wax Y, Black M, Funaro M, Shitrit A. A case-control study of caffeine and methylxanthines in benign breast disease. JAMA 1985; 253: 2388–2392.

148. Marshall J, Graham S, Swanson M. Caffeine consumption and benign breast disease: a case-control comparison. Am J Public Health 1982; 72:610–612.

149. Owens GR, Tannenbaum R. Theophylline-induced urinary retention. Ann Intern Med 1981; 94:212–213.

150. McPherson ML, Prince SR, Atamer ER, Maxwell DB, Ross-Clunis H, Estep HL. Theophylline-induced hypercalcemia. Ann Intern Med 1986; 105:52–54.

151. Rumpf KW, Wagner H, Criee CP, Schwarck H, Klein H, Kreuzer H, Scheler F. Rhabdomyolysis after theophylline overdose. Lancet 1985; 1:1451–1452.

152. Enzenauer RW, Bass JW, McDonnell JT. Esophageal ulceration associated with oral theophylline. N Engl J Med 1984; 310:261.

153. Hardebo JE, Edvinsson L. Adenine compounds: cerebrovascular effects in vitro with reference to their possible involvement in migraine. Stroke 1979; 10:58–62.

154. Petrozzi JW, Shore RN. Generalized exfoliative dermatitis from ethylenediamine. Arch Dermatol 1976; 112:525–526.

155. Elias JA, Levinson AI. Hypersensitivity reactions to ethylenediamine in aminophylline. Am Rev Respir Dis 1981; 123:550–552.

156. Upton RA, Sansom L, Guentert TW, Powell JR, Thiercelin JF, Shah VP, Coates PE, Riegelman S. Evaluation of the absorption from 15 commercial theophylline products indicating deficiencies in currently applied bioavailability criteria. J Pharmacokinet Biopharm 1980; 8:229–242.

157. Heimann G, Murgescu J, Bergt U. Influence of food intake on bioavailability of theophylline in premature infants. Eur J Clin Pharmacol 1982; 22:171–173.

158. Welling PG, Lyons LL, Craig WA, Trochta GA. Influence of diet and fluid on bioavailability of theophylline. Clin Pharmacol Ther 1975; 17:475–480.

159. Arnold LA, Spurbeck GH, Shelver WH, Henderson WM. Effect of antacid on gastrointestinal absorption of theophylline. Am J Hosp Pharm 1979; 36:1059–1062.

160. Shargel L, Stevens JA, Fuchs JE, Yu AB. Effect of antacid on bioavailability of theophylline from rapid and timed-release drug products. J Pharm Sci 1981; 70:599–602.

161. Scott PH, Kramer WG, Smolensky MH, Harrist RB, Hiatt PW, Baenziger JC, Klank BJ, Eigen H. Day-night differences in steady-state theophylline pharmacokinetics in asthmatic children. Chronobiol Int 1989; 6:163–171.

162. Kishida M, Hukushima K, Iikura Y. Posture and circadian variations in serum theophylline concentrations. Arerugi 1990; 39:1422—1426.
163. Milavetz G, Weinberger M, Vaughan L. Dose dependency for absorption and elimination rates of theophylline: implications for studies of bioavailability. Pharmacotherapy 1984; 4:216–220.
164. Lesko LJ, Brousseau D, Canada AT, Eastwood G. Temporal variations in trough serum theophylline concentrations at steady-state. J Pharm Sci 1980; 69:358–359.
165. Scott PH, Tabachnik E, MacLeod S, Correia J, Newth C, Levison H. Sustained release theophylline for chldhood asthma: evidence for circadian variation of theophylline pharmacokinetics. J Pediatr 1981; 99:476–479.
166. Sallent J, Hill M, Stecenko A, McKenzie M, Hendeles L. Bioavailability of a slow-release theophylline capsule given twice daily to preschool children with chronic asthma: comparison with liquid theophylline. Pediatrics 1988; 81: 116–120.
167. Waxler SH, Schack JA. Administration of aminophylline (theophylline ethylenediamine). JAMA 1950; 143:736–739.
168. Mason WD, Lanman RC, Amick EN, Arnold J, March L. Bioavailability of theophylline following a rectally administered concentrated aminophylline solution. J Allergy Clin Immunol 1980; 66:119–122.
169. Bolme P, Edlund PO, Eriksson M, Paalzow L, Winbladh B. Pharmacokinetics of theophylline in young children with asthma: Comparison of rectal enema and suppositories. Eur J Clin Pharmacol 1979; 16:133–139.
170. Ridolfo AS, Kohlstaedt KG. A simplified method for the rectal instillation of theophylline. Am J Med Sci 1959; 237:585–589.
171. Weinberger M, Hendeles L, Bighley L. The relation of product formulation to absorption of oral theophylline. N Engl J Med 1978; 299:852–857.
172. Hendeles L, Iafrate RP, Weinberger M. A clinical and pharmacokinetic basis for the selection and use of slow-release theophylline products. Clin Pharmacokinet 1984; 9:95–135.
173. Spangler DL, Kalof DD, Bloom FL, Wittig JH. Theophylline bioavailability following oral administration of six sustained-release preparations. Ann Allergy 1978; 40:6–11.
174. Upton RA, Thiercelin J, Guentert TW, Thiercelin JF, Sansom L, Coates PE, Riegelman S. Evaluation of the absorption from some commercial sustained-release theophylline products. J Pharmacokinet Biopharm 1980; 8:131–149.
175. Weinberger MM, Hendeles L, Wong L. Relationship of formulation and dosing interval to fluctuation of serum theophylline concentration in children with chronic asthma. J Pediatr 1981; 99:145–152.
176. Hendeles L, Weinberger M, Milavetz G, Hill M 3d, Vaughan L. Food-induced "dose-dumping" from a once-a-day theophylline product as a cause of theophylline toxicity. Chest 1985; 87:758–765.
177. Pedersen S, Moeller-Petersen J. Erratic absorption of a slow-release theophylline sprinkle product. Pediatrics 1984; 74:534–538.
178. Sips AP, Edelbroek PM, Kulstad S, de Wolff FA, Dijkman JH. Food does not affect bioavailability of theophylline from Theolin Retard. Eur J Clin Pharmacol 1984; 26:405–407.

179. Weinberger M, Milavetz G. Influence of formulation on oral drug delivery: considerations for generic substitution and selection of slow-release products. Iowa Med 1986; 76:24–28.

180. Karim A, Burns T, Wearley L, Streicher J, Palmer M. Food-induced changes in theophylline absorption from controlled-release formulations. Part I. Substantial increased and decreased absorption with Uniphyl tablets and Theo-Dur Sprinkle. Clin Pharmacol Ther 1985; 38:77–83.

181. Milavetz G, Vaughan LM, Weinberger MM, Harris JB, Mullenix TA. Relationship between rate and extent of absorption of oral theophylline from Uniphyl brand of slow-release theophylline and resulting serum concentrations during multiple dosing. J Allergy Clin Immunol 1987; 80:723–729.

182. Lagas M, Jonkman JH. Greatly enhanced bioavailability of theophylline on postprandial administration of a sustained-release tablet. Eur J Clin Pharmacol 1983; 24:761–767.

183. Pedersen S. Delay in the absorption rate of theophylline from a sustained release theophylline preparation caused by food. Br J Clin Pharmacol 1981; 12:904–905.

184. Pedersen S, Moeller-Petersen J. Influence of food on the absorption rate and bioavailability of a sustained release theophylline preparation. Allergy 1982; 37:531–534.

185. Thompson PJ, Kemp MW, McAllister WA, Turner-Warwick M. Slow-release theophylline in patients with airway obstruction with particular reference to the effects of food upon serum levels. Br J Dis Chest 1983; 77:293–298.

186. Shaw LM, Fields L, Mayoc R. Factors influencing theophylline serum protein binding. Clin Pharmacol Ther 1982; 32:490–496.

187. Koysooko R, Ellis EF, Levy G. Relationship between theophylline concentration in plasma and saliva of man. Clin Pharmacol Ther 1974; 15:454–460.

188. Lesko LJ, Tabor KJ, Johnson BF. Theophylline serum protein binding in obstructive airways disease. Clin Pharmacol Ther 1981; 29:776–781.

189. Rohrbaugh TM, Danish M, Ragni MC, Yaffe SJ. The effect of obesity on apparent volume of distribution of theophylline. Pediatr Pharmacol (New York) 1982; 2:75–83.

190. Zell M, Curtis RA, Troyer WG, Fischer JH. Volume of distribution of theophylline in acute exacerbations of reversible airway disease. Effect of body weight. Chest 1985; 87:212–216.

191. Ellis EF, Koysooko R, Levy G. Pharmacokinetics of theophylline in children with asthma. Pediatrics 1976; 58:542–547.

192. Loughnan PM, Sitar DS, Ogilvie RI, Eisen A, Fox Z, Neims AH. Pharmacokinetic analysis of the disposition of intravenous theophylline in young children. J Pediatr 1976; 88:874–879.

193. Mitenko PA, Ogilvie RI. Pharmacokinetics of intravenous theophylline. Clin Pharmacol Ther 1973; 14:509–513.

194. Aranda JV, Sitar DS, Parsons WD, Loughnan PM, Neims AH. Pharmacokinetic aspects of theophylline in premature newborns. N Engl J Med 1976; 295:413–416.

195. Piafsky KM, Sitar DS, Rangno RE, Ogilvie RI. Theophylline disposition in patients with hepatic cirrhosis. N Engl J Med 1977; 296:1495–1497.

196. Mangione A, Imhoff TE, Lee RV, Shum LY, Jusko WJ. Pharmacokinetics of theophylline in hepatic disease. Chest 1978; 73:616–622.

197. Vallner JJ, Speir WA Jr, Kolbeck RC, Harrison GN, Bransome ED Jr. Effect of pH on the binding of theophylline to serum proteins. Am Rev Respir Dis 1979; 120:83–86.

198. Antal EJ, Kramer PA, Mercik SA, Chapron DJ, Lawson IR. Theophylline pharmacokinetics in advanced age. Br J Clin Pharmacol 1981; 12:637–645.

199. Zarowitz B, Shlom J, Eichenhorn MS, Popovich J. Alterations in theophylline protein binding in acutely ill patients with COPD. Chest 1985; 87:766–769.

200. Gardner MJ, Schatz M, Cousins L, Zeiger R, Middleton E, Jusdo WJ. Longitudinal effects of pregnancy on the pharmacokinetics of theophylline. Eur J Clin Pharm 1987; 32:289–295.

201. Arwood LL, Dasta JF, Friedman C. Placental transfer of theophylline: Two case reports. Pediatrics 1979; 63:844–846.

202. Yeh TF, Pildes RS. Transplacental aminophylline toxicity in a neonate (letter). Lancet 1977; 1:910.

203. Yurchak AM, Jusko WJ. Theophylline secretion into breast milk. Pediatrics 1976; 57:518–520.

204. Stec GP, Greenberger P, Ruo TI, Henthorn T, Morita Y, Atkinson AJ Jr, Patterson R. Kinetics of theophylline transfer to breast milk. Clin Pharmacol Ther 1980; 28:404–408.

205. Somani SM, Khanna NN, Bada HS. Caffeine and theophylline: serum/CSF correlation in premature infants. J Pediatr 1980; 96:1091–1093.

206. Auritt WA, McGeady SJ, Mansmann HC. The relationship of cerebrospinal fluid and plasma theophylline concentrations in children and adolescents taking theophylline. J Allergy Clin Immunol 1985; 75:731–735.

207. Levy G, Ellis EF, Koysooko R. Indirect plasma-theophylline monitoring in asthmatic children by determination of theophylline concentration in saliva. Pediatrics 1974; 53:873–876.

208. Hendeles L, Burkey S, Bighley L, Richardson R. Unpredictability of theophylline saliva measurements in chronic obstructive pulmonary disease. J Allergy Clin Immunol 1977; 60:335–338.

209. Cornish HH, Christman AA. A study of the metabolism of theobromine, theophylline and caffeine in man. J Biol Chem 1957; 228:315–323.

210. Tang-Liu DDS, Williams RL, Riegelman S. Non-linear theophylline elimination. Clin Pharmacol Ther 1982; 31:358–369.

211. Sarkar MA, Hunt C, Guzelian PS, Karnes HT. Characterization of human liver cytochromes P-450 involved in theophylline metabolism. Drug Metab Dispos 1992; 20:31–37.

212. Monks TJ, Caldwell J, Smith RL. Influence of methylxanthine-containing foods on theophylline metabolism and kinetics. Clin Pharmacol Ther 1979; 26:513–524.

213. Grygiel JJ, Wing LM, Farkas J, Birkett DJ. Effects of allopurinol on theophylline metabolism and clearance. Clin Pharmacol Ther 1979; 26:660–667.

214. Tang-Liu D, Riegelman S. Metabolism of theophylline to caffeine in adults. Res Commun Chem Pathol Pharmacol 1981; 34:371–380.

215. Ogilvie RI. Clinical pharmacokinetics of theophylline. Clin Pharmacokinet 1978; 3:267–293.
216. Levy G, Koysooko R. Renal clearance of theophylline in man. J Clin Pharmacol 1976; 16:329–332.
217. Bauer LA, Bauer SP, Blouin RA. The effect of acute and chronic renal failure of theophylline clearance. J Clin Pharmacol 1982; 22:65–68.
218. Bonati M, Latini R, Marra G, Assael BM, Parini R. Theophylline metabolism during the first month of life and development. Pediatr Res 1981; 15:304–308.
219. Tserng K, King KC, Takieddine FN. Theophylline metabolism in premature infants. Clin Pharmacol Ther 1981; 29:594–600.
220. Grygiel JJ, Birkett DJ. Effect of age on patterns of theophylline metabolism. Clin Pharmacol Ther 1980; 28:456–462.
221. Bada HS, Khanna NN, Somani SM, Tin AA. Interconversion of theophylline and caffeine in newborn infants. J Pediatr 1979; 94:993–995.
222. Bory C, Baltassat P, Porthault M, Bethenod M, Frederich A, Aranda JV. Metabolism of theophylline to caffeine in premature newborn infants. J Pediatr 1979; 94:988–993.
223. Ginchansky E, Weinberger M. Relationship of theophylline clearance to oral dosage in children with chronic asthma. J Pediatr 1977; 91:655–660.
224. Asmus MJ, Weinberger MM, Milavetz G, Marshik P, Teresi ME, Hendeles L. Apparent decrease in population clearance of theophylline: implications for dosage. Clin Pharm Ther 1997; 62:483–489.
225. Weinberger MM, Ginchansky E. Dose-dependent kinetics of theophylline disposition in asthmatic children. J Pediatr 1977; 91:820–824.
226. Sarrazin E, Hendeles L, Weinberger M, Muir K, Riegelman S. Dose-dependent kinetics for theophylline: Observations among ambulatory asthmatic children. J Pediatr 1980; 97:825–828.
227. Butcher MA, Frazer LA, Reddel HK, Marlin GE. Dose-dependent pharmacokinetics with single daily dose slow release theophylline in patients with chronic lung disease. Br J Clin Pharmacol 1982; 13:241–243.
228. Pancorbo S, Benson J, Goetz D, Moore K, Vaida A, Johnson D. Evaluation of the effect of nonlinear kinetics on dosage adjustments of theophylline. Ther Drug Monit 1983; 5:173–177.
229. Milavetz G, Vaughan L, Weinberger M. Stability of theophylline elimination rate. Clin Pharmacol Ther 1987; 41:388–391.
230. Nassif EG, Weinberger MM, Shannon D, Guiang SF, Hendeles L, Jimenez D, Ekwo E. Theophylline disposition in infancy. J Pediatr 1981; 98:158–161.
231. Cary J, Hein K, Dell R. Theophylline disposition in adolescents with asthma. Ther Drug Monit 1991; 13:309–313.
232. Gal P, Jusko WJ, Yurchak AM, Franklin BA. Theophylline disposition in obesity. Clin Pharmacol Ther 1978; 23:438–444.
233. Blouin RA, Elgert JF, Bauer LA. Theophylline clearance. Effect of marked obesity. Clin Pharmacol Ther 1980; 28:619–623.
234. Koup JR, Vawter TK. Theophylline pharmacokinetics in an extremely obese patient. Clin Pharm 1983; 2:181–183.

235. Slaughter RL, Lanc RA. Theophylline clearance in obese patients in relation to smoking and congestive heart failure. Drug Intell Clin Pharm 1983; 17: 274–276.

236. Nielsen-Kudsk F, Magnussen I, Jakobsen P. Pharmacokinetics of theophylline in ten elderly patients. Acta Pharmacol Toxicol 1978; 42:226–234.

237. Shin S, Juan D, Rammohan M. Theophylline pharmacokinetics in normal elderly subjects. Clin Pharmacol Ther 1988; 44:522–530.

238. Hendeles L, Vaughn L, Weinberger M, Smith G. Influence of gender on theophylline dosage requirements in children with chronic asthma. Drug Intell Clin Pharm 1981; 15:338–340.

239. Jusko WJ, Gardner MJ, Mangione A, Schentag JJ, Koup JR, Vance JW. Factors affecting theophylline clearances: Age, tobacco, marijuana, cirrhosis, congestive heart failure, obesity, oral contraceptives, benzodiazepines, barbiturates, and ethanol. J Med Bord 1979; 68:1358–1366.

240. Gardner MJ, Jusko WJ. Effect of age and sex on theophylline clearance in young subjects. Pediatr Pharmacol 1982; 2:157–169.

241. Staib AH, Schuppan D, Lissner R, Zilly W, von Bomhard G, Richter E. Pharmacokinetics and metabolism of theophylline in patients with liver diseases. Int J Clin Pharmacol Ther Toxicol 1980; 18:500–502.

242. Piafsky KM, Sitar DS, Rangno RE, Ogilvie RI. Theophylline kinetics in acute pulmonary edema. Clin Pharmacol Ther 1977; 21:310–316.

243. Jenne JW, Chick TW, Miller BA, Strickland RD. Apparent theophylline half-life fluctuations during treatment of acute left ventricular failure. Am J Hosp Pharm 1977; 34:408–409.

244. Powell JR, Vozeh S, Hopewell P, Costello J, Sheiner LB, Riegelman S. Theophylline disposition in acutely ill hospitalized patients: the effect of smoking, heart failure, severe airway obstruction, and pneumonia. Am Rev Respir Dis 1978; 118:229–238.

245. Vicuna N, McNay JL, Ludden TM, Schwertner H. Impaired theophylline clearance in patients with cor pulmonale. Br J Clin Pharmacol 1979; 7:33–37.

246. Pokrajac M, Simic D, Varagic VM. Pharmacokinetics of theophylline in hyperthyroid and hypothyroid patients with chronic obstructive pulmonary disease. Eur J Clin Pharmacol 1987; 33:483–486.

247. Toft P, Heslet L, Hansen M, Klitgaard NA. Theophylline and ethylenediamine pharmacokinetics following administration of aminophylline to septic patients with multiorgan failure. Intensive Care Med 1991; 17:465–468.

248. Kraemer MJ, Furukawa CT, Koup JR, Shapiro GG, Pierson WE, Bierman CW. Altered theophylline clearance during an influenza B outbreak. Pediatrics 1982; 69:476–480.

249. Fleetham JA, Nakatsu K, Munt PW. Theophylline pharmacokinetics and respiratory infections (letter). Lancet 1978; 2:898.

250. Clark CJ, Boyd G. Theophylline pharmacokinetics during respiratory viral infection (letter). Lancet 1979; 1:492.

251. Matthay RA, Matthay MA, Weinberger MM. Grand mal seizure induced by oral theophylline. Thorax 1976; 31:470–471.

252. Elin RJ, Vesell ES, Wolff SM. Effects of etiocholanolone-induced fever on plasma antipyrine half-lives and metabolic clearance. Clin Pharmacol Ther 1975; 17:447–457.

253. Anolik R, Kolski GB, Schaible DH, Ratner J. Transient alteration of theophylline half-life: possible association with herpes simplex infection. Ann Allergy 1982; 49:109–111.

254. Bachmann K, Schwartz J, Martin M, Jauregui L. Theophylline clearance during and after mild upper respiratory infection. Ther Drug Monit 1987; 9: 279–282.

255. Muslow HA, Bernard L, Brown D, Jamison RM, Manno JE, Bocchini JA, Wilson JT. Lack of effect of respiratory syncytial virus infection on theophylline disposition in children. J Pediatr 1992; 121:466–471.

256. Hunt SN, Jusko WJ, Yurchak AM. Effect of smoking on theophylline disposition. Clin Pharmacol Ther 1976; 19:546–551.

257. Kappas A, Anderson KE, Conney AH, Alvares AP. Influence of dietary protein and carbohydrate on antipyrine and theophylline metabolism in man. Clin Pharmacol Ther 1976; 20:643–653.

258. Feldman CH, Hutchinson VE, Pippenger CE, Blumenfeld TA, Feldman BR, Davis WJ. Effect of dietary protein and carbohydrate on theophylline metabolism in children. Pediatrics 1980; 66:956–962.

259. Kappas A, Alvares AP, Anderson KE, Pantuck EJ, Pantuck CB, Chang R, Conney AH. Effect of charcoal-broiled beef on antipyrine and theophylline metabolism. Clin Pharmacol Ther 1978; 23:445–450.

260. Juan D, Shin SG, Holmes T, Hughes RL. Diet-induced changes in trough theophylline concentrations in an elderly asthmatic patient. Chest 1988; 93:1113–1114.

261. Cusack BJ, Crowley JJ, Mercer GD, Charan NB, Vestal RE. Theophylline clearance in patients with severe chronic obstructive pulmonary disease receiving supplemental oxygen and the effect of hypoxemia. Am Rev Respir Dis 1986; 133:1110–1114.

262. Jonkman JH, van der Boon WJ, Schoenmaker R, Holtkamp AH, Hempenius J. Clinical pharmacokinetics of amoxicillin and theophylline during cotreatment with both medicaments. Chemotherapy 1985; 31:329–335.

263. Jonkman JH, van der Boon WJ, Schoenmaker R, Holtkamp A, Hempenius J. Lack of effect of amoxicillin on theophylline pharmacokinetics. Br J Clin Pharmacol 1985; 19:99–101.

264. Cazzola M, Santangelo G, Guidetti E, Mattina R, Caputi M, Girbino G. Influence of sulbactam plus ampicillin on theophylline clearance. Int J Clin Pharmacol Res 1991; 11:11–15.

265. Kadlec GJ, Ha LT, Jarboe CH, Richards D, Karibo JM. Effect of ampicillin on theophylline half-life in infants and young children. South Med J 1978; 71:1584.

266. Jonkman JH, van der Boon WJ, Schoenmaker R, Holtkamp A, Hempenius J. No effect of cefaclor on theophylline pharmacokinetics. Eur J Respir Dis 1985; 66:47–49.

267. Bachmann K, Schwartz J, Forney RB Jr, Jauregui L. Impact of cefaclor on the pharmacokinetics of theophylline. Ther Drug Monit 1986; 8:151–154.

268. Reitberg DP, Klarnet JP, Carlson JK, Schentag JJ. Effect of metronidazole on theophylline pharmacokinetics. Clin Pharm 1983; 2:441–444.

269. Lo KF, Nation L, Sansom LN. Lack of effect of co-trimoxazole on the pharmacokinetics of orally administered theophylline. Biopharm Drug Dispos 1989; 10:573–580.

270. Mathis J, Prince RA, Weinberger MM, McElnay JC. The effect of tetracycline hydrochloride on theophylline kinetics. Clin Pharm 1982; 1:446–448.

271. Hopkins S. Clinical toleration and safety of azithromycin. Am J Med 1991; 91:40S–45S.

272. Luskin SG, Fitzsimmons WE, MacLeod CM, Luskin AT. Pharmacokinetic evaluation of the terfenadine-theophylline interaction. J Allergy Clin Immunol 1989; 83:406–411.

273. Gregoire SL, Grasela TH Jr, Freer JP, Tack KJ, Schentag JJ. Inhibition of theophylline clearance by coadministered ofloxacin without alteration of theophylline effects. Antimicrob Agents Chemother 1987; 31:375–378.

274. Al-Turk WA, Shaheen OM, Othman S, Khalaf RM, Awidi AS. Effect of ofloxacin on the pharmacokinetics of a single intravenous theophylline dose. Ther Drug Monit 1988; 10:160–163.

275. Ho G, Tierney MG, Dales RE. Evaluation of the effect of norfloxacin on the pharmacokinetics of theophylline. Clin Pharmacol Ther 1988; 44:35–38.

276. Davis RL, Kelly HW, Quenzer RW, Standefer J, Steinberg B, Gallegos J. Effect of norfloxacin on theophylline metabolism. Antimicrob Agents Chemother. 1989; 33:212–214.

277. Sano M, Yamamoto I, Ueda J, Yoshikawa E, Yamashina H, Goto M. Comparative pharmacokinetics of theophylline following two fluoroquinolones co-administration. Eur J Clin Pharmacol 1987; 32:431–432.

278. Staib AH, Harder S, Fuhr U, Wack C. Interaction of quinolones with the theophylline metabolism in man: investigations with lomefloxacin and pipemidic acid. Int J Clin Pharmacol Ther Toxicol 1989; 27:289–293.

279. Nix DE, Norman A, Schentag JJ. Effect of lomefloxacin on theophylline pharmacokinetics. Antimicrob Agents Chemother 1989; 33:1006–1008.

280. Robson RA, Begg EJ, Atkinson HC, Saunders DA, Frampton CM. Comparative effects of ciprofloxacin and lomefloxacin on the oxidative metabolism of theophylline. Br J Clin Pharmacol 1990; 29:491–493.

281. LeBel M, Vallee F, St-Laurent M. Influence of lomefloxacin on the pharmacokinetics of theophylline. Antimicrob Agents Chemother 1990; 34: 1254–1256.

282. Kamali F, Edwards C, Rawlins MD. Lack of effect of flosequinan on the pharmacokinetics of theophylline. Br J Clin Pharmacol 1991; 32:124–126.

283. Verdiani P, DiCarlo S, Baronti A. Famotidine effects on theophylline pharmacokinetics in subjects affected by COPD. Comparison with cimetidine and placebo. Chest 1988; 94:807–810.

284. Kelly HW, Powell JR, Donohue JF. Ranitidine at very large doses does not inhibit theophylline elimination. Clin Pharmacol Ther 1986; 39:577–581.

285. Secor JW, Speeg KV, Meredith CG, Johnson RF, Snowdy P, Schenker S. Lack of effect of nizatidine on hepatic drug metabolism in man. Br J Clin Pharmac 1985; 20:710–713.

286. Albin H, Vincon G, Bezier M, Pehourcq F, Cabanieu G. Pharmacocoinetique de la theophylline par voie oral chez des malades asthmatiques sous cortotherapie au long cours (Pharmacokinetics of oral theophylline in asthmatic patients on long-term corticoid therapy). Therapie 1983; 38:333–339.

287. Anderson J, Ayres JW, Hall CA. Potential pharmacokinetic interaction between theophylline and prednisone. Clin Pharm 1984; 3:187–189.

288. Upton RA. Pharmacokinetic interactions between theophylline and other medication (Part I). Clin Pharmacokinet 1991; 20:66–80.

289. Upton RA. Pharmacokinetic interactions between theophylline and other medication (Part II). Clin Pharmacokinet 1991; 20:135–150.

290. Hendeles L, Jenkins J, Temple R. Revised FDA labeling guideline for theophylline oral dosage forms. Pharmacotherapy 1995; 15:409–427.

291. Paulsen O, Höglund P, Nilsson LG, Bengtsson HI. The interaction of erythromycin with theophylline. Eur J Clin Pharmacol 1987; 32:493–498.

292. Thomsen K, Schou M. Renal lithium excretion in man. J Physiol 1968; 215:823–827.

293. Bonfiglio MF, Dasta JF. Clinical significance of the benzodiazepine-theophylline interaction. Pharmacother 1991; 11:85–87.

294. Doll DC, Rosenberg H. Antagonism of neuromuscular blockage by theophylline. Anesth Analg 1979; 58:139–140.

295. Billing B, Dahlqvist R, Garle M, Hornblad Y, Ripe E. Separate and combined use of terbutaline and theophylline in asthmatics: effects related to plasma levels. Eur J Respir Dis 1982; 63:399–409.

296. Roizen MF, Stevens WC. Multiform ventricular tachycardia due to the interaction of aminophylline and halothane. Anesth Analg 1978; 57:738–741.

297. Hirshman CA, Krieger W, Littlejohn G, Lee R, Julien R. Ketamine-aminophylline induced decrease in seizure threshold. Anesthesiology 1982; 56:464–467.

298. Bukowskyj M, Munt PW, Wigle R, Nakatsu K. Theophylline clearance. Lack of effect of influenza vaccination and ascorbic acid. Am Rev Respir Dis 1984; 129:672–675.

299. Grabowski N, May JJ, Pratt DS, Richtsmeier WJ, Bertino JS, Bertino JS Jr. The effect of split virus influenza vaccination on theophylline pharmacokinetics. Am Rev Respir Dis 1985; 131:934–938.

300. Renton KW, Gray JD, Hall RI. Decreased elimination of theophylline after influenza vaccination. Can Med Assoc J 1980; 123:288–290.

301. Meredith CG, Christian CD, Johnson RF, Troxell R, Davis GL, Schenker S. Effects of influenza virus vaccine on hepatic drug metabolism. Clin Pharmacol Ther 1985; 37:396–401.

302. Gomolin IH, Chapron DJ, Luhan PA. Lack of effect of influenza vaccine on theophylline levels and warfarin anticoagulation in the elderly. J Am Geriatr Soc 1985; 33:269–272.

303. Winstanley PA, Tija J, Back DJ, Hobson D, Breckenridge AM. Lack of effect of highly purified subunit influenza vaccination on theophylline metabolism. Br J Clin Pharmacol 1985; 20:47–53.

304. Hannan SE, May JJ, Pratt DS, Richtsmeier WJ, Bertino JS, Bertino JS Jr. The effect of whole virus influenza vaccination on theophylline pharmacokinetics. Am Rev Respir Dis 1988; 137:903–906.

305. Jonkman JH, Wymenga AS, de Zeeuw RA, van der Boon WV, Beugelink JK, Ossterhuis B, Jedema JN. No effect of influenza vaccination on theophylline pharmacokinetics as studied by ultraviolet spectrophotometry, HPLC, and EMIT assay methods. Ther Drug Monit 1988; 10:345–348.

306. Kramer P, McClain CJ. Depression of aminopyrine metabolism by influenza vaccination. N Engl J Med 1981; 305:1262–1264.

307. Walker S, Schreiber L, Middelkamp JN. Serum theophylline levels after influenza vaccination. Can Med Assoc J 1981; 125:243–244.

308. Goldstein RS, Cheung OT, Seguin R, Lobley G, Johnson AC. Decreased elimination of theophylline after influenza vaccination (letter). Can Med Assoc J 1982; 126:470.

309. Stults BM, Hashiasaki PA. Influenza vaccination and theophylline pharmacokinetics in patients with chronic obstructive lung disease. West J Med 1983; 139:651–654.

310. Fischer RG, Booth BH, Mitchell DQ, Kibbe AH. Influence of trivalent influenza vaccine on serum theophylline levels. Can Med Assoc J 1982; 126:1312–1313.

311. Britton L, Ruben FL. Serum theophylline levels after influenza vaccination. Can Med Assoc J 1982; 126:1375.

312. Patriarca PA, Kendal AP, Stricof RL, Weber JA, Meissner MK, Dateno B. Influenza vaccination and warfarin or theophylline toxicity in nursing home residents. N Engl J Med 1983; 308:1601–1602.

313. Mitenko PA, Ogilvie RI. Rapidly achieved plasma concentration platueaus with observations on theophylline kinetics. Clin Pharmacol Ther 1972; 13:329–335.

314. Schudt C, Tenor H, Hatzelmann A. PDE isoenzymes as targets for anti-asthma drugs. Eur Respir J 1995; 8:1179–1183.

315. Nicholson CD, Shahid M, Bruin J, Barron E, Spiers I, de Boer J, van Amsterdam RG, Zaagsma J, Kelly JJ, Dent G. Characterization of ORG 20241, a combined phosphodiesterase IV/III cyclic nucleotide phosphodiesterase inhibitor for asthma. J Pharmacol Exp Ther 1995; 274:678–687.

316. Gozzard N, Herd CM, Blake SM, Holbrook M, Hughes B, Higgs GA, Page CP. Effects of theophylline and rolipram on antigen-induced airway responses in neonatally immunized rabbits. Br J Pharmacol 1996; 117:1405–1412.

317. Hughes P, Howat D, Lisle H, Holbrook M, James T, Gozzard N, Blease K, Hughes P, Kingaby R, Warrellow G, et al. The inhibition of antigen-induced eosinophilia and bronchoconstriction by CDP840, a novel stereo-selective inhibitor of phosphodiesterase type 4. Br J Pharmacol 1996; 118:1183–1191.

318. Myou S, Fujimura M, Kamio Y, Ishiura Y, Tachibana H, Hirose T, Hashimoto T, Matsuda T. Bronchodilator effect of inhaled olprinone, a phosphodiesterase 3 inhibitor, in asthmatic patients. Am J Respir crit Care Med 1999; 160:817–820.

319. Myou S, Fujimura M, Kamio Y, Hirose T, Kita T, Tachibana H, Ishiura Y, Watanabe K, Hashimoto T, Nakao S. Bronchodilator effects of intravenous

olprinone, a phosphodiesterase 3 inhibitor, with and without aminophylline in asthmatic patients. Br J Clin Pharmacol 2003; 55:341–346.

320. Giembycz MA. Cilomilast: a second generation phosphodiesterase 4 inhibitor for asthma and chronic obstructive pulmonary disease. Expert Opin Investig Drugs 2001; 10:1361–1379.

321. Timmer W, Leclerc V, Birraux G, Neuhauser M, Hatzelmann A, Bethke T, Wurst W. The new phosphodiesterase 4 inhibitor roflumilast is efficacious in exercise-induced asthma and leads to suppression of LPS-stimulate TNF-alpha ex vivo. J Clin Pharmacol 2002; 42:297–303.

322. Spina D. Phosphodiesterase-4 inhibitors in the treatment of inflammatory lung disease. Drugs 2003; 63:2575–2594.

7

Cromolyn and Nedocromil

MARGARET LOWERY

Department of Pediatrics (Allergy/
   Immunology), Medical College of
   Wisconsin
Milwaukee, Wisconsin, U.S.A.

KEVIN J. KELLY

Department of Pediatrics, Children's Mercy
   Hospital, University of Missouri Kansas
   City
Kansas City, Missouri, U.S.A.

I. Introduction

The current consensus in the scientific medical community is that asthma is a chronic inflammatory condition of the bronchial mucosa that may lead to basement membrane thickening, collagen deposition, and airway remodeling. It is a disease characterized by airflow obstruction and bronchial hyper-responsiveness. In 2002, the National Institutes of Health National Heart, Lung, and Blood Institute revised the asthma guidelines (1). The revised guidelines recommend daily use of a low-dose inhaled corticosteroid (ICS) or an alternative inhaled anti-inflammatory medication including cromolyn or a leukotriene receptor antagonist for the management of mild persistent asthma in children <5 years. For adults and children ≥ 5 years the recommendations include the additional alternative use of nedocromil or sustained-release theophylline treatment for mild persistent asthma.

Traditionally many physician who have treated pediatric patients used cromolyn sodium (CS) as a first-line treatment in mild persistent asthma. Several studies have demonstrated the benefit of cromolyn and nedocromil in the daily symptom control of asthma. In many cases this course of treatment

195

was chosen secondary to concerns by medical practitioners and parents of children with asthma because of the theoretic risk of untoward effects that ICS might have on longitudinal growth and development. More recently several studies have demonstrated that the use of ICS does not have any long-term effects on growth despite short-term reductions in growth velocity. As a result, the widespread use of cromolyn has been supplanted by ICS and the availability of leukotriene antagonists.

Cromolyn is available in multiple delivery devices or forms, including an oral inhaler, nebulization solution, nasal inhaler, ocular eye drops, and oral capsules. Thus, cromolyn has been available for use in the treatment of asthma, allergic rhinitis, allergic conjunctivitis, chronic idiopathic urticaria, mastocytosis, and idiopathic anaphylaxis. Nedocromil has only been available as a metered dose inhaler (MDI), which has limited its use to primary pulmonary problems of asthma and chronic cough. In addition, exercise-induced bronchospasm and allergen-induced early- and late-phase declines in expiratory airflow may be prevented with the use of cromolyn and nedocromil. The action of these agents can be categorized as effects on mast cells, neuromodulatory actions, and anti-inflammatory activity. This chapter will review the chemistry, mechanisms of action, physiochemical properties, clinical trials and comparative trials, clinical administration, toxicity, benefits, and limitations of cromolyn and nedocromil.

II. Historical Background

Cromolyn and nedocromil are members of the chromone group of chemical compounds. The chemical formula for chromone is 5:6 benz-1:4 pyrone (2) (Fig. 1). In 1968, disodium cromoglycate (DSCG) or CS combined with isoproterenol was introduced in the United Kingdom as the first anti-inflammatory medication used in asthma (3–5). The addition of the bronchodilator was done to prevent bronchoconstriction that can occur with inhalation of a sodium salt (4). By 1973, cromolyn was approved by the Food and Drug Administration (FDA) for the treatment of asthma and in 1983 for the treatment of allergic rhinitis (5). Khellin (2) was the first identified chromone, which was extracted from seeds of the plant *Amni visnaga*, the same plant from which cromolyn was derived. It was used as a diuretic and smooth muscle relaxant, especially for the relief of ureteric colic. In 1947, Anrep et al. (6) reported the clinical utility of khellin for the treatment of asthma. Multiple compounds were synthesized using the khellin molecular structure as a starting point. Two other chromones, K18 and GR4 (Fig. 2), used in the sensitized guinea pig lung with antigen challenge prevented the release of histamine and slow-releasing substances of anaphylaxis (SRS-A) (7).

Dr. Roger Altounyan discovered cromolyn in 1964 after many trials with other chromone compounds. As a young child he had a history of atopy

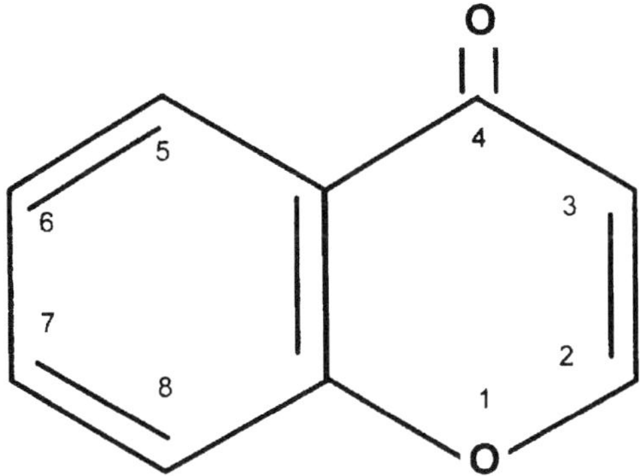

Figure 1 The chromone chemical structure.

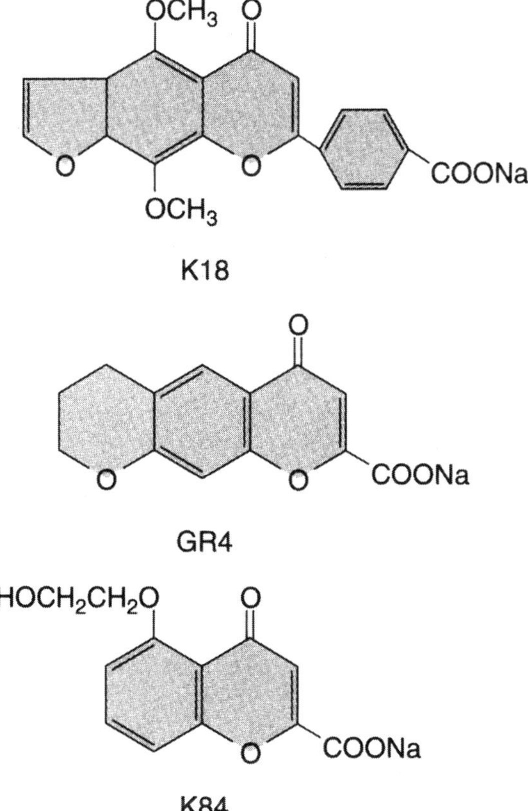

Figure 2 Chemical structure of early chromones: K18, GR4, and K84.

and eczema, and later he developed severe chronic asthma (2). In his early experiments he performed bronchial allergen challenges on himself to induce bronchoconstriction. Pretreatment of himself with K18 and GR4 demonstrated a 50% and 70% protection, respectively, against allergen challenge. In 1963, a K84 compound provided 57% protection when administered one hour prior to allergen challenge, but subsequent studies failed to reproduce these observations. This discovery led to a desire to perform human trials aimed at clarifying any therapeutic effectiveness of this compound to treat asthmatics. Since the drug was effective prior to inhalation of antigen in the preliminary observations, the first human trial involved prolonged administration of K84 prior to antigen challenge. Disappointingly, this trial of K84 in one adult patient showed no improvement in his asthma symptoms. Further analysis determined that the protection from allergen challenge in the initial K84 experiments might be due to an "impurity" in the compound. Eventually it was determined that two K84 molecules, joined

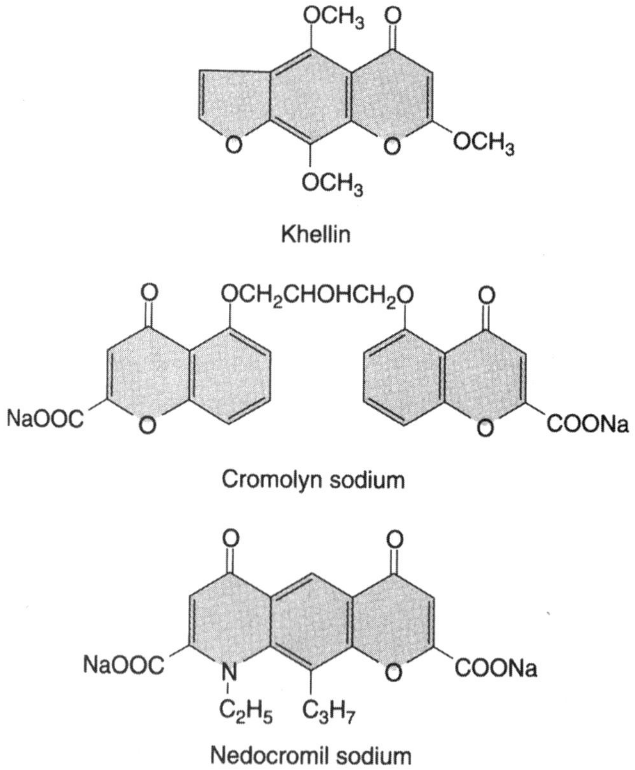

Figure 3   Chemical structure of khellin, cromolyn sodium, and nedocromil sodium.

at the -5 position (Fig. 3), were responsible for the clinical observations. Thus, a new bischromone, CS, was brought to clinical medicine (7). A second molecule known as GR4 was the starting compound that led to the synthesis of the monochromone, nedocromil sodium.

III. Pharmacokinetics

A. Cromolyn

At physiological pH both cromolyn and nedocromil are small, water-soluble, highly ionized compounds with negligible fat solubility that are poorly absorbed from the gastrointestinal (GI) tract (8). These properties are responsible for the inability of these drugs to enter the intracellular space of cells leading to their excretion in the urine (80%) and feces after biliary secretion (20%) (8). CS binding to plasma proteins is poor and reversible, which accounts for the extremely low incidence of adverse drug interactions (7). Less than 1% of an oral dose of CS is absorbed from the gastrointestinal tract, but approximately 7% to 9% of an inhaled dose reaches the systemic circulation with peak plasma levels achieved 10 to 15 minutes after inhalation (9). Relatively rapid clearance occurs from the lung with up to 75% of the inhaled dose being removed by two hours. Only 2% of the inhaled dose may remain in the lung for 24 hours (7–9). Plasma half-life is less than two hours and is nearly undetectable for four hours, suggesting that a rapid clearance from the vascular space occurs.

B. Nedocromil

Nedocromil belongs to the structural class of pyranoquinolines (3). As noted above nedocromil is water soluble, rapidly absorbed from the lung, has negligible fat accumulation, and has minimal absorption from the GI tract. Similar to CS, adverse drug reactions occur infrequently due to the low to moderate protein binding capacity of nedocromil. Drugs that do bind proteins readily are not displaced by nedocromil, resulting in no changes in half-life or clearance of these other compounds. Nedocromil has only one available vehicle of medication-inhalation, a 2 mg per actuation MDI, with <10% deposition of the total dose in the lung. The peak plasma concentration is reached at 15 minutes in asthmatic patients and the drug is excreted after pulmonary absorption in the urine and GI tract from swallowing (90%) and biliary excretion (7,10).

IV. Drug Distribution in the Lung

The total delivered dosage and distribution of chromones in the lung are important factors in determining efficacy in the treatment of asthma.

The inhalation airflow rate as well as the method of inhalation will determine the amount of drug reaching the lung (7). Cromolyn is available as an MDI (1 mg and 5 mg), Spinhaler® and nebulizer solution (20 mg/2 mL). An inhalation rate of 30 L/min delivers a dose of 5.5% and 11.8% with the 5 mg and 1 mg MDI, respectively, to the lung (11,12). This proportion increases to 16.1% with the addition of a 10 cm spacer using the 1 mg MDI. Therefore, using a large volume spacer will increase the amount of drug delivered to the lung. Laube et al. (13) reported an increase of 8.6% to 11.8% (a nearly 40% increase) of drug delivery to the lung when the inhalation rate was reduced from 70 L/min to 30 L/min. This increased drug deposition in the lung resulted in protection against allergen challenge. The use of a spinhaler at lower rates of inspiratory airflow reduces deposition in the lung. This requires the clinician to give specific instruction on the use of each delivery device for optimal drug effect.

The peak plasma level reflects the dose of drug delivered to the lung (7). The peak plasma concentration with 1% aqueous cromolyn solution in healthy volunteers was 8.8 ng/mL using 2 mL cromolyn alone, 17.2 ng/mL with 5 mL of cromolyn and isotonic saline, and 24.5 ng/mL with 0.3 mL of a β_2-agonist (procaterol), cromolyn, and isotonic saline (14). The addition of a β_2-agonist to cromolyn increased drug delivery to the lung. This has been interpreted that the bronchodilation effect will enhance drug deposition into the lung.

The amount of cromolyn delivered to the lung can be measured by the 24-hour urinary excretion of DSCG. The addition of a large-volume spacer with DSCG MDI increased from 1.82% to 6.13% of the delivered dose as measured by the 24-hour urinary excretion of DSCG (15). The 24-hour urinary excretion of DSCG increased by a factor of 1.53 with the addition of salbutamol in children with moderate to severe asthma (16).

V. Cromone Mechanism of Action

The exact mechanism of action of cromolyn and nedocromil has not been determined. Multiple mechanisms involving ion channel blockade, blockade of signaling of heat shock protein or G-protein, or even blockade of capsaicin receptor have been identified. However, the final common mechanism appears to be an inhibition of mast cell activation.

Studies have reported that the phosphorylation of a 78-kDa-molecular-weight protein prevents mediator release in mast cells (17). More specifically in rat peritoneal mast cells, both medications are reported to phosphorylate a 78-kDa protein from the β and γ subunits of the IgE binding protein (FCϵRI), which may impair a cell volume–dependent chloride current (17,18). Wang et al. (19) reported that protein kinase C inhibitors prevented phosphorylation of the 78-kDa protein by cromolyn and that this protein was insensitive to protein kinase C activators and Ca^{2+}. This suggests that regulation of an atypical protein kinase C may be involved as an additional mechanism where cromolyn inhibits mast cell activation. The protein kinase C isoenzymes are an important step in signaling cascade involved in the process of mast cell degranulation. Other proteins with molecular weights of 42, 59, and 68-kDa are activated in 10 seconds after the mast cell is challenged with allergen or compound 48/80, whereas the 78-kDa protein responds after 30 to 60 seconds (8). It is possible that termination of mediator release may be associated with phosphorylation of this 78-kDa protein (7). More recently this 78-kDa protein has been identified as moesin, a member of the 4.1 ERM superfamily, which includes ezrin, radixin, and merlin (20,21). These ERM proteins possess actin-binding domains and co-localize with actin at the plasma membrane surface (2). Thus, it is possible that moesin may interact with the cytoskeleton and prevent mast cell activation and secretion of mediators (7).

Furthermore, Garland and Mongor reported that cromolyn inhibited histamine release from rat peritoneal mast cells using phosphatidylserine and calcium (22). Both calcium and phosphatidylserine are required for the action of protein kinase C (8). This suggests that cromolyn may inhibit protein kinase C, which prevents mediator release in the mast cell.

Another study reported that chromones act to inhibit the activation of a chloride current in cells undergoing shape and volume changes (23). Both cromolyn and nedocromil can inhibit chloride transport (24). In rat mucosal mast cells cromolyn has been reported to block an "intermediate conductance" chloride channel, which may inhibit the antigen-induced mediator secretion (25). In addition Heinke et al. (23) reported that both medications inhibit chloride current in activated pulmonary endothelial cells exposed to hypotonic saline and reduce open-channel availability of single chloride channels in sheep airway epithelial cells (Fig. 4). Thus if the chloride current isn't activated the membrane will not be hyperpolarized to allow for subsequent mast cell degranulation.

Kay et al. (27) have reported that cromolyn can prevent extracellular calcium influx into the cytoplasm of the mast cell. The calcium channel activation that occurs after cross-linking membrane-bound IgE by antigen can be inhibited when mast cells are incubated with cromolyn (28). Thus, by inhibiting calcium influx and mediator release cromolyn may prevent allergic inflammatory responses.

As previously described, cromolyn and nedocromil do not enter the intracellular space due to their physiochemical properties. It is likely that the effects of cromolyn are due to the binding of a membrane receptor at the cell surface. A specific binding site has been reported on rat basophil leukemia cells (RBL-2H3) for cromolyn by Mazurek et al. (28). Later work by other investigators reported that these RBL-2H3 cells were insensitive to the inhibitory effects of CS (8).

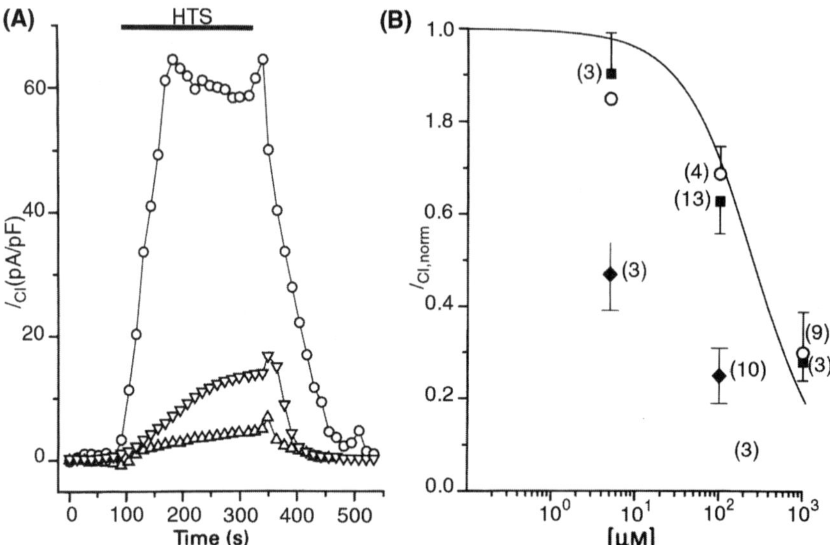

Figure 4 Concentration-dependence of the effects of intracellular and extracellular sodium cromoglycate. (**A**) Hypotonic saline (HTS)-activated current from three different cells under control conditions (○) and after intracellular loading with 5 (∇) and 50 μM (Δ) sodium cromoglycate. Currents are expressed per unit membrane capacitance (measured before HTS). Note the slower activation of the current in the presence of sodium cromoglycate. (**B**) Synopsis of the data with extracellular sodium cromoglycate (SCG ■) and nedocromil sodium (○), as well as those by intracellular loading with sodium cromoglycate (♦). For extracellular sodium cromoglycate, a K_1 value of 310 μM was obtained (see text). The value for intracellular sodium cromoglycate is in the range of 5–10 μM, i.e., nearly two orders of magnitude smaller.

The inhalation of adenosine results in bronchoconstriction in asthmatic patients. Tamaoki et al. (29) reported that inhaled adenosine also caused microvascular leakage in sensitized rats. Pretreatment with capsaicin or the tachykinin neurokinin-1 receptor antagonist FK888 prevents this microvascular leakage with inhaled adenosine. Moreover, cromolyn also prevents this adenosine-induced vascular extravasation of fluid (29).

Okada et al. (30) reported that cromolyn inhibited part of the heat shock protein 90 (Hsp 90) complex in vitro. The Hsp90 protein may be involved in signaling cascade, leading to mast cell degranulation. This protein can act to prevent protein aggregation and promote refolding in vitro.

Both morphine and certain anesthetic muscle relaxants are known mast cell activators, but the mechanism of this effect has not been completely elucidated. One possible mechanism of morphine and d-Tubocurarine mast cell activation may be through activation of G-proteins. At concentrations of 10 μM and 100 μM DSCG reduced the stimulation of these

G-proteins by morphine by 50% and 80%, respectively, possibly through direct inhibition of the G-proteins and resultant suppression of mast cell activation (31).

Another possible mechanism for cromolyn may involve guanosine 3′, 5′ cyclic monophosphate (cGMP). A study with rat peritoneal mast cells showed that exogenously applied cGMP and treatment with DSCG produced a potent inhibition of histamine release (32).

VI. Immunoregulatory Effects

Cromolyn and nedocromil have a wide spectrum of activity that includes: inhibition of mediator release from mast cells, eosinophils, and neutrophils; protection against allergen-induced and exercise-induced bronchospasm; and prevention of the early- and late-phase asthmatic response (3).

Sheard and Blair were the first to report that CS prevented the antigen-induced release of histamine and SRS-A (leukotrienes) from passively sensitized human lung (33). More recently, pretreatment of rat peritoneal mast cells with DSCG prior to anti-DNP exposure resulted in significant inhibition of histamine release in a dose-dependent manner (34) (Fig. 5).

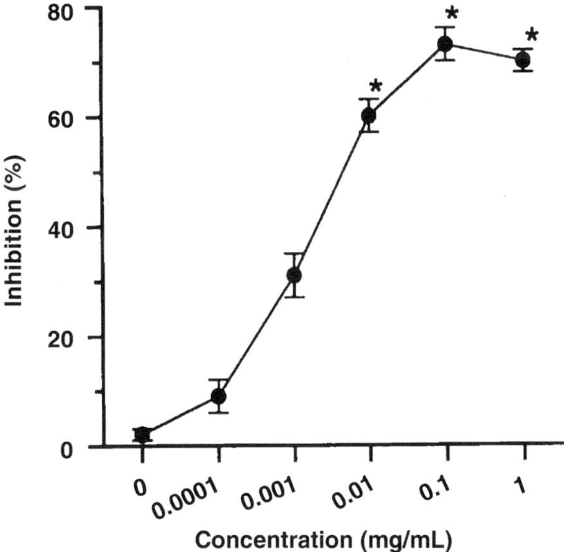

Figure 5 Effect of disodium cromoglycate (DSCG) on IgE production by T cell-depleted, B cell-enriched populations of cells in the presence of IL-4 (50 μg/mL) and anti-CD40 mAb (5 μg/mL). Cells were cultured at a concentration of 10^6 cells/mL for 10 days with different concentrations of DSCG. Supernatants were harvested after 10 days and IgE levels were measured by radioimmunoassay. Results represent mean ± SE net synthesis IgE (pg/mL) of five experiments.

Both cromolyn and nedocromil inhibit histamine and PGD2 release from human mast cells; block activation of human eosinophils; inhibit activation, chemotaxis, and mediator release from neutrophils; inhibit IgE antibody function from mononuclear cells; inhibit the S_μ to S_ε switch; inhibit TNF-α release; and reduce mRNA for TNF-α from rat peritoneal cells (Table 1, Fig. 6) (27, 36–42).

When atopic asthmatic patients are stimulated with *Dermatophagoides farinae*, cromolyn has been shown to inhibit the production of IL-5 and IFN-γ by sensitized human peripheral blood mononuclear cells (43). A significant decrease in TNF-α and IL-5 was reported in sensitized human lung specimens from atopic patients (43). In addition to IL-5, Oh et al. (44) reported that DSCG reduced secretion of IL-4 and IL-13 in PBMC from atopic patients. In bronchoalveolar lavage (BAL) and nasal lavage fluid, cromolyn reduced the increase in neutrophils, myeloperoxidase, soluble intercellular adhesion molecule-1 (ICAM-1), IL-6, and TNF-α (46) (Fig. 7). In patients with bronchopulmonary dysplasia (BPD), cromolyn was reported to decrease TNF-α and IL-8 in lung lavage fluid (45,46). Shin et al. (34) reported significant inhibition of TNF-α release in the rat mast cell line RBL-2H3 pretreated with DSCG prior to antigen challenge.

In 1969, Kennedy reported a reduction in sputum eosinophils with cromolyn treatment compared to placebo (48). More recently bronchial biopsy specimens had a reduction in EG2+ eosinophils, AA1+ mast cells, and CD4+, CD8+, CD3+, and CD68+ lymphocytes in patients treated with 12 weeks of cromolyn (49) (Fig. 8). Furthermore, a reduced expression of ICAM-1 and vascular cell adhesion molecule-1 (VCAM-1) were seen on bronchial epithelium and vascular endothelium after treatment with cromolyn (49).

CS has been beneficial in the treatment of aspirin-sensitive asthma (ASA) subjects. Amayasu et al. (50) reported that ASA patients treated with cromolyn for one week resulted in an improvement in asthma symptoms, and demonstrated a significant decrease in blood and sputum eosinophils and sputum eosinophilic cationic protein (ECP) levels compared with placebo. Furthermore, there was an improvement in bronchial hypersensitivity in almost all patients.

In addition to their effects on mast cells, cromolyn and nedocromil inhibit the expression of membrane receptors for complement (C3b) and IgG (Fc) in human neutrophils (8). Both medications have been reported to inhibit activation of human neutrophils by platelet-activating factor (PAF) or zymosan-activated serum (51). Cromolyn treatment decreases oxygen radical production in guinea-pig alveolar macrophages in response to zymosan in a concentration-dependent manner by 72% (52). The combination medication reproterol (β_2-agonist) and DSCG is used in Europe for the treatment of asthma. The combined reproterol and DSCG showed a significant inhibition of histamine release compared to another β_2-agonist (salbutamol) in rat mast cells (53).

Table 1 Immunologic Effects of Cromolyn and Nedocromil

Action (Ref.)	Cromolyn	Nedocromil
Inhibits histamine (35)	✓	✓
Inhibit PGD2 release from human mast cells (36)	✓	✓
Inhibit TNFα release and decrease mRNA for TNFα from peritoneal rat mast cells (37)	✓	
Inhibit production of IL-5 from human PBMCs (43)	✓	
Reduce the increase in neutrophils, myeloperoxidase, ICAM-1, IL-6, TNFα in BAL and nasal lavage fluid (46)		
Decrease TNFα and IL-8 in lung lavage fluid of BPD patients (47)	✓	
Decrease in IL-6 in human airway macrophages (166)		✓
Decreases lysosomal enzyme release from human alveolar macrophages (56)		✓
Decreases oxygen radical release from human monocytes (56)		✓
Block activation of human blood eosinophils (27,39)	✓	✓
Inhibits release of pre-formed (granule-associated) newly generated eicosanoid medications (51,54)		✓
Blocks chemotactic response of eosinophils to PAF and LTB4 (57)		✓
Blocks survival of eosinophils in presence of IL-5 (167)		✓
Inhibits release of ECP from eosinophils (168)		✓
Decreases the release of TNFα, IL-8, soluble ICAM-1 from human bronchial epithelial cells (169)		✓
Inhibits GMCSF and IL-8 (170,171)		✓
Inhibits cell surface ICAM-1 expression (172)		✓
Inhibits release of cytotoxic mediators from platelets taken from patient with ASA (173)		✓
Inhibits urinary LTE4 in ASA patients (174)	✓	
Inhibits generation of TBX2 and IP3 from thromboxane stimulated patients (175)		
Inhibits activation, chemotaxis, and mediator release from neutrophils (56,176–179)	✓	✓
Inhibit IgE antibody function from mononuclear cells (38,39)	✓	✓
Inhibits s$_\mu$ to s$_\varepsilon$ switch (41)	✓	✓
Inhibits allergen-induced and mitogen induced proliferation and IL-2 release from mouse lymphocytes (180)		✓

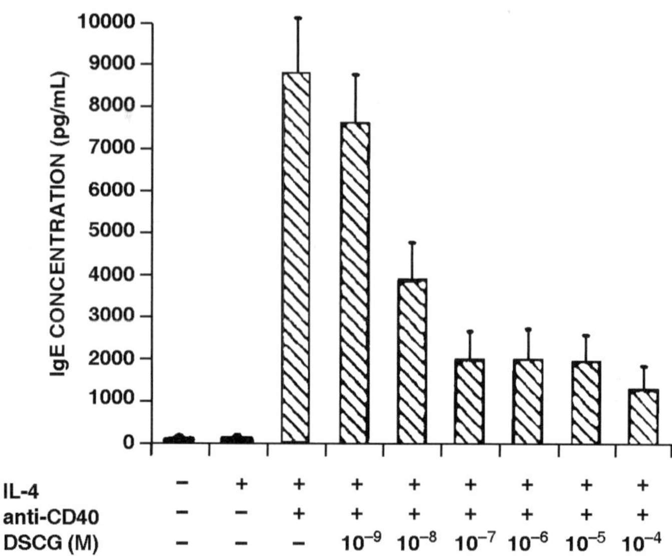

Figure 6 Effect of cramolyn sodium on immunoglobulin E (IgE) production by T cell-depleted, B cell-enriched populations of cells (10^6 cells/mL) in the presence of interleukin-4 (IL-4, 50 U/mL) and anti-CD40 monoclonal antibody (mAb, 5 μg/mL). Results represent mean ± SE for net synthesis of IgE (pg/mL) from five experiments. *Source*: From Ref. 41.

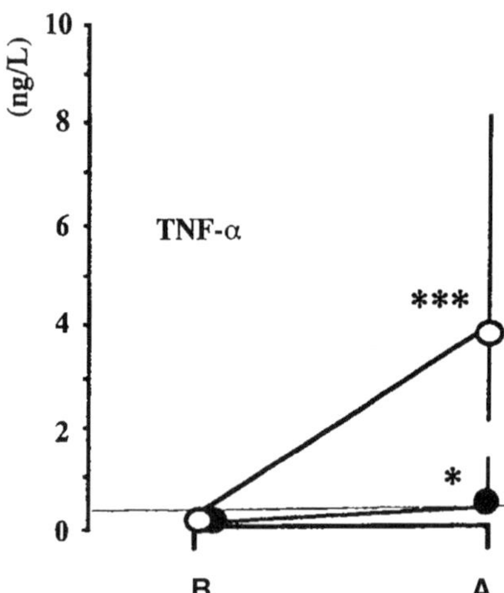

Figure 7 Effect of concentration of tumor necrosis factor alpha (TNF-α) in BAL fluid after two weeks of treatment with cramolyn sodium ($n = 16$) or placebo ($n = 16$) before (*B*) and after (*A*) exposure to swine dust; median values and 25th to 75th percentiles. Difference between groups is significant ($p = 0.0003$). *Source*: From Ref. 46.

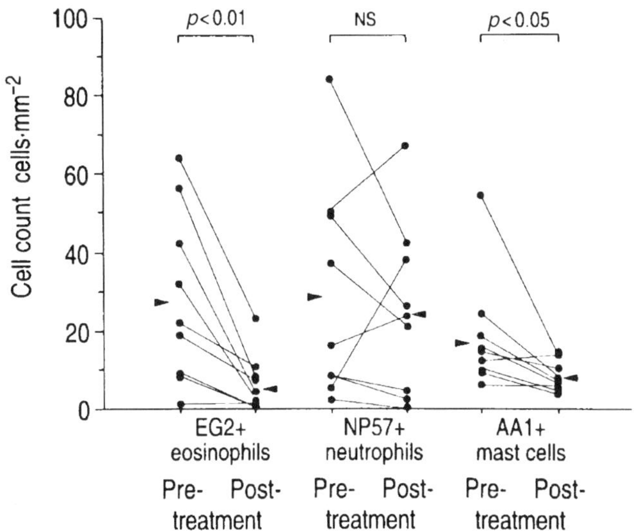

Figure 8 Effect of cromolyn sodium (CS) on individual cell counts of EG2+ eosinophils, NP 57+ neutrophils, and AA1+ mast cells expressed as number of cells per square millimeter of lamina propria in bronchial mucosa before and after treatment with CS. *Symbol*: →, mean values. *Abbreviation*: NS, not significant. *Source*: From Ref. 49.

A study in human lung mast cells demonstrated that CS is a weak inhibitor of histamine release when given 15 minutes before allergen challenge. CS effectiveness is inversely related to the intensity of immunologic stimulation (8). At a concentration of $1000 \mu M$, cromolyn inhibits histamine release by 25% and PGD2 release by 85%. Since PGD2 is a potent bronchoconstrictor, this may be an important effect of cromolyn. Church et al. (8) reported that the inhibitory effects of cromolyn on human mast cells are increased with a longer preincubation time. However, human skin mast cells are unresponsive to cromolyn, which is further supported by previous observations that cromolyn does not inhibit mast cell degranulation or the wheal and flare response in vivo.

Nedocromil and cromolyn have been shown to inhibit the release of preformed (granule associated) and newly generated eicosanoid mediators from activated eosinophils. These specific proteins are eosinophil granule-associated peroxidase and eosinophilic cationic protein (54). In rat monocytes and peritoneal macrophages, as well as in human monocytes and alveolar macrophages, nedocromil has been reported to inhibit FcεR2-mediated activation (55,56). Bruijnzeel et al. (57) reported that nedocromil blocked the chemotactic response of eosinophils to PAF and leukotriene B4 (LTB4). In the human airway, nedocromil has been reported to decrease IL-6 and lysosomal enzyme release from alveolar macrophages (7). In addition, nedocromil reduces histamine and tryptase release five minutes after allergen challenge in bronchial segments of allergic asthmatic patients. This is accompanied by a reduction of eosinophils in BAL fluid 48 hours after challenge (58). A longer-term study comparing 16 weeks of treatment with nedocromil versus regular albuterol showed a reduction in the number of activated eosinophils in those patients treated with nedocromil on bronchial biopsy (59). Furthermore, nedocromil decreases the release of TNF-α, IL-8, and soluble ICAM-1 from human bronchial epithelial cells (7).

VII. Neurogenic Mechanisms of Chromones

The bronchoconstriction induced by sulfur dioxide and bradykinin is inhibited by both cromolyn and nedocromil (Table 2) (60). Inhaled sodium metabisulfate generates sulfur dioxide in the airways with both of these agents causing bronchoconstriction in asthma subjects. The mechanism of action of sulfur dioxide may be through stimulation of laryngeal afferent nerve fibers in experimental animals (61). Nedocromil has been shown to prevent the bronchial hyper-responsiveness in dogs exposed to sulfur dioxide (62). Bradykinin may have broader effects than sulfur dioxide by causing vascular vasodilatation and increased vascular permeability in addition to the bronchoconstrictor effect. The cough and dyspnea induced by bradykinin is blocked by cromolyn and nedocromil (63). In experimental animals, bradykinin has been reported to stimulate afferent C-fibers to release substance P (a mast cell histamine releaser), neurokinin A, and calcitonin gene-related peptide, which all have bronchoconstrictor properties (64). In fact, Chatterjee et al. (65) reported that nedocromil decreased cough in asthmatic patients and was initially marketed specifically for cough-related asthma. The angiotensin-converting enzyme (ACE) inhibitor–induced cough, a known complication of this class of medications, is inhibited by CS (66).

Table 2 Neurogenic Mechanisms of Chromone Action

Action (Ref.)	Cromolyn	Nedocromil
Inhibits bronchoconstriction induced by sulfur dioxide and bradykinin (60,63)	✓	✓
Blocks myelinated and non-myelinated fiber transmission is canine airways (64,71)	✓	
Decreases cough and dyspnea induced by bradykinin (63)	✓	✓
Inhibits ACE inhibitor cough (66)	✓	
Inhibits substance-P induced histamine release from human mast cells (67)		✓

Thus, the inhibition of bradykinin by chromones is likely to be the mechanism of action in preventing ACE inhibitor–induced cough. The substance P–induced histamine release from human mast cells is inhibited with nedocromil (67).

There are a few case reports of successful treatment of ACE inhibitor–induced cough with inhaled cromolyn. The case reports involve a total of 13 patients of whom most had cromolyn added and continued on the ACE inhibitor (68). Four of the 13 patients had the ACE inhibitor stopped and were given cromolyn for seven days before the ACE inhibitor was resumed. The cough resolved in three of these patients (68). Only one trial evaluated the efficacy of cromolyn for treatment of the ACE inhibitor–induced cough. This was a double-blind crossover study of 10 patients. The median cough score decreased significantly in the cromolyn treated group (69). Alternatively, another small study with six diabetic patients on ACE inhibitors treated with nedocromil reported only one patient with cough relief (70).

In canine airways, cromolyn has been shown to block both myelinated and non-myelinated (C) fibers (64,71). It is important to note that C-fibers respond to chemical irritants rather than mechanical stimulation and this may be a factor in the nonspecific irritation of the airways in asthma (8). Jackson (72) reported that the stimulation of the cough reflex with inhalation of citric acid in a dog model is blocked by nedocromil but not cromolyn. In contrast, nedocromil was ineffective in the inhibition of citric acid–induced cough in asthmatic patients (73).

Adenosine and adenosine 5' monophosphate (AMP) result in broncho-constriction in asthmatic patients by not normal subjects (8). Both CS and nedocromil inhibit adenosine-induced bronchoconstriction, although various studies show nedocromil to be more effective (8).

The inhalation of hypertonic saline (5–15%) produced microvascular leakage in rat trachea (9). Yamawaki et al. (74) reported that pretreatment with DSCG reduced this extravasation in a dose-dependent manner. In addition, pretreatment with DSCG inhibited the microvascular extravasation from inhaled substance P in this study.

VIII. Allergen Challenge Clinical Trials

Both cromolyn and nedocromil have been shown to have a protective effect in exercise-induced bronchospasm in both children and adults (75,76). Also, these medications have an equal protective effect in response to cold air and bradykinin, substance P, neurokinin A, adenosine, and hypertonic saline (61,77–82). However, nedocromil has been shown to be more effective against sulfur dioxide and sodium metabisulfate (60). On the other hand, Altounyan showed that 10 times the dose of cromolyn is needed to provide

50% protection against sulfur dioxide challenge as compared to the dose needed for allergen challenge (83). An important clinical observation, potentially useful to allergic asthma subjects acutely exposed to allergen, was demonstrated when three doses of nedocromil given acutely over 90 minutes prior to antigen challenge resulted in the inhibition of the late asthmatic response (84). Furthermore, neither cromolyn nor nedocromil prevent the bronchoconstrictor response to inhaled histamine or methacholine. However, prolonged treatment may reduce bronchial hyper-reactivity (3).

The use of cromolyn in allergen challenge studies has given variable results. As previously described in this chapter, Laube et al. CI,13 reported greater protection to allergen challenge (76% vs. 43%) with a slower inspiratory rate and use of a spacer device when cromolyn was taken 30 minutes before allergen challenge. This is likely to due to a dose-dependent delivery of active drug. Similarly, exercise challenge studies have produced variable results. Tullett et al. (85) showed a protective effect with cromolyn of 38%, 56%, and 68% with doses of two puffs of 1 mg, two puffs of 5 mg, and four puffs of 5 mg, respectively, given 30 minutes before exercise (85), whereas no difference between the 1 mg and 5 mg dose of cromolyn was demonstrated in another study (86). Alternatively, Schoeffel et al. (87) showed that two puffs of the 1 mg cromolyn dose provided >50% protection in nine patients, which increased to 13 patients when four puffs of the 1 mg dose were given.

IX. Cromolyn for Asthma

Several studies have shown that ICS are more effective than cromolyn in patients with severe asthma (88–90). However, some studies in mild to moderate asthmatics have shown either comparable efficacy (91–93) or an even better response to ICS (94,95). On the other hand, the addition of cromolyn to ICS failed to show any beneficial effect (96). A more recent review of 24 placebo-controlled trials of cromolyn concluded, "there is insufficient evidence for a beneficial effect of CS as maintenance treatment in children with asthma." Further review of this study shows that cromolyn is more effective in older children (97). In addition, a recent review reported no significant difference between DSCG and placebo in children with asthma (98). The use of cromolyn versus placebo administered via face mask with spacer device in 167 children aged one to four years found no difference in the primary outcome measure of symptom-free asthma days between the two groups (99). Long-term studies with cromolyn have reported good asthma control and improvement in lung function with a lower dosage of cromolyn (100,101).

Konig and Shaffer reported that children on cromolyn and ICS for prolonged periods had no evidence of irreversible airway changes in a retrospective study in 175 infants in three treatment groups (102).

One group of mild asthmatics was treated with as needed bronchodilators, moderate asthmatics were treated with CS, and the severe asthmatics were treated with ICS (102). In this study the final pulmonary function tests (PFT) improved in both the cromolyn and ICS groups compared to bronchodilators alone (Fig. 9) (102). However, the overall change in pulmonary function from start to end of a study showed a significant improvement of FVC only in the ICS group (Fig. 10) (103). Overall, the clinical outcomes showed improvements in the frequency of hospitalizations ($p < 0.05$) in both the cromolyn group and the ICS-treated group. Likewise, a reduction in emergency department (ED) visits ($p < 0.05$) was observed in the ICS-treated group when compared to the bronchodilator group, despite the perceived mild severity of the latter group. Furthermore, a delay in starting cromolyn was associated with an unfavorable effect in clinical outcomes, whereas no effects were observed with delay of initiation of ICS (102).

A Finnish cross-sectional study of school children was divided into three groups—bronchodilators only, cromolyn, and ICS—reported improved PFT in the cromolyn group (104). This study involved 297 children: 60/297 (20%) on bronchodilators as needed for symptoms, 169/297 (57%) on cromolyn (97/169) or nedocromil (72/169), and 68/297 (23%) or ICS with budesonide (65/68) or beclomethasone (3/68). Thus, the majority of children in this study were on chromones medication. The decrease in at least one of the parameters of pulmonary function (PEF, FVC, FEV_1,

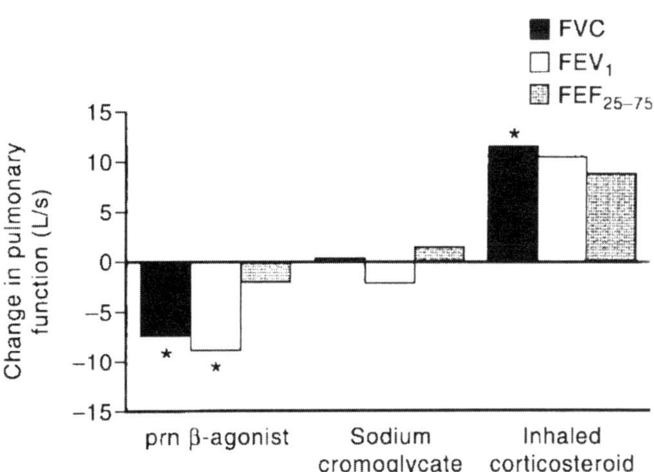

Figure 9 Change in pulmonary function from start to end of initial treatment with either β-agonists, sodium cromolyn, or inhaled cartiosteroid. All values are pre-bronchodilator use. *Abbreviations*: FVC, forced vital capacity; FEF_{25-75}, forced expiratory flow; PRN, as needed. *Source*: From Ref. 103.

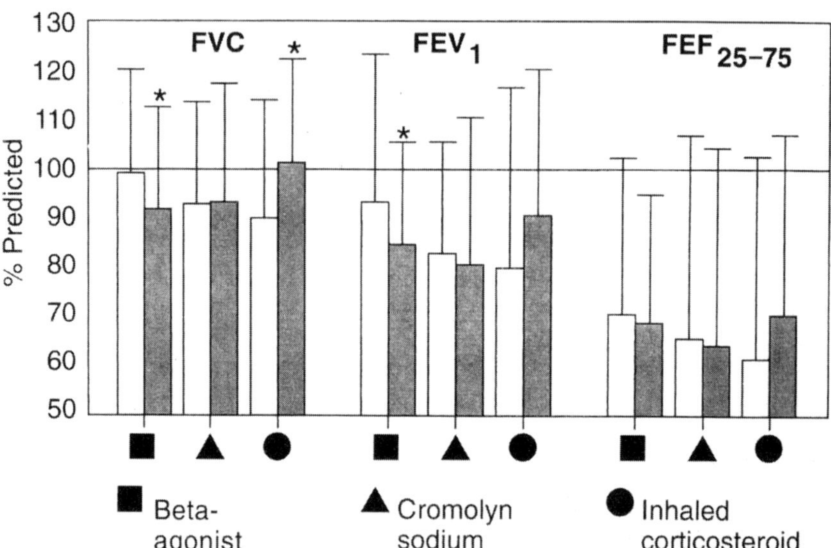

Figure 10 Mean (±SD) within treatment changes in prebronchodilator pulmonary function test results reported as percentage of predicted normal value. Data represent start to end of treatment, regardless of whether the end of treatment was the end of the study or represented a change in therapeutic agent, β-agonist, $n = 44$; cramolyn sodium, $n = 28$; inhaled cartiosteroid, $n = 26$. *Open bars*, start of treatment results; *shaded bars*, end of treatment test results. $^{*}p < 0.05$. *Source*: From Ref. (102).

or the MMEF) was highest in the ICS group and lowest in the chromone group (104). Analysis of the chromone group demonstrated that the FVC and FEV_1 were higher in the cromoglycate group ($p < 0.05$). This study only followed spirometry over one year and had disproportionate numbers of participants in the study groups. Today the ICS have proven to be beneficial and asthma guidelines have changed. The percentage of patients with mild, moderate, and severe asthma on ICS has steadily increased in the last decade.

De Baets et al. (105) compared cromolyn to budesonide in a small double-blind crossover study. This study involved 13 subjects (43–66 months) given inhaled cromolyn 10 mg tid or budesonide 100 μg tid for two months. A significant difference in morning peak flows was demonstrated in the ICS group [160 L/min vs. 150 L/min ($p < 0.03$)]. Fewer asthma exacerbations were reported in the ICS group as well, 7 versus 16 on cromolyn ($p < 0.005$). However, there were no differences in bronchial hyper-responsiveness observed.

The use of cromolyn therapy in early infancy and childhood has given conflicting data. While some studies have suggested that cromolyn may not be effective in the first year of life, one report verified that children under one year did show improvement with cromolyn (106–108). A reduction in symptoms and bronchodilator use has been observed with the use of cromolyn in a group of premature infants and children (109). In contrast, a recent review by the Cochrane database concluded that "cromolyn sodium cannot be recommended for the prevention of chronic lung disease in preterm infants" (110). The enigma of persistent wheezing after bronchiolitis has led investigators to experiment with preventive therapy during active disease. Reijonen et al. (111) reported that a single subsequent wheezing episode was lower in a group of children with bronchiolitis treated with cromolyn or budesonide. Prevention of the high cost of care from hospitalization favored the use of both medications in a subgroup of atopic children.

Another method used to assess the efficacy of therapy is to match pharmacy records to outcomes of emergency visits or need for hospitalization. Such investigations are fraught with numerous confounding variables but point out important trends in subjects using medication. One study reviewed inhaled anti-inflammatory medication dispensing through an analysis of automated pharmacy records of 11,195 children ages 3 to 15 years with a diagnosis of asthma (112). The outcome measures were ED visits and hospitalization for asthma. The adjusted relative risk (RR) for ED visits with the use of either cromolyn or ICS were 0.4 (95% CI 0.3, 0.5) and 0.5 (95% CI 0.4, 0.6), respectively. For hospitalizations, the adjusted RR with cromolyn and ICS were 0.6 (95% CI 0.4, 0.9) and 0.4 (95% CI 0.3, 0.7), respectively. Thus, a record of the patient obtaining one of these agents (use can not be demonstrated) is highly associated with prevention of ED visits and hospitalization for asthma (112).

A second investigation of pharmacy records analyzed the number of hospitalizations for asthma in 16,941 members from a Health Maintenance Organization (HMO) related to the use of ICS, cromolyn, and β-agonists (113). The primary outcome measure was time to the first hospitalization for asthma after dispensing. Dispensing one cromolyn inhaler was associated with a significant decreased RR of hospitalization of 0.8 (95% CI 0.6–0.9) for ages 0 to 17 years but was not protective in adults with RR of 0.8 (95% CI 0.6–1.1) for ages 18 to 44 years and RR of 0.8 (95% CI 0.6–1.3) for ages >45 years. For ICS the overall RR was 0.5 (95% CI 0.4–0.6). Furthermore, the RR for the dispensing of >8 canisters of β-agonists was 4.3 (95% CI 3.1–6.0). This study was limited to one specific HMO and excluded patients on Medicaid/Medicare (113).

Recently a study done by the Severe Asthma Research Committee in Japan compared cromolyn to salbutamol (114). This study investigated 232 children with persistent asthma classified as either severe (64%) or moderate (35%). DSCG (20 mg) nebulized solution mixed with salbutamol was compared to either agent of DSCG and salbutamol alone. The primary outcome measure was the change in daily asthma symptom score.

The combination medication improved this score by 39% when compared to salbutamol and 38% compared to DSCG. Although the individual agents resulted in improvement, the combination was superior.

Similar studies with DSCG and bronchodilators also showed an improvement in asthma symptoms. DSCG powder combined with isoprenaline resulted in a 59% improvement with the combination medication compared to only a 44% improvement with isoprenaline alone (115). A reduction of 33% to 35% in asthma severity classification was observed in 189 patients treated with cromolyn ($p < 0.00005$) (116).

For adult patients there were two critical clinical trials involving cromolyn performed through the Medical Research Council (MRC) and the Drug Committee of the American Academy of Allergy (AAA). The MRC trial involved 103 patients in four groups—cromolyn, isoproterenol, cromolyn and isoproterenol, and placebo—for 12 months (117). After eight weeks, the dose of cromolyn was reduced from 20 mg tid to a twice-daily dosage and finally to a daily dose. At the end of the study no outcome difference was found between patients receiving the full or reduced dosage. Although pivotal, the power of the study to make this observation may be problematic given the low number of subjects and multiple treatment arms.

The AAA trial involved 252 patients comparing cromolyn with placebo in a crossover design over eight weeks (118). The investigators observed a significant treatment effect in 80% of the patients receiving the placebo first.

Blumenthal et al. (119) reported on a group of patients controlled on cromolyn spincaps that were switched to placebo. After four weeks, the patients with worsening asthma were treated with cromolyn or placebo. The patients treated with cromolyn had significant improvement in their daily symptom scores for overall asthma severity and pulmonary function parameter of FVC and PEF when compared to the placebo treated subjects (119).

Ideally, inhaled chromone therapy would reduce the need for oral corticosteroid use in asthma. In an early study, the addition of cromolyn to oral corticosteroids resulted in a 41% reduction in dose after six months and withdrawal of steroids in 25% of patients after 1.5 years (120).

X. Nedocromil for Asthma

As nedocromil is a newer agent when compared to cromolyn and comes in only a single form, there is less information to draw conclusions from. Most of the studies show a beneficial effect of nedocromil when compared to placebo. Children with grass pollen asthma responded better to nedocromil compared to placebo (121). In a study by Konig et al. (122), the use of nedocromil did not prevent viral-induced bronchospasm but did improve their recovery, overall symptoms, and PEFR on nedocromil. A third investigation that compared nedocromil to placebo resulted in an advantage to nedocromil with total symptom score reduction of 50% (123). In addition, significant improvement in daytime and nighttime asthma, morning and evening PEF, and use of rescue bronchodilators was shown with the regular use of nedocromil (124).

Currently there is only one study comparing nedocromil to the use of ICS. Children treated with beclomethasone dipropionate had a significant improvement in nonspecific bronchial hyper-reactivity but no difference in symptom scores, bronchodilator use, or pulmonary function changes (125).

At least three studies have demonstrated beneficial outcomes of pulmonary function improvement, symptom scores, bronchodilator use, and even corticosteroid sparing effect. Foo et al. (126) reported an improvement in FEV_1/FVC when nedocromil was added to ICS in 120 children. In 76 asthmatic adults an improvement in symptoms, bronchodilator use, and PEFR was observed when nedocromil was added to ICS (127). Furthermore, Bone reported a reduction in the dosage of ICS with the use of a nedocromil inhaler in adults (128).

The CAMP study measured several variables related to childhood asthma treatment between four study groups: 311 patients on budesonide compared with 208 patients on placebo, 312 patients on nedocromil compared with 210 patients on placebo (129). The outcome measures included: spirometry, AM/PM peak flows, methacholine challenge, use of study medication, albuterol use, courses of prednisone, physician office visits, ED visits, hospitalizations, and height. Overall the spirometry showed no significant differences in either the budesonide or nedocromil groups. However, there were some exceptions. In the nedocromil group the FVC before bronchodilation was lower than in the placebo group, 0.6 versus 2.4, respectively ($p = 0.02$). In the budesonide group the FEV_1/FVC before bronchodilation was 0.2 versus 1.8 in the placebo group ($p = 0.001$). Four months after discontinuation of the study medication, the nedocromil group had a smaller decrease in the baseline FEV_1/FVC before and after bronchodilation: 1.1 versus 2.5 ($p = 0.01$) and 1.2 versus 2.2 ($p = 0.03$), respectively. The budesonide group had a 43% lower rate of hospitalizations ($p = 0.04$) compared with nedocromil, which showed no significant difference compared to placebo. Urgent visits and prednisone courses were reduced in the budesonide group by 45% ($p < 0.001$) and 43% ($p < 0.001$), respectively. The nedocromil group showed a reduction of 27% ($p = 0.02$) and 16% ($p = 0.01$), respectively, compared to placebo (129).

In 1993, a multistudy analysis of 4723 patients in 127 trials reported that nedocromil was better than placebo in multiple variables: daytime and nighttime asthma symptoms, cough, daily mean PEF, and FEV_1, rescue bronchodilator use, and patient satisfaction (130). This analysis showed a 50% reduction in ICS dose when a higher nedocromil dose was used.

XI. Cromolyn and Nedocromil Comparison Trials

A few studies have compared cromolyn to nedocromil, whereas others have compared cromolyn, nedocromil, and ICS. No differences in PFT could be found in 195 children treated with cromolyn, nedocromil, or ICS (131). Similarly, there were no differences found in efficacy when comparing cromolyn to nedocromil in another paper (132). Review of the Cochrane database also could find no difference in efficacy between DSCG and nedocromil during the post-exercise pulmonary functions in either the maximum percent decrease in FEV_1 or complete protection (133).

An additional study by Lal et al. (134) reported a 50% reduction of ICS dose with the addition of cromolyn or nedocromil in adults. They reported that nedocromil was more effective than cromolyn in symptom control and reduction of bronchodilator use.

Orefice et al. found nedocromil superior in controlling symptoms; however, both cromolyn and nedocromil were effective with decreasing non-specific bronchial hyper-reactivity and the need for rescue bronchodilators (135). Similarly, Altounyan et al. (136) found that nedocromil was more effective against sulfur dioxide challenge, but that there was no difference between cromolyn and nedocromil with protection against inhaled allergen. This suggests that nedocromil may be superior in controlling neuronal-induced mechanisms of bronchospasm when compared to cromolyn. In contrast, another study involving 306 younger, milder allergic asthmatics found the use of cromolyn to produce improved results when compared to nedocromil (137). Exercise-challenge induced bronchospasm was controlled with both of the two chromones and both were more effective than placebo (138).

A comparison of nebulized cromolyn to nebulized nedocromil in children <2 years was conducted in 23 asthmatic children (19/23 males), treated for two months with cromolyn, nedocromil, then placebo. No significant differences in symptom scores between the treatment groups were reported. However, in the cromolyn group there was a trend for older children to respond to cromolyn (16.4 months) versus nedocromil (12.1 months) (139).

Both medications have been used to treat patients with ASA. Robuschi et al. (140) compared nedocromil and DSCG in 10 patients with ASA who were treated with lysine acetylsalicylate. They reported that DSCG and nedocromil use resulted in a maximal decrease in FEV_1 to 20% ± 3% and 18% ± 4%, respectively ($p < 0.01$) during challenge without a significant difference between the two medications (140).

In vitro comparisons of basophil histamine release after stimulation with anti-IgE, anti-IgE + IL-3, and ryegrass allergen showed unexpected findings. Nedocromil augmented histamine release only with ryegrass and cromolyn did not affect histamine release (141).

XII. Cromolyn for Allergic Rhinitis

In recent years, the one airway hypothesis linking disease and therapy in the lung and nose simultaneously suggests a need to briefly review the effect of the chromones on nasal allergy. Intranasal cromolyn is available over the counter as an aqueous preparation topical spray. Several studies have reported that intranasal cromolyn is superior to placebo in the treatment of seasonal allergic rhinitis (SAR) (5). In particular, a decrease in mouth breathing, nasal congestion, rhinorrhea, postnasal drip, and sneezing in 66 patients treated with intranasal cromolyn for ragweed rhinitis was observed (142). Similarly, a decrease in rhinitis symptoms and, in this case, ocular symptoms, was observed in 88 patients treated with cromolyn for pollen-induced SAR (143). A decrease in rhinitis symptoms measured by the average daily rhinitis symptom score resulted in decreased antihistamine use with cromolyn in a small study of 47 patients ($p < 0.01$) (144). Perennial allergic rhinitis symptoms were decreased with cromolyn in a study by Cohan et al. (145). In contrast, two studies showed that intranasal cromolyn was equivalent to placebo (146,147).

Intranasal cromolyn and nedocromil were equivalent in reducing allergic rhinitis symptoms compared to placebo in a study by Schuller et al. involving 233 patients. Overall, rhinitis symptoms were significantly reduced with nedocromil as recorded by the symptom summary card ($p = 0.02$) (148). A comparison of terfenadine, a non-sedating antihistamine, with cromolyn was found to be equivalent (149). Terfenadine was subsequently withdrawn from the market due to cardiac dysrhythmia problems. This study cannot be extrapolated to other antihistamines. This study also showed that cromolyn had a significant reduction in the number of eosinophils ($p = 0.025$) measured by nasal cytology scores, whereas terfenadine patients showed no significant differences.

When cromolyn is compared to nasal corticosteroids, both flunisolide and beclomethasone have shown greater efficacy (150,151). However, both nasal corticosteroids and intranasal cromolyn are more effective than placebo for allergic rhinitis (152).

XIII. Dosing

Cromolyn is available for use in allergic disease and asthma as a single-dose vial for oral nebulization, metered dose inhaler (oral and nasal), and ophthalmic preparation. Oral cromolyn, although poorly absorbed from the GI tract, has been used in the treatment of mastocytosis, chronic idiopathic urticaria, and GI-associated anaphylaxis with anecdotal success.

CS for oral inhalation is available as 1 and 5 mg per actuation MDI, 20 mg 1% aqueous solution, and 20 mg capsules for use with the Spinhaler or E-haler (Eclipse) (7). The 1 mg per actuation MDI and 20 mg 1% aqueous solution are available in the United States.

Intranasal cromolyn is available over the counter as a 4% solution. The recommended dosage is one spray per nostril four times daily.

When cromolyn was first developed it was combined with isoprenaline to prevent the bronchoconstriction associated with the inhalation of the sodium salt (2). The blood levels of cromolyn can be increased by the addition of a β_2-agonist (15). Furthermore, the clinical response of cromolyn is improved with addition of a β_2-agonist (114). In light of the favorable outcomes with ICS compared to cromolyn alone, new research may be needed to compare the use of cromolyn in combination with a β_2-agonist compared to ICS to ascertain the correct circumstances and delivery method in asthma therapy.

Nedocromil sodium is available as a 2 mg MDI. Two studies on the nedocromil dosing frequencies reported no overall difference, but Wells (130) reported that patients in the higher dose frequency required few courses of oral steroids (127,130). The CAMP study evaluated long-term use of nedocromil and reported a reduction in urgent care visits and fewer courses of prednisone (129). However, another study with short-term use of nedocromil reported significant differences compared with placebo (136).

Compliance with medication regimens remains an issue with all patients. Traditionally, inhaled cromolyn is dosed four times daily while nedocromil is dosed twice daily. Furukawa et al. studied the same children on cromolyn four, three, or twice daily for one-month intervals. They reported that pulmonary function during the twice-daily use for a month showed a trend toward deterioration compared with the month of dosing three times daily (153). In a similar study with adults, no difference in those patients allowed to reduce their cromolyn dose (2.5 doses/day) compared to those on four daily doses was seen (154). In general, cromolyn is started four times daily and is often reduced to twice daily when asthma has been controlled. Whether there would be equal efficacy if the same total mg dose was delivered twice daily versus four times daily is unclear.

XIV. Safety

Overall, both oral inhaled cromolyn and nedocromil are well tolerated with minimal side effects. The side effects reported with cromolyn include: throat irritation, cough, nasal congestion, mild bronchospasm, urticaria, angioedema, anaphylaxis, anaphylactoid reaction, and pulmonary infiltration with eosinophilia (PIE), cardiac tamponade and eosinophilia, dysuria, dermatitis, and myositis (155). One patient experienced a near-death exacerbation as he tried to use DSCG during an asthma attack (156).

The adverse effects of intranasal cromolyn include: sneezing, nasal burning or stinging (3). It has been reported that ocular cromolyn can result in contact dermatitis, allergic conjunctivitis, and chemosis (157,158). A 63-year-old male treated with DSCG ophthalmic solution developed allergic conjunctivitis and IgE antibodies to DSCG were demonstrated in serum by RAST (158).

Anti-CS antibodies have been documented by intracutaneous and RAST testing (159–161). Furthermore, Sheffer et al. (162) reported increased lymphocyte proliferation and elevated production of migration inhibition factor in response to cromolyn stimulation and increased serum immunoglobulin G binding of cromolyn in one patient with PIE compared to cromolyn-tolerant patients.

Drug interactions have not been documented with cromolyn. Overall, cromolyn can be used safely in elderly patients with hypertension, heart disease, seizure disorders, or prostate disease. Cromolyn is classified as category B in pregnancy. Patients who will benefit from intranasal cromolyn include: children >2 years, elderly patients, patients with comorbidities, patients reluctant to take medications, patients and athletes who undergo drug monitoring to avoid corticosteroids (3).

In general, nedocromil is well tolerated with a good safety record. On the other hand, nedocromil has been associated with an unpleasant taste, nausea, and vomiting (3).

There has been a concern with growth rate and the use of ICS in children. A recent study compared bone mineral density in children on fluticasone propionate (FP) versus nedocromil for two years (163). No significant difference in growth was observed between the groups; adjusted mean growth rates were 6.1 cm/yr with FP and 5.8 cm/yr with nedocromil (163).

Both cromolyn and nedocromil have no effect on normal host defense, no known teratogenic effects, and do not influence the development of neoplastic disease (164,165). A 10-year follow-up study with cromolyn showed no adverse effects (101).

In summary, both cromolyn and nedocromil can be useful as adjuvant therapy in the treatment of asthma. Their benefits have been seen in a reduction in ED visits and hospitalizations for asthma, and a decrease in allergen/exercise-induced bronchospasm and frequency of prednisone use. Furthermore, cromolyn has been useful in the treatment of allergic rhinitis and allergic conjunctivitis, with occasional use in other systemic diseases.

References

1. Expert Panel Report. Guidelines for the diagnosis and management of asthma—update on selected topics. JACI 2002; 110(5):appendix A1.
2. Edwards AM, Howell JB. The chromones: history, chemistry and clinical development. A tribute to the work of Dr R. E. C. Altounyan. Clin Exp Allergy 2000; 30:756–774.

3. Konig P, Grigg CF. Cromolyn sodium or nedocromil in childhood asthma: does it matter? Clin Exp Allergy 2000; 30:164–171.

4. Edwards AM. Editorial, Optimizing the use of chromones in the management of asthma: attention to detail over delivered dose and method of administration is essential. Clin Exp Allergy 2002; 32:1543–1545.

5. Ratner PH, Ehrlich PM, Fineman SM, Meltzer EO, Skoner DP. Use of intranasal cromolyn sodium for allergic rhinitis. Mayo Clin Proc 2002; 77:350–354.

6. Anrep GV, Kenawy MR, Barsoum GS, Misrahy G. Therapuetic uses of khellin. Lancet 1947; i:557.

7. Edwards, AM, Holgate ST. The Chromones: Cromolyn Sodium and Nedocromil Sodium in Principles and Practice of Allergy. St. Louis: Mosby 2003: 915–927.

8. Church MK, Polosa R, Rimmer SJ. Cromolyn sodium and nedocromil sodium: mast cell stabilizers, neuromodulators, or anti-inflammatory drugs? In: Kaliner MA, Barnes PJ, Persson CG, eds. Pharmacotherapy of Asthma. New York: Marcel Dekker Inc., 1991:561–593.

9. Moss G, Jones K, Ritchie J, Cox S. Plasma levels and urinary excretion of disodium cromoglycate after inhalation by human volunteers. Toxicol Appl Pharmacol 1971; 20:147–156.

10. Neale MG, Brown K, Foulds RA, Lai S, Morris DA, Thomas D. The pharmokinetics of nedocromil sodium, an new drug for the treatment of reversible obstructive airways disease, in human volunteers and patients with reversible obstructive airways disease. Br J Clin Pharmacol 1987; 24:493.

11. Newman SP, Clark AR, Talaee N, Clarke SW. Lung deposition of 5 mg of Intal from a pressurized metered dose inhaler assessed by radiotracer technique. Int J Pharm 1991; 74:203.

12. Newman SP, Clark AR, Talaee N, Clarke SW. Pressurized aerosol deposition in the human lung with and without an "open" spacer device. Thorax 1989; 44:706.

13. Laube BL, Edwards AM, Dalby RN, Creticos PS, Norman PS. The efficacy of slow versus faster inhalation of cromolyn sodium in protecting against allergen challenge in patients with asthma. J Allergy Clin Immunol 1998; 101:475.

14. Kato Y, Muraki K, Fujitaka M, Sakura N, Ueda K. Plasma concentrations of disodium cromoglycate after various inhalation methods in healthy subjects. Br J Clin Pharmacol 1999; 48:154.

15. Aswania O, Chrystyn H. Relative lung bioavailability of generic sodium cromoglycate inhalers used with and without a spacer device. Pulm Pharmacol Ther 2001; 14:129–133.

16. Hirota T. Efficacy and limitations of inhaled antiallergic therapy in asthma. In: Shinomiya K, ed. Current Advances in Pediatric Allergy and Clinical Immunology. Tokyo: Churchill Livingstone, 1996:125–128.

17. Theoharides TC, Sieghart W, Greengard P, Douglas WW. Anti-allergic drug cromolyn may inhibit histamine secretion by regulating phosphorylation of a mast cell protein. Science 1980; 207:80–82.

18. Wells E, Mann J. Phosphorylation of a mast cell protein in response to treatment with anti-allergic compounds: implications for the mode of action of sodium cromoglycate. Biochem Pharmacol 1983; 32:837.

19. Wang L, Correia I, Basu S, Theoharides TC. Ca2+ and phorbol ester effect on the mast cell phosphorylation induced by cromolyn. Eur J of Pharmacol 1999; 371:241–249.

20. Theoharides TC, Wang L, Pang X, Letourneau R, Culm KE, Basu S, Wang Y, Correia I. Cloning and cellular localization of the rat mast cell 78 kDa protein phosphorylated in response to the mast cell "stabilizer" cromolyn. J Pharmacol Exp Ther 2000; 294:810.

21. Pestonjamasp K, Amieva MR, Strassel CP, Nauseef WM, Furthmayr H, Luna EJ. Moesin, ezrin, and p205 are actin-binding proteins associated with neutrophil plasma membranes. Mol Biol Cell 1995; 6:247.

22. Garland LG, Mongar JL. Inhibition by cromoglycate of histamine release from rat Peritoneal mast cells induced by mixtures of dextran, phosphatidylserine and Calcium ions. Br J Pharmacol 1974; 50:137–143.

23. Heinke S, Szucs G, Norris AA, Droogmans G, Nilius B. Inhibition of volume activated chloride currents in endothelial cells by chromones. Br J Pharmacol 1995; 115:1393–1398.

24. Norris AA, Alton EW. Chloride transport and the action of sodium cromoglycate and nedocromil sodium in asthma. Clin Exp Allergy 1996; 26:250.

25. Romanin C, Reinsprecht M, Pecht I, Schindler H. Immunologically activated chloride channels involved in degranulation of rat mucosal cells. EMBO J 1991; 10:3603.

26. Alton EW, Kingsleigh-Smith DJ, Munkonge FM, Smith SN, Lindsay AR, Gruenert DC, Jeffery PK, Norris A, Geddes DM, Williams AJ. Asthma prophylaxis agents alter the function of an airway epithelial chloride channel. Am J Respir Cell Mol Biol 1996; 14:380.

27. Kay AB, Walsh GM, Moqbel R, MacDonald AJ, Nagakura T, Carroll MP, Richerson HB. Disodium cromoglycate inhibits activation of human inflammatory cells in vitro. J Allergy Clin Immunol 1987; 80:1–8.

28. Mazurek N, Schindler H, Schurholz T, Pecht I. The cromolyn binding protein constitutes the Ca^{2+} channel of basophils opening upon immunological stimulus. Proc Natl Acad Sci USA 1984; 81:6841.

29. Tamaoki J, Yamawaki I, Taira M, Nagano Y, Nakata J, Nagai A. Effect of cromolyn on adenosine-induced airway microvascular leakage in sensitized rats. Eur Respir J 1999; 14:1082–1087.

30. Okada M, Itoh H, Hatakeyama T, Tokumitsu H, Kobayashi R. Hsp 90 is a direct target of the anti-allergic drugs disodium cromoglycate and amlexanox. Biochem J 2003; 374:433–441.

31. Klinker JF, Seifert R. Morphine and muscle relaxants are receptor-independent G-protein activators and cromolyn is an inhibitor of stimulated G-protein activity. Inflamm Res 1997; 46:46–50.

32. Mackay GA, Pearce FL. Extracellular guanosine 3'5'-cyclic monophosphate and disodium cromoglycate share a similar spectrum of activity in the inhibition of histamine release from isolated mast cells and basophils. Int Arch of Allergy Immunol 1996; 109:258–265.

33. Sheard P, Blair AM. Disodium cromoglycate: activity in three in vitro models of the immediate hypersensitivity reaction in lung. Int Arch Allergy Appl Immunol 1970; 38:217.

34. Shin, H, Kim J, An N, Park R, Kim H. Effect of disodium cromoglycate on mast cell-mediated immediate type allergic reactions. Life Sci 2004; 74:2877–2887.

35. Leung KB, Flint KC, Brostoff J, Hudspith BN, Johnson NM, Lau HY, Liu WL, Pearce FL. Effects of sodium cromoglycate and nedocromil sodium on histamine secretion from human lung mast cells. Thorax 1988; 43:756.

36. Okayama Y, Benyon RC, Rees PH, Lowman MA, Hillier K, Church MK. Inhibition profiles of sodium cromoglycate and nedocromil sodium on mediator release from mast cells of human skin, lung, tonsil, adenoid and intestine. Clin Exp Allergy 1992; 22:401.

37. Bissonnette EY, Enciso JA, Befus AD. Inhibition of tumor necrosis factor-alpha (TNF-α) release from mast cells by the anti-inflammatory drugs, sodium cromoglycate and nedocromil sodium. Clin Exp Immunol 1995; 102:78.

38. Moqbel R, Cromwell O, Walsh GM, Wardlaw AJ, Kurlak L, Kay AB. Effects of nedocromil sodium (Tilade) on the activation of human eosinophils and neutrophils and the release of histamine from mast cells. Allergy 1988; 43:268.

39. Kimata H, Yoshida A, Ishioka C, Mikawa H. Disodium cromoglycate (DSCG) selectively inhibits IgE production and enhances IgG4 production by human B cell in vitro. Clin Exp Immunol 1991; 84:395.

40. Kimata H, Mikawa H. Nedocromil sodium selectively inhibits IgE and IgG4 production in human B cells stimulated with IL-4. J Immunol 1993; 151:6723.

41. Loh RK, Jabara HH, Geha RS. Disodium cromoglycate inhibits $S\mu \rightarrow S\varepsilon$ deletional switch recombination and IgE synthesis in human B cells. J Exp Med 1994; 180:663.

42. Loh RK, Jabara HH, Geha RS. Mechanisms of inhibition of IgE synthesis by nedocromil sodium: nedocromil sodium inhibits deletional switch recombination in human B cells. J Allergy Clin Immunol 1996; 97:1141.

43. Matsuse H, Shimoda T, Matsuo N, Obase Y, Fukushima C, Asai S, Kohno S. Sodium cromoglycate inhibits antigen induced cytokine production by peripheral blood mononuclear cells from atopic asthmatics in vitro. Ann Allergy Asthma Immunol 1999; 83:511.

44. Oh JW, Lee HB, Chung YH, Choi Y. The effect of disodium cromoglycate, budesonide, and cyclosporine A on interleukin-4, interleukin-5, and interleukin-secretions in Der p I-stimulated T cells from house dust mite sensitive atopic and nonatopic individuals. Allergy Asthma Proc 2002; 23:109–115.

45. Matsuo N, Shimoda T, Matsuse H, Obase Y, Asai S, Kohno S. Effects of sodium cromoglycate on cytokine production following antigen stimulation of a passively sensitized human lung model. Ann Allergy Immunol 2000; 84:72–78.

46. Larsson K, Larsson BM, Sandstrom T, Sundblad BM, Palmberg L. Sodium cromoglycate attenuates pulmonary inflammation without influencing bronchial responsiveness in health subjects exposed to organic dust. Clin Exp Allergy 2001; 31:1356.

47. Viscardi RM, Hasday JD, Gumpper KF, Taciak V, Campbell AB, Palmer TW. Cromolyn sodium prophylaxis inhibits pulmonary proinflammatory cytokines in infants at high risk for bronchopulmonary dysplasia. Am J Respir Crit Care Med 1997; 156:1523.

48. Kennedy MC. Disodium cromoglycate in the control of asthma: a double-blind trial. B J Dis Chest 1969; 63:96.

49. Hoshino M, Nakamura Y. The effect of inhaled sodium cromoglycate on cellular infiltration into the bronchial mucosa and the expression of adhesion molecules in asthmatics. Eur Respir J 1997; 10:858.

50. Amayasu H, Nakabayashi M, Akahori K, Ishizaki Y, Shoji T, Nakagawa H, Hasegawa H, Yoshida S. Cromolyn sodium suppresses eosinophilic inflammation in patients with aspirin-intolerant asthma. Ann Allergy Immunol 2001; 87:146–150.

51. Bruijnzeel PL, Hamelink ML, Kok PT, Kreukniet J. Nedocromil sodium inhibits the A23187 and opsonized zymosan-induced leukotriene formation by human eosinophils but not by human neutrophils. Br J Pharmacol 1989; 96:631.

52. Sadeghi-Hashjin G, Nijkamp FP, Henricks PA, Folkerts G. Sodium cromoglycate and doxantrazole are oxygen radical scavengers. Eur Respir J 2002; 20:867–872.

53. Eleno N, Gajate E, Macias J, Garay RP. Enhancement by reproterol of the ability of disodium cromoglycate to stabilize rat mastocytes. Pulm Pharmacol Therapeut 1999; 12:55–60.

54. Spry CJF, Kumaraswami V, Tai PC. The effect of nedocromil sodium on secretion from human eosinophils. Eur J Respir Dis 1986; 69:241.

55. Joseph M, Capron A, Thorel T, Tonnel AB. Nedocromil sodium inhibits IgE-dependent activation of rat macrophages and platelets as measured by schistosome killing, chemiluminescence and enzyme release. Eur J Respir Dis 1986; 147:220–222.

56. Thorel T, Joseph M, Tsicopoulos A, Tonnel AB, Capron A. Inhibition by nedocromil sodium of IgE-mediated activation of human mononuclear phagocytes and platelets in Allergy. Int Arch Allergy Appl Immunol 1988; 85:232–237.

57. Bruijnzeel PL, Warringa RA, Kok PT, Kreukniet J. Inhibition of neutrophil and eosinophil induced chemotaxis by nedocromil sodium and sodium cromoglycate. Br J Pharmacol 1990; 99:798.

58. Calhoun, WJ, Jarjour, NN, Gleich, GJ, Schwartz, LB, Busse, WW. Effects of nedocromil sodium pretreatment on the immediate and late responses of the airway to segmental antigen challenge. J Allergy Clin Immunol 1996; 98:S46.

59. Manolitsas, ND, Wang, J, Devalia, JL, Trigg, CJ, McAulay, AE, Davies, RJ. Regular albuterol, nedocromil sodium, and bronchial inflammation in asthma. Am J Respir Crit Care Med 1995; 151:1925.

60. Dixon CM, Ind PW. Inhaled sodium metabisulphite-induced bronchoconstriction: inhibition by nedocromil sodium and sodium cromoglycate. Br J Clin Pharmacol 1990; 30:371.

61. Boushey, HA, Richardson, PS, Widdicombe, JG, Wise, JC. The response of laryngeal afferent fibres in mechanical and chemical stimuli. J Physiol 1974; 240:153–175.

62. Jackson DM, Eady RP. Acute transient SO2-induced airway hyperreactivity: effects of nedocromil sodium. J Appl Physiol 1988; 65:1119–1124.

63. Dixon CM, Barnes PJ. Bradykinin-induced bronchoconstriction inhibition by nedocromil sodium and sodium cromoglycate. Br J Clin Pharmacol 1989; 27:831.

64. Dixon M, Jackson DM, Richards IM. The action of sodium cromoglycate on "C" fibre endings in the dog lung. Br J Pharmacol 1980; 70:11.

65. Chatterjee PC, Fyans PG, Chatterjee SS. A trial comparing nedocromil sodium (Tilade) and placebo in the management of perennial bronchial asthma. Eur J Respir Dis 1986; 69:314–316.

66. Hargreaves M. Sodium cromoglycate: a remedy for ACE inhibitor-induced cough. Br J Clin Pract 1993; 47:319.

67. Louis RE, Radermecker MF. Substance P-induced histamine release from human basophils, skin and lung fragments: effect of nedocromil sodium and theophylline. Int Arch Allergy Appl Immunol 1990; 92:329.

68. Allen TL, Gora-Harper ML. Cromolyn Sodium for ACE Inhibitor-Induced Cough. Ann Pharm 1997; 31:773–775.

69. Hargreaves MR, Benson MK. Inhaled sodium cromoglycate in angiotensin converting enzyme inhibitor cough. Lancet 1995; 345:13–16.

70. Puolijoki H, Rekiaro M, Cleland JG. Lack of effect of nedocromil sodium in ACE inhibitor induced cough. Lancet 1995; 345:394–395.

71. Jackson DM, Richards IM. The effects of sodium cromoglycate on histamine aerosol-induced reflex bronchoconstriction in the anesthetized dog. Br J Pharmacol 1977; 61:257.

72. Jackson DM. The effects of nedocromil sodium, sodium cromoglycate and codeine phosphate on citric acid-induced cough in dogs. Br J Pharmacol 1988; 93:609–612.

73. Lowry RH, Higenbottam TW. Antitussive effect of nedocromil sodium on chemically induced cough. Thorax 1988; 43:256.

74. Yamawaki I, Tamaoki J, Takeda Y, Nagai A. Inhaled cromoglycate reduces airway neurogenic inflammation via tachykinin antagonism. Res Com Mol Path Pharmacol 1997; 98:265–272.

75. Konig P, Jordvik NL, Kreutz C. The preventive effect and duration of action of nedocromil sodium and cromolyn sodium on exercise-induced asthma (EIA) in adults. J Allergy Clin Immunol 1987; 79:64–68.

76. de Benedictis FM, Tuteri G, Pazzelli P, Bertotto A, Bruni L, Vaccaro R. Cromolyn versus nedocromil: duration of action in exercise-induced asthma in children. J Allergy Clin Immunol 1995; 96:510–514.

77. Juniper EF, Kline PA, Morris MM, Hargreaves FE. Airway constriction by isocapnic hyperventilation of cold, dry air: comparison of magnitude and duration of protection by nedocromil sodium and sodium cromoglycate. Clin Allergy 1987; 17:523–528.

78. Crimi N, Palermo F, Oliveri R, Vancheri C, Palermo B, Polosa R, Mistretta A. Bronchospasm induced by inhalation of substance P: effect of sodium cromoglycate. Respiration 1988; 54(suppl 1):95.

79. Crimi N, Palermo F, Oliveri R, Vancheri C, Palermo B, Polosa R, Mistretta A. Protection of nedocromil sodium on bronchoconstriction induced by inhaled neurokinin A (NKA) in asthmatic patients. Clin Exp Allergy 1992; 22:75.

80. Richards R, Phillips GD, Holgate ST. Nedocromil sodium is more potent than sodium cromoglycate against AMP-induced bronchoconstriction in atopic asthmatic subjects. Clin Exp Allergy 1989; 19:285.

81. Anderson SD, du Toit JI, Rodwell LT, Jenkins CR. Acute effect of sodium cromoglycate in airway narrowing induced by 4.5 percent saline aerosol: outcome before and during treatment with aerosol corticosteroids in patients with asthma. Chest 1994; 105:673.

82. Rodwell LT, Anderson SD, Du Toit J, Seale JP. Nedocromil sodium inhibits the airway response to hyperosmolar challenge in patients with asthma. Am Rev Respir Dis 1992; 146:1149.

83. Altounyan RE. Review of clinical activity and mode of action of sodium cromoglycate. Clin Allergy 1980; 10(suppl):481.

84. Pelikan Z, Knottnerus I. Inhibition of the late asthmatic response by nedocromil sodium administered more than two hours after allergen challenge. J Allergy Clin Immunol 1993; 92:19.

85. Tullett WM, Tan KM, Wall RT, Patel KR. Dose-response effect of sodium cromoglycate pressurized aerosol in exercise induced asthma. Thorax 1985; 40:41.

86. Storm van's Gravesande K, Mattes J, Grossklauss E, Zurmuhl A, Moseler M, Kuhr J. Preventive effect of 2 and 10 mg of sodium cromoglycate on exercise-induced bronchoconstriction. Eur J Pediatr 2000; 159:759.

87. Schoeffel RE, Anderson SD, Lindsay DA. Sodium cromoglycate as a pressurized aerosol (Vicrom) in exercise-induced asthma. Aust NZ J Med 1983; 13:157.

88. Francis RS, McEnery G. Disodium cromoglycate compared with beclomethasone dipropionate in juvenile asthma. Clin Allergy 1984; 14:537–540.

89. Sarsfield JK, Sugden E. A comparative study of betamethasone valerate aerosol and sodium cromoglycate in children with severe asthma. Practioner 1977; 218:128–132.

90. Hiller EJ, Milner AD. Betamethasone 17-valerate aerosol and disodium cromoglycate in severe childhood asthma. Br J Dis Chest 1975; 69:103–106.

91. Mitchell I, Patterson IC, Cameron SJ, Grant IWB. Treatment of childhood asthma with sodium cromoglycate and beclomethasone dipropionate aerosol singly and in combination. Br Med J 1976; 2:457–458.

92. Shapiro GG, Sharpe M, DeRouen TA, Pierson WE, Furukawa CT, Virant FS, Bierman CW. Cromolyn versus triamcinolone acetonide for youngsters with moderate asthma. J Allergy Clin Immunol 1991; 88:742–748.

93. Petersen W, Karup-Pedersen F, Friis B, Howitz P, Nielsen F, Stromquist LH. Sodium cromoglycate as a replacement for inhaled corticosteroids in mild-to-moderate childhood asthma. Allergy 1996; 51:870–875.

94. Ng SH, Dash CH, Savage SJ. Betamethasone valerate compared with sodium cromoglycate in asthmatic children. Postgrad Med J 1977; 53:315–320.

95. Price JF, Weller PH. Comparison of fluticasone propionate and sodium cromoglycate for the treatment of childhood asthma (an open parallel group study). Respir Med 1995; 89:363–368.

96. Toogood JH, Jennings B, Lefcoe NM. A clinical trial of combined cromolyn / beclomethasone treatment for chronic asthma. J Allergy Clin Immunol 1981; 67:317–324.

97. Tasche, MJ, Uijen, JH, Bernsen, RM, de Jongste, JC, van der Wouden, JC. Inhaled disodium cromoglycate (DSCG) as maintenance therapy in children with asthma: a systematic review. Thorax 2000; 55:913.

98. Tasche MJ, van der Wouden JC, Uijen JH, Ponsioen BP, Bernsen RM, van Suijlekom-Smit LW, de Jongste JC. Randomised placebo-controlled trial of inhaled sodium cromoglycate in 1–4-year-old children with moderate asthma. Lancet 1997; 350:1060.

99. van der Wouden JC, Tasche MJ, Bernsen RM, Uijen JH, de Jongste JC, Ducharme FM. Inhaled sodium cromoglycate for asthma in children. Cochrane Data Sys Rev 2004; 2.

100. Godfrey S, Balfour-Lynn L, Konig P. The place of cromolyn sodium in the long-term management of childhood asthma based on a 3- to 5-year follow-up. J Pediatr 1975; 87:465.

101. Dickson W, Cole M. Severe asthma in children: a 10 year follow-up. In: Pepys J, Edwards AM, eds. The Mast Cell: Its Role in Health and Disease. London: Pitman Medical, 1979:343.

102. Konig P, Shaffer J. The effect of drug therapy on long-term outcome of childhood asthma: a possible preview of the international guidelines. J Allergy Clin Immunol 1996; 98(6):1103–1111.

103. Konig P. Evidence for benefits of early intervention with non-steroidal drugs in asthma. Pediatr Pulm 1997; 15:34–39.

104. Korppi M, Remes K. Asthma treatment in school children: lung function in different therapeutic groups. Acta Paediatr 1996; 85:190–194.

105. De Baets F, Van Daele S, Franckx H, Vinaimont F. Inhaled steroids compared with disodium cromoglycate in preschool children with episodic viral wheeze. Pediatr Pulm 1998; 25:361.

106. Geller-Bernstein C, Levin S. Nebulized sodium cromoglycate in the treatment of wheezy bronchitis in infants and young children. Respiration 1982; 43: 294–298.

107. Furfaro S, Spier S, Drblik SP, Turgeon JP, Robert M. Efficacy of cromoglycate in persistently wheezing infants. Arch Dis Child 1994; 71: 331–334.

108. Henry RL, Hiller EJ, Milner AD, Hodges IGC, Stokes GM. Nebulized ipratropium bromide and sodium cromoglycate in the first two years of life. Arch Dis Child 1984; 59:54–57.

109. Yuksel B, Greenough A. The effect of sodium cromoglycate on upper and lower respiratory symptoms in children born prematurely. Eur J Pediatr 1993; 152:615–618.

110. Ng GY, Ohlsson A. Cromolyn sodium for the prevention of chronic lung disease in preterm infants. Cochrane Data Sys Rev 2005, 3.

111. Reijonen T, Korppi M, Kuikka L, Remes K. Anti-inflammatory therapy reduces wheezing after bronchiolitis. Arch Pediatr Adolesc Med 1996; 150: 512–517.

112. Adams RJ, Fuhlbrigge A, Finkelstein JA, Lozano P, Livingston JM, Weiss KB, Weiss ST. Impact of inhaled anti-inflammatory therapy on hospitalization and emergency department visits for children with asthma. Pediatrics 2001; 107:706–711.

113. Donahue JG, Weiss ST, Livingston JM, Goetsch MA, Greineder DK, Platt R. Inhaled steroids and the risk of hospitalization for asthma. JAMA 1997; 277:887–891.

114. Furusho K, Nishikawa K, Sasaki S, Akasaka T, Arita M, Edwards A. The combination of nebulized sodium cromoglycate and salbutamol in the treatment of moderate-to severe asthma in children. Pediatr Allergy Immunol 2002; 13:209–216.

115. Silverman M, Connolly NM, Balfour-Lynn L, Godfrey S. Long-term trial of disodium cromoglycate and isoprenaline in children with asthma. Br Med J 1972; 3:378–381.

116. Berman BA, Fenton MM, Girsch LS, Haddad ZH, Sellars WA, Strem EL, Thompson HC, Wall LE. Cromolyn sodium in the treatment of children with severe, perennial asthma. Pediatrics 1975; 55(5):621–629.

117. Long-term study of disodium cromoglycate in treatment of severe extrinsic or intrinsic bronchial asthma in adults. Brompton hospital-medical research council collaborative trial. Br Med J 1972; 4:383.

118. Bernstein IL, Siegel SC, Brandon ML, Brown EB, Evans RR, Feinberg AR, Friedlaender S, Krumholz RA, Hadley RA, Handelman NI, Thurston D, Yamate M. A controlled study of cromolyn sodium sponsored by the Drug Committee of the American Academy of Allergy. J Allergy Clin Immunol 1972; 50:235.

119. Blumenthal MN, Selcow J, Spector S, Zeiger RS, Mellon M. A multicenter evaluation of the clinical benefits of cromolyn sodium aerosol by metered-dose inhaler in the treatment of asthma. J Allergy Clin Immunol 1988; 81:681.

120. Engstrom I, Kraepelien S. The corticosteroid sparing effect of sodium cromoglycate in children and adolescents with bronchial asthma. Acta Allergol 1971; 26:90–100.

121. Businco L, Cantani A, Di Fazio A, Bernardini L. A double-blind, placebo-controlled study to assess the efficacy of nedocromil sodium in the management of childhood grass-pollen asthma. Clin Exp Allergy 1990; 20(6): 683–638.

122. Konig P, Eigen H, Ellis MH, Ellis E, Blake K, Geller D, Shapiro G, Welch M, Scott C. The effect of nedocromil sodium on childhood asthma during the viral season. Am J Respir Crit Care Med 1995; 152:1879–1886.

123. Armenio L, Baldini G, Bardare M, Boner A, Burgio R, Cavagni G, La Rosa M, Marcucci F, Miraglia del Giudice M, Pulejo MR. Double blind, placebo controlled study of nedocromil sodium in asthma. Arch Dis Child 1993; 66:193.

124. Edwards AM, Lyons J, Weinberg E, Weinberg F, Gillies JD, Reid G, Robertson CF, Robinson P, Dalton M, Van Asperen P, Wilson C, Mullineux J, Mullineux A, Sly PD, Cox M, Isles AF. Early use of inhaled nedocromil sodium in children following an acute episode of asthma. Thorax 1999; 54:308.

125. Capristo AF, Miraglia del Guidice M, Alfaro C, Maiello N. Corticosteroid-sparing effect of cromoglycate sodium and nedocromil. Med Inflam 1994; 3:S25–S30.

126. Foo AL, Lanteri CJ, Burton PR, Sly PD. The effect of nedocromil sodium on histamine responsiveness in clinically stable asthmatic children. J Asthma 1993; 30:381–390.

127. Wells A, Drennan C, Holst P, Jones D, Rea H, Thornley P. Comparison of nedocromil sodium at two dosage frequencies vs. placebo in the management of chronic asthma. Respir Med 1992; 86:311–316.

128. Bone MF, Kubik MM, Keaney NP, Summers GD, Connolly CK, Burge PS, Dent RG, Allan GW. Nedocromil sodium in adults with asthma dependent on inhaled corticosteroids: a double-blind placebo controlled study. Thorax 1989; 44:654–659.

129. Childhood Asthma Management Program Research Group. Long-term Effects of Budesonide or Nedocromil in Children with Asthma, NEJM 2000; 343:1054–1062.

130. Edwards AM, Stevens MT. The clinical efficacy of inhaled nedocromil sodium (Tilade®) in the treatment of asthma. Eur Respir J 1993; 6:35.

131. Korhonen L, Korppi M, Remes ST, Reijonen TM, Remes K. Lung function in school aged asthmatic children: with inhaled cromoglycate, nedocromil and corticosteroid therapy. Eur Respir J 1999; 13:82–86.

132. Hakim EA, Hide D, Kuzemko J. Can nedocromil sodium substitute for sodium cromoglycate in children with asthma? Eur Respir J Supplement 1994; 18:139S.

133. Kelly K, Spooner CH, Rowe BH. Nedocromil sodium versus sodium cromoglycate for preventing exercise-induced bronchoconstriction in asthmatics. Cochrane Data Sys Rev 2005, 3.

134. Lal S, Dorow PD, Venho KK, Chatterjee SS. Nedocromil is more effective than cromolyn sodium for the treatment of chronic reversible obstructive airway disease. Chest 1993; 104:438–447.

135. Orefice U, Struzzo P, Dorigo R, Peratoner A. Long-term treatment with sodium cromoglycate, nedocromil sodium and beclomethasone dipropionate reduces bronchial hyperresponsiveness in asthmatic subjects. Respiration 1992; 59(2):97–101.

136. Novembre E, Frongia GF, Veneruso G, Vierucci A. Evaluation of the efficacy of nedocromil sodium in clinical pharmacological models of asthma. Atem Lungen 1986; 12:1593.

137. Schwartz HJ, Blumenthal M, Brady R, Braun S, Lockey R, Myers D, Mansfield L, Mullarkey M, Owens G, Ratner P, Repsher L, van As A. A comparative study on the clinical efficacy of nedocromil sodium and placebo: How does cromolyn sodium compare as an active control treatment? Chest 1996; 109:945–952.

138. Novembre E, Frongia GF, Veneruso G, Vierucci A. Inhibition of exercise-induced asthma (EIA) by nedocromil sodium and sodium cromoglycate in children. Pediatr Allergy Immunol 1994; 5:107.

139. Henry RL, Hiller EJ, Milner AD, Hodges IG, Stokes GM. Nebulized ipratropium bromide and sodium cromoglycate in the first two years of life. Arch Dis Child 1984; 59:54–57.

140. Robuschi M, Gambaro G, Sestini P, Pieroni MG, Refini RM, Vaghi A, Bianco S. Attenuation of aspirin-induced bronchoconstriction by sodium

cromoglycate and nedocromil sodium. Am J Respir Crit Care Med 1997; 155: 1461–1464.

141. Kivity S, Agami O, Topilsky M, Fireman E. Effect of nedocromil and cromolyn sodium on atopic basophil function. Int J Immunopharm 1996; 18:75–78.

142. Welsh PW, Yunginger JW, Kern EB, Gleich GJ. Preseasonal IgE ragweed antibody level as a predictor of response to therapy of ragweed hay fever with intranasal cromolyn sodium solution. J Allergy Clin Immunol 1977; 60: 104–109.

143. Handelman NI, Friday GA, Schwartz HJ, Kuhn FS, Lindsay DE, Koors PG, Moyer RP, Smith CS, Kemper CF, Nagel JR, Rosch J, Murphey S, Miller DL. Cromolyn sodium nasal solution in the prophylactic treatment of pollen-induced seasonal allergic rhinitis. J Allergy Clin Immunol 1977; 59:237–242.

144. Chandra RK, Heresi G, Woodford G. Double-blind controlled crossover trial of 4% intranasal sodium cromoglycate solution in patients with seasonal allergic rhinitis. Ann Allergy 1982; 49:131–134.

145. Cohan RH, Bloom FL, Rhoades RB, Wittig HJ, Haugh LD. Treatment of perennial allergic rhinitis with cromolyn sodium: double-blind study on 34 adult patients. J Allergy Clin Immunol 1976; 58(1 pt 2):121–128.

146. Craig S, Rubinstein E, Reisman RE, Arbesman CE. Sodium cromolyn nasal solution for the treatment of seasonal ragweed hay fever (abstract). J Allergy Clin Immunol 1976; 57:240–241 [abst 126].

147. Posey WC, Nelson HS. Controlled trials with four per cent cromolyn spray in seasonal allergic rhinitis. Clin Allergy 1977; 7:485–496.

148. Schuller DE, Selcow JE, Joos TH, Hannaway PJ, Hirsch SR, Schwartz HJ, Filley WV, Fink JN. A multicenter trial of nedocromil sodium, 1% nasal solution, compared with cromolyn sodium and placebo in ragweed seasonal allergic rhinitis. J Allergy Clin Immunol 1990; 86(4 pt 1):554–561..

149. Orgel HA, Meltzer EO, Kemp JP, Ostrom NK, Welch MJ. Comparison of intranasal cromolyn sodium 4%, and oral terfenadine for allergic rhinitis: childhood grass-pollen asthma. Clin Exp Allergy 1990; 20:683–688.

150. Reed CE, Marcoux JP, Welsh PW. Effects of topical nasal treatment on asthma symptoms. J Allergy Clin Immunol 1988; 81(5 pt 2):1042–1047.

151. Welsh PW, Stricker WE, Chu CP, Naessens JM, Reese ME, Reed CE, Marcoux JP. Superiority of beclomethasone over cromolyn in the self-treatment of seasonal allergic rhinitis (abstract). Pharmacotherapy 1998; 18:1165 [abst 174].

152. Welsh PW, Stricker WE, Chu CP, Naessens JM, Reese ME, Reed CE, Marcoux JP. Efficacy of beclomethasone nasal solution, flunisolide, and cromolyn in relieving symptoms of ragweed allergy. Mayo Clin Proc 1987; 62:125–134.

153. Furukawa CT, Shapiro GG, Bierman CW, Kraemer MJ, Ward DJ, Pierson WE. A double-blind study comparing the effectiveness of cromolyn sodium and sustained-release theophylline in childhood asthma. Pediatrics 1984; 74:453–459.

154. Turner-Warwick M, Batten JC. Brompton Hospital/Medical Research Council participants. Long-term study of disodium cromoglycate in treatment of severe extrinsic or intrinsic bronchial asthma in adults. Br Med J 1972; 4: 383–388.

155. Lester MR, Bratton DL. Adverse reactions to cromolyn sodium: patient report and review of the literature. Clin Ped 1997; 36:707–710.

156. Katayama H, Yokoyama A, Fujino S, Kondo K, Abe M, Nishida W, Kohara K, Kohno N, Hiwada K. Near-death asthmatic reaction induced by disodium cromoglycate. Int Med 1996; 35:967–968.

157. Camarasa JG, Serra-Baldrich E, Monreal P, Soller J. Contact dermatitis from sodium-cromoglycate-containing eye drops. Cont Derm 1997; 36: 160–161.

158. Valdivieso R, Subiza J, Varela-Losada S, Subiza JL, Narganes MJ, Cabrera M, Serrano L. Severe allergic conjunctivitis and chemosis caused by disodium cromoglycate. J Invest Allergo Clin Immunol 1998; 8:58–60.

159. Menon M, Das A. Asthma and urticaria during disodium cromoglycate treatment: a case report. Scand J Resp Dis 1977; 58:145–150.

160. Wass U, Plaschke P, Bjorkander J, Belin L. Assay of specific IgE antibodies to disodium cromoglycate in serum from a patient with an immediate hypersensitivity reaction. J Allergy Clin Immunol 1988; 81:750–757.

161. Ibanez M, Laso T, Martinez-San IM, Alonso E. Anaphylaxis to disodium cromoglycate. Ann Allergy Asthma Immunol 1996; 77:185–186.

162. Sheffer A, Rocklin R, Goetzl E. Immunologic components of hypersensitivity reactions to cromolyn sodium. N Engl J Med 1975; 293:1220–1224.

163. Roux C, Kolta S, Desfougeres JL, Minini P, Bidat E. Long-term safety of fluticasone propionate and nedocromil sodium on bone in children with asthma. Pediatrics 2003; 111:1427 [abstr].

164. Cox JS, Beach JE, Blair AM, Clarke AJ, King J, Lee TB, Loveday DE, Moss GF, Orr TS, Ritchie JT, Sheard P. Disodium cromoglycate (Intal®). Adv Drug Res 1970; 5:115.

165. Clark B. General pharmacology, pharmokinetics, and toxicology of nedocromil sodium. J Allergy Clin Immunol 1993; 92:200.

166. Borish L, Williams J, Johnson S, Mascali JJ, Miller R, Rosenwasser LJ. Anti-inflammatory effects of nedocromil sodium: inhibition of alveolar macrophage function. Clin Exp Allergy 1992; 22:984.

167. Resler B, Sedgwick JB, Busse WW. Inhibition of interleukin-5 effects on human eosinophils by nedocromil sodium. J Allergy Clin Immunol 1992; 89:235.

168. Devalia JL, Sapsford RJ, Rusznak C, Toumbis MJ, Davies RJ. The effect of human eosinophils on cultured human nasal epithelial cell activity and the influence of nedocromil sodium in vitro. Am J Respir Cell Mol Biol 1992; 7:270.

169. Rusznak C, Devalia JL, Sapsford RJ, Davies RJ. Ozone-induced mediator release from human bronchial epithelial cells in vitro and the influence of nedocromil sodium. Eur Resp J 1996; 9:2298.

170. Marini M, Soloperto M, Zheng Y, Mezzetti M, Mattoli S. Protective effect of nedocromil sodium on the IL-1 induced release of GM-CSF from cultured human bronchial epithelial cells. Pulm Pharmacol 1992; 5:61.

171. Vittori E, Sciacca F, Colotta F, Mantovani A, Mattoli S. Protective effect of nedocromil sodium on the interleukin-1-induced production of interleukin-8 in human bronchial epithelial cells. J Allergy Clin Immunol 1992; 90:76.

172. Vignola AM, Chanez P, Lacoste P, Campbell AM, Norris A, Michel FB, Bousquet J, Godard P. Nedocromil modulates the histamine induced expression of ICAM-1 and HLA-DR molecules on human bronchial epithelial cells. Am Rev Resp Dis 1993; 147:A45.

173. Marquette CH, Joseph M, Tonnel AB, Vorng H, Lassalle P, Tsicopoulos A, Capron A. The Abnormal in vitro response to aspirin of platelets from aspirin-sensitive asthmatics is inhibited after inhalation of nedocromil sodium but not of sodium cromoglycate. Br J Clin Pharmacol 1990; 29:525.

174. Yoshida S, Amayasu H, Sakamoto H, Onuma K, Shoji T, Nakagawa H, Tajima T. Cromolyn sodium prevents bronchoconstriction and urinary LTE_4 excretion in aspirin-induced asthma. Ann Allergy Asthma Immunol 1998; 80:171.

175. Roth M, Soler M, Lefkowitz H, Emmons LR, Anstine D, Hornung M, Perruchoud AP. Inhibition of receptor-mediated platelet activation by nedocromil sodium. J Allergy Clin Immunol 1993; 91:1217.

176. Moqbel R, Walsh GM, Macdonald AJ, Kay B. Effect of disodium cromoglycate on activation of human eosinophils and neutrophils following reversed (anti-IgE) anaphylaxis. Clin Allergy 1986; 16:73.

177. Bruijnzeel PL, Warringa RA, Kok PT. Inhibition of platelet activating factor and zymosan-activated serum-induced chemotaxis of human neutrophils by nedocromil sodium, BN 52021 and sodium cromoglycate. Br J Pharmacol 1989; 97:1251.

178. Rubin RP. On the mode of action of the anti-asthmatic drug nedocromil sodium on neutrophil function. Einstein Q J Biol Med 1991; 9:1251.

179. White MV, Phillips RL, Kaliner MA. Neutrophils and mast cells: nedocromil sodium inhibits the generation of neutrophil-derived histamine-releasing activity (HRA-N). J Allergy Clin Immunol 1991; 87:812.

180. Mekori YA, Baram D, Goldberg A, Hershkoviz R, Reshef T, Sredni D. Nedocromil sodium inhibits T-cell function in vitro and in vivo. J Allergy Clin Immunol 1993; 91:817.

8

Systemic Corticosteroids in Asthma

RUTH H. GREEN and ANDREW J. WARDLAW

Department of Respiratory Medicine and Thoracic Surgery, Institute for Lung Health, Glenfield Hospital
Leicester, U.K.

I. Introduction

The vast majority of patients achieve adequate asthma control with regular inhaled corticosteroids and bronchodilators. A subgroup will require additional therapy or combinations of treatment, but a small percentage of patients have refractory disease with poorly controlled symptoms, recurrent exacerbations, and/or persistent airflow obstruction despite such treatment (1). The regular use of systemic corticosteroids may be required to achieve improvements in asthma control in these patients. Additionally, systemic corticosteroids remain the treatment of choice for the management of acute severe exacerbations of asthma. This chapter will discuss the pharmacology and mechanisms of action of systemic corticosteroids, review the evidence for their clinical effectiveness and adverse effects, and offer recommendations for their use in asthma.

II. Review of Pharmacology

A. Chemical Structure

The basic chemical structure of systemically active corticosteroids is given
in Figure 1. A number of different preparations are available but all contain
the key features of a double-carbon chain and hydroxyl group at carbon 17,
methyl groups at carbons 18 and 19, ketones at carbons 3 and 20, a double
bond between carbons 4 and 5, and a hydroxyl group at carbon 11 (Fig. 1).
Modifications to this basic chemical structure alter the half-life and relative
potency of the molecule (Table 1).

B. Pharmacokinetics and Pharmacodynamics

Corticosteroids are highly lipophilic molecules that are generally well
absorbed from the gastrointestinal tract, resulting in systemic bioavailability
of 50% to 90% in healthy controls (2) and in patients with asthma, even in
those with a poor clinical response to treatment (3). Enteric-coated prednisolone tablets were developed in the 1950s in an attempt to minimize the
incidence of gastric ulceration and irritation seen with prednisolone by releasing the active corticosteroid molecule in the lower gastrointestinal tract (4).

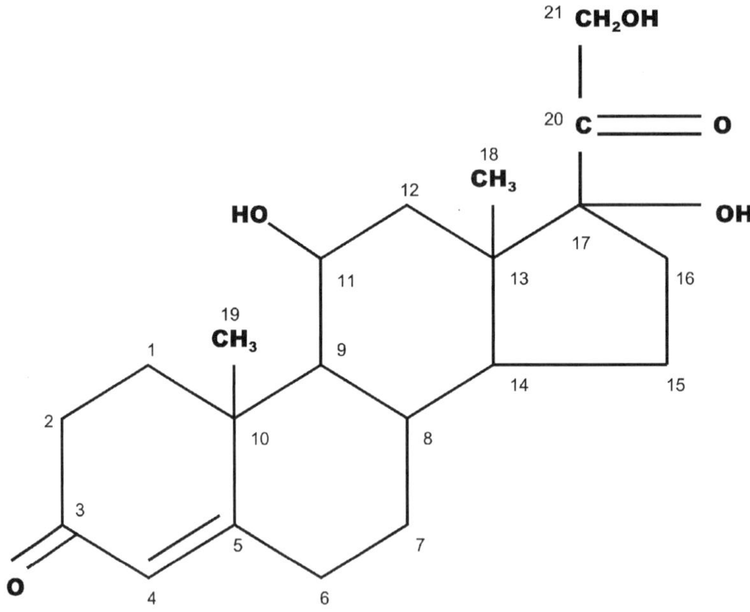

Figure 1   Chemical structure of hydrocortisone (cortisol) demonstrating the features common to all glucocorticoid molecules.

Table 1 Common Systemic Corticosteroids: Modifications to Basic Corticosteroid Structure and Relative Potencies

Drug	Modifications	Relative potency
Hydrocortisone	—	1
Prednisolone	Double bond between carbons 1 and 2	4
Methylprednisolone	Double bond between carbons 1 and 2 Methyl group at carbon 6	5
Dexamethasone	Double bond between carbons 1 and 2 Flourination of carbon 9 Methyl group at carbon 16	30
Triamcinolone	Double bond between carbons 1 and 2 Flourination of carbon 9 Hydroxyl group at carbon 16	5
Prednisone (prodrug)	Substitution of ketone group for hydroxyl group at carbon 11[a]	3.5

[a]Requires metabolism of 11-ketone group to 11-hydroxyl group for conversion to its active form (Prenisolone).

Systemic bioavailability following administration of such enteric-coated preparations in patients with asthma has not been fully studied although there is some evidence to suggest that absorption is delayed (5), more erratic (6), and affected to a greater extent by the presence of food (7). Prednisone is absorbed at a similar rate to prednisolone undergoing rapid first-pass metabolism in the liver to convert the ketone group at carbon 11 to a hydroxyl group. In general, absorption and bioavailability of systemic corticosteroids does not appear to be significantly affected by age, smoking, or the presence of disease (7).

Corticosteroids are distributed as free molecules and also bound to the proteins transcortin, albumin, and α_1-acid glycoprotein. Transcortin has a particularly high affinity for prednisolone, while other corticosteroids such as methylprednisolone and dexamethasone preferentially bind to albumin (8). Protein binding is concentration dependent such that at high concentrations there is a relatively greater free corticosteroid fraction. This leads to greater plasma clearance at high doses and an apparent increase in the volume of distribution (9), one factor leading to the non-linear pharmacokinetics observed with prednisolone (10). The free, unbound corticosteroid molecules are thought to be responsible for the effects of these drugs, and differences in the relative concentrations of free and bound corticoste-

Table 2 Important Drug Interactions with Systemic Corticosteroids

---

Impaired clearance of corticosteroids with increased risk of adverse effects
  Oral contraceptive pill
  Ketoconazole
  Cyclosporin
Accelerated clearance of corticosteroids with reduced therapeutic effects
  Rifampicin
  Anticonvulsants: carbemazepine, phenobarbital, and phenytoin
Increased risk of hypokalaemia
  Amphotericin
  High dose β_2-agonists
  Theophylline
  Diuretics

---

roids may account for the differences in clinical effects observed between patients treated with similar doses. While corticosteroids are metabolized in the liver, chronic liver disease does not appear to significantly alter the effects of systemic corticosteroids, since glucuronidation is maintained even in the face of advanced hepatic failure (2). A number of drugs given in addition to corticosteroids lead to inhibition of microsomal liver enzymes, resulting in impaired clearance and the potential for greater adverse effects. Conversely, drugs such as anticonvulsants may result in accelerated corticosteroid clearance due to induction of liver enzymes (2) (Table 2).

While the effect of systemic corticosteroids on circulating eosinophils and glucose is observed within minutes, improvements in airflow obstruction occur much later. Following a single dose of oral prednisolone, a significant improvement in lung function can be seen at three hours, reaching a maximal effect between 9 and 12 hours (11). Animal models have suggested that the administration of higher doses results in an increase in the duration of action rather than improvements in the maximum response (12) and support the suggestion that smaller doses given frequently may be preferable to larger single doses (13).

It has been suggested that abnormalities of steroid pharmacokinetics may account for the apparent lack of response to systemic corticosteroids in some individuals. Studies in patients with severe asthma, however, have shown relatively little variability in prednisolone absorption, distribution, and clearance between individuals (14). Nevertheless, pharmacokinetic studies may have a useful role in the clinical evaluation of individual patients with chronic corticosteroid-dependent asthma to identify abnormalities in absorption or clearance (15), and serum prednisolone concentrations interpreted alongside plasma cortisol levels may give useful evidence of non-compliance in patients failing to respond to treatment.

III. Mechanisms of Action

A. Effects at the Molecular Level

Circulating corticosteroid molecules cross the cell membrane to bind to the glucocorticoid receptor α located in the cytoplasm in a protein-bound form. The corticosteroid-receptor complex then translocates to the nucleus, where it binds to sequences of DNA in the promoter region of steroid-sensitive genes, known as the glucocorticoid response element (GRE). Such binding leads to alterations in the transcription of target genes (16). Corticosteroids also bind to coactivator molecules, which also activate gene transcription by activating histone deacetylase. These mechanisms result in the activation of a number of genes encoding anti-inflammatory proteins, including annexin-1, interleukin-10, and secretory leukoprotease inhibitor (17). The major anti-inflammatory effects of corticosteroids are thought to result from the suppression of genes that code for inflammatory proteins, but the precise mechanism is not fully understood since GREs have not been widely demonstrated in the promoter regions of inflammatory genes that are known to be suppressed by corticosteroids in asthma (17). Recent work has suggested that suppression of the transcription of inflammatory genes may occur via the modification of core histones, e.g., by histone deacetylation, resulting in disruption of chromatin structure (17,18). Whatever the precise mechanism, a wide range of inflammatory genes appear to be suppressed, including cytokines (e.g., IL-4, IL-5, IL-13, TNF-α, and GM-CSF), chemokines (e.g., IL-8, RANTES, and eotaxin), adhesion molecules (e.g., ICAM-1, VICAM-1, and E-selectin), and a number of other inflammatory enzymes and receptors. This broad effect on a number of components of the anti-inflammatory pathway appears key to the therapeutic effects of corticosteroids in asthma, since more selective agents have not had the same success (19).

B. Effects at the Cellular Level

As a result of the molecular interactions outlined above, corticosteroids have a range of effects on inflammatory cells in asthma, including a reduction in the number of eosinophils, T lymphocytes, mast cells, and dendritic cells. The inhibition of key cytokines, including IL-5 and GM-CSF, leads to increased eosinophil apoptosis (20) and a dramatic reduction in eosinophil survival. Mediator release from eosinophils is also directly inhibited and circulating eosinophil numbers may be reduced by a direct action on the production of eosinophils in the bone marrow. Corticosteroids are also able to inhibit the proliferation of T lymphocytes and their cytokine production, particularly of the T-cell growth factor IL-2 (21,22). In contrast, corticosteroids do not appear to inhibit neutrophilic inflammation and actually increase circulating numbers of neutrophils, possibly by preventing neutrophil apoptosis (23).

Systemic corticosteroids also have important effects on structural components of the asthmatic airway. These include inhibition of the release of cytokines and mediators from epithelial cells (24), prevention of plasma leakage through vascular endothelium (25), and reduction of mucous secretion from airway mucosal glands (26). Additionally, important effects on airway smooth muscle may occur via the suppression of inflammatory mediator release and also by the up-regulation of the number of β-adrenoceptors in individuals with β_2-agonist–induced desensitization (27,28).

IV. Clinical Effects in Asthma

A. Anti-inflammatory Effects

That systemic corticosteroids are thought to exert their therapeutic effects in asthma largely by suppressing airway inflammation has already been discussed. Perhaps surprisingly, there is rather more convincing evidence supporting the anti-inflammatory effects of inhaled rather than systemic corticosteroids in individual patients with asthma.

The few bronchoscopy studies evaluating the anti-inflammatory effects of systemic corticosteroids in vivo have not had entirely consistent results. In a double-blind, placebo-controlled study, Djukanovic et al. (29) studied the anti-inflammatory effects of prednisolone at a dose of 20 mg for two weeks followed by 10 mg for four weeks. Compared to placebo, treatment with prednisolone lead to significant reductions in submucosal eosinophils (by 81%) and mast cells (by 62%). Significant improvements in asthma symptoms and FEV_1 were also seen. In similar studies, Robinson et al. (30) and Bentley AM et al. (31) randomized 18 patients with moderately severe asthma to 0.6 mg/kg/day of prednisolone or placebo for two weeks and took bronchial biopsies before and after treatment. Compared to placebo, prednisolone resulted in reductions in the number of cells expressing mRNA for IL-4 and IL-5 and an increase in IFN-γ expressing cells in bronchial biopsies and bronchoaleveolar lavage, although the interpretation of this data is complicated by significant baseline differences in these markers between the placebo and prednisolone treated groups. Prednisolone treatment lead to a fall in the number of CD3+ T cells, eosinophils, and mucosal-type mast cells in bronchial biopsies and in BAL eosinophils, but only the latter differed significantly from placebo.

The development of noninvasive markers of airway inflammation, particularly induced sputum eosinophil counts and exhaled nitric oxide (NO), has provided further opportunities to assess the anti-inflammatory activity of asthma treatments, but again few studies have used oral corticosteroids. Claman et al. (32) performed a randomized, placebo-controlled, double-blind study of the effects of six days of treatment with prednisone 0.5 mg/ kg/day in 24 patients with chronic stable asthma. Compared to placebo, prednisolone lead to significant reductions in the percentage and absolute numbers of eosinophils in induced sputum and in sputum eosinophil cationic protein (ECP) levels. These changes correlated with significant increases in peak expiratory flow. Other studies have shown similar changes in sputum eosinophil and ECP levels with both inhaled and oral corticosteroids (33,34). Pizzichini et al. (35) demonstrated a significant reduction in sputum eosinophils and ECP levels in 10 patients treated with oral prednisone for a severe asthma exacerbation, although a placebo group was not included for ethical reasons. The improvements in sputum eosinophils and ECP levels began 48 hours after treatment (and correlated with increases in FEV_1) while symptoms, lung function, and blood eosinophil and ECP levels improved more quickly, within 24 hours of treatment.

Systemic corticosteroids have also been shown to reduce the elevated exhaled NO levels seen in asthma (36,37), although a number of subjects demonstrate persistently elevated NO levels despite treatment with oral prednisolone (38,39). This suggests that some aspects of the underlying airway inflammation seen in asthma are resistant to systemic corticosteroids, at least in subgroups of patients, although the dose and route of administration may be important. A recent study by ten Brinke et al. (40) showed that the intramuscular use of triamcinolone acetate was associated with marked suppression of induced sputum eosinophilic airway inflammation in patients who had persistently elevated sputum eosinophil counts despite high doses of inhaled and/or oral corticosteroids. We have found similar results in patients with oral corticosteroid–dependent asthma attending our clinic, where sputum eosinophil counts significantly improved in all patients given intramuscular triamcinalone.

While systemic corticosteroids clearly do not completely remove airway inflammation in asthma and heterogeneity to their anti-inflammatory response occurs, the overall evidence from clinical studies does support the theory that these agents exert their therapeutic effects largely by suppressing airway inflammation, particularly eosinophilic inflammation. This leads to the suggestion that exposure to the potential toxic effects of systemic corticosteroids should be confined to patients who have uncontrolled eosinophilic airway inflammation despite treatment with inhaled corticosteroids, and there is some evidence to support this. We have previously identified a group of non-eosinophilic patients with symptomatic asthma and have associated the absence of sputum eosinophils with a poor response to short-term treatment with inhaled corticosteroids (41). Little et al. (36) have similarly demonstrated that the response to a two-week course of oral prednisolone in patients with chronic stable asthma is greatest in those patients with evidence of airway inflammation demonstrated by raised sputum eosinophil counts or elevated NO concentrations. The presence of a sputum eosinophilia has also been found to predict the short-term response to oral prednisolone in patients with chronic obstructive pulmonary disease (42).

Finally, we have recently reported the results of a randomized, controlled trial of a management strategy that aimed to normalize the induced sputum eosinophil count using appropriate doses of inhaled and oral corticosteroids in patients with moderate to severe asthma (43). Compared to traditional management following British Thoracic Society guidelines, treatment directed at minimizing eosinophilic inflammation resulted in significantly fewer severe asthma exacerbations and hospital admissions. The dramatic improvement occurred despite similar overall corticosteroid doses between the two groups. In effect, in the sputum guided group, treatment was targeted to those patients with eosinophilic inflammation to prevent exacerbations, while systemic corticosteroids were required in the control group to treat exacerbations. Additionally, a subset of patients with predominantly non-eosinophilic airway inflammation was identified and in this group corticosteroids were successfully withdrawn without loss of asthma control. This study identifies sputum eosinophilia as a marker of exacerbation frequency in asthma and emphasizes the close relationship between the beneficial effect of corticosteroids and the presence of eosinophilic airway inflammation.

B. Effects on Airway Hyper-Responsiveness (AHR)

Airway hyper-responsiveness (AHR) is one of the characteristic clinical features of asthma leading to variable airflow obstruction and asthma symptoms. While AHR generally occurs along with airway inflammation, it is becoming increasingly clear that the relationship between inflammation, AHR, and clinical expression of the disease is complex. This is supported by the identification of a group of patients with eosinophilic bronchitis who have a similar corticosteroid responsive immunopathology to that seen in asthma with sputum and submucosal eosinophilia, basement membrane thickening, and increased Th2 cytokine expression, but unlike asthma is characterized by the absence of AHR (44,45). Evidence from a recent study comparing the immunopathology of eosinophilic bronchitis with asthma has suggested that microlocalization of mast cells within the airway smooth muscle is the key abnormality associated with AHR in asthma (45). It cannot therefore be assumed that systemic corticosteroids attenuate airway hyper-responsiveness in asthma via their anti-inflammatory effects. The effect of systemic corticosteroids on AHR has been assessed in a number of studies.

Bhagat and Grunstein (46) compared the effect of a one-week course of prednisolone to placebo in 10 children with atopic asthma. Prednisolone resulted in significant improvements in AHR measured as the PD20-FEV$_1$ to methacholine, which were not seen with placebo. The improvement in PD20-FEV$_1$ correlated with increases in the FEV$_1$, and the greatest improvements were demonstrated in those with lower values of FEV$_1$ before treatment.

Similar improvements in AHR in adults treated with oral prednisolone have lead to somewhat conflicting results. In a study of 12 patients with well-controlled asthma, no improvements in methacholine PC_{20} were observed eight hours after a single dose of intravenous methylprednisolone or after eight days treatment with oral methylprednisolone (32 mg daily) (47). Jenkins and Woolcock performed a randomized, double-dummy, single-blind, cross-over study comparing the effects of three weeks treatment with inhaled beclomethasone diproprionate (BDP) 1200 µg daily with oral prednisolone 12.5 mg daily in 18 adults with asthma. No significant changes in histamine PD_{20} were seen with prednisolone, while inhaled BDP lead to an approximately 2.5 doubling dose improvement (48). In the bronchoscopy study of Djukanovic et al. (29) discussed earlier, subjects treated with oral prednisolone demonstrated significant improvements in methacholine PC_{20} but these did not differ from placebo. In contrast, the study of Robinson et al. (30) demonstrated a fourfold increase in methacholine PC_{20}, which was significant compared to placebo. This improvement occurred despite the fact that the fall in submucosal eosinophil numbers was not significantly different from placebo, again supporting the idea that disordered airway physiology in asthma is disassociated from eosinophilic inflammation.

Meijer et al. (33) measured AHR to both methacholine and adenosine $5'$ monophosphate (AMP) before and after two weeks of treatment with three corticosteroid regimes: 2000 µg/day of inhaled fluticasone, 500 µg/day of inhaled fluticasone, and 30 mg/day of oral prednisone. Changes in serum and sputum eosinophils and ECP levels were also assessed. Mean PC_{20} methacholine and PC_{20} AMP improved significantly with all three treatment regimes, but the improvements following prednisolone were significantly lower than with high-dose fluticasone. In contrast, oral prednisolone had a significantly greater effect on suppression of peripheral blood eosinophils and ECP than either dose of inhaled steroid. Greater improvements in PC_{20} AMP compared to PC_{20} methacholine were seen for all three treatment regimes, possibly reflecting differences in the timescale of the response to corticosteroids at different parts of the inflammatory cascade. Oral prednisolone and high-dose fluticasone had similar effects on sputum eosinophils and ECP in this study, and further analysis showed that the improvement in AHR significantly correlated with reductions in sputum eosinophil counts, particularly the PC_{20} AMP (49).

Overall the results of these studies highlight the complexity of the relationship between airway inflammation and AHR in asthma and suggest that the dose–response to corticosteroids varies between the different outcome parameters.

C. Effects on Acute Exacerbations of Asthma

Systemic corticosteroids are widely accepted as essential in the management of patients presenting with acute severe exacerbations of asthma, and failure to prescribe them in this situation has been identified as a risk factor for asthma deaths (50). The first randomized, controlled trial of systemic corticosteroids in patients admitted to the hospital with acute severe asthma reported significant improvements in symptoms, respiratory rate, heart rate, and airflow obstruction in patients given a reducing dose of cortisone acetate compared to those treated conventionally (with subcutaneous adrenaline, inhaled isoprenaline, oxygen, antibiotics, and sedatives) (51). These initial findings have been confirmed by a number of subsequent studies. A double-blind, placebo-controlled comparison by Loren et al. (52) compared treatment with prednisolone 2 mg/kg/day to placebo in 16 patients presenting with an acute asthma exacerbation. Patients given prednisolone required less nebulized or intravenous β_2-agonist and demonstrated significant improvements in PEF compared to placebo-treated patients. Fanta et al. (53) performed a double-blind, placebo-controlled study of intravenous hydrocortisone (given as a 2 mg/Kg bolus followed by an infusion of 0.5 mg/kg/hr for 24 hours) in 20 patients who had persistent symptoms and signs of an acute severe asthma exacerbation despite eight hours of conventional treatment. Steroid-treated patients had significant improvements in lung function compared to placebo, although the improvements were not seen until 12 hours after the onset of treatment (FEV increase $118\pm25\%$ from baseline compared to $35\pm22\%$ with placebo). Littenberg and Gluck (54) performed a similar placebo-controlled study of a bolus of 125 mg intravenous methylprednisolone, given in addition to standard treatment, in 97 patients presenting to the emergency room with acute severe asthma. While a nonsignificant trend in greater improvements in FEV_1 among the steroid treated patients was seen, significantly fewer patients treated with methylprednsiolone required admission to the hospital for further treatment (19% vs. 47%, $p < 0.003$). A contrasting study by Stein and Cole (55) was unable to demonstrate a reduction in the number of patients requiring hospital admission following treatment with an identical dose of intravenous methylprednisolone compared to placebo. The reasons for this negative finding are not obvious, but measurements of lung function were not performed, and the study included a requirement to admit patients when treatment time exceeded 12 hours.

The route of administration and dose of systemic corticosteroid in the management of acute severe asthma have been a source of debate, particularly since side effects such as myopathy are more likely to occur with high-dose regimes (56). An early study by Haskell et al. (57) suggested that 40 or 125 mg of intravenous methylprednisolone was associated with better improvements in lung function than low-dose treatment (15 mg methylprednisolone). A number of subsequent studies, however, have failed to confirm this finding (58–60). One problem is that the majority of studies of this kind have been confined to a small number of patients, and a recent meta-analysis of nine randomized, controlled trials comparing different doses of corticosteroids in adults hospitalized for acute severe asthma was undertaken (61). This pooled analysis of over 300 patients concluded that doses of systemic corticosteroids in excess of 80 mg/day of methylprednisolone (equivalent to 400 mg of hydrocortisone or 100 mg of prednisolone) offered no therapeutic benefit. Further subgroup analysis suggested that oral treatment was as efficacious as the intravenous route, although data was included from only two studies (62). Overall the evidence suggests that low-dose oral treatment will be sufficient for the majority of patients presenting with acute severe asthma, although none of the studies have included patients presenting in respiratory failure, and intravenous treatment may be warranted in a subgroup at risk of failure of absorption via the oral route, e.g., due to vomiting.

Following hospitalization due to acute severe asthma, patients are at significant risk of relapse with one study estimating that 45% of patients relapse by eight weeks following discharge (63). A number of studies have therefore addressed the use of systemic corticosteroids in the prevention of subsequent relapse. Chapman et al. (64) recruited 93 patients discharged from the emergency room following treatment for acute severe asthma and randomized them to receive either a tapering course of prednisolone (from 40 to 0 mg over eight days) or placebo. Compared to placebo, the prednisolone-treated group had significantly fewer symptoms and less use of rescue bronchodilators during the first week and had a significantly lower rate of relapse (3 of 48 compared to 11 of 45, $p < 0.05$). A number of other studies have shown similar results, both for short courses of oral prednisolone (65,66) and for intramuscular corticosteroid (67). A meta-analysis of the available studies concluded that as few as 13 patients needed to be treated with systemic corticosteroids on discharge to prevent relapse requiring additional emergency care (68). There is little evidence to support the theory that the dose of corticosteroid should be slowly tapered with studies showing that the abrupt cessation of treatment after 7 to 10 days does not lead to a rebound deterioration in symptoms or airflow obstruction (69,70). It is generally recommended that the precise treatment regime be tailored to the individual patient; in some cases longer courses of systemic corticosteroids may be needed.

D. Effects in Chronic Asthma

The highly effective anti-inflammatory properties of inhaled corticosteroids mean that the vast majority of patients with asthma achieve adequate control without the need for systemic corticosteroid treatment, except perhaps for the occasional severe exacerbation. The introduction of inhaled corticosteroids enabled many patients with chronic asthma to stop or dramatically reduce their dose of oral treatment (71,72). A small number of patients, however, have persistent symptoms, airflow obstruction, and/or recurrent severe exacerbations of asthma despite the use of high-dose inhaled corticosteroids and additional therapy such as long-acting β_2-agonists, methylxanthines, and leukotriene modifiers. In this group of patients the regular use of maintenance doses of oral corticosteroids requires careful consideration in view of the unfavorable therapeutic ratio. There are surprisingly few studies supporting the use of maintenance oral corticosteroids in these circumstances, with placebo-controlled evidence dating back to the original Medical Research Council trial (51). This was a randomized, placebo-controlled study in 96 patients with chronic symptomatic asthma comparing the effects of oral cortisone acetate at a dose of 300 mg/day, reducing to 100 mg/day after one week then tapered according to clinical need. Attempts were made to withdraw treatment after 24 weeks. Compared to placebo, patients receiving cortisone had fewer symptoms and physical signs, better exercise tolerance, and were less likely to be withdrawn from the study due to poor asthma control (73). Despite this, few patients in either group were able to withdraw their study medication, and by three months the differences in the two groups were no longer significant. The majority of cortisone-treated patients experienced side effects, most commonly weight gain, hypertension, and edema.

Subsequent clinical studies have largely compared the use of maintenance oral corticosteroids with alternative anti-inflammatory treatments, particularly inhaled corticosteroids. The British Thoracic and Tuberculosis Association published the results of a double-blind, placebo-controlled, cross-over study comparing the effects of oral prednisolone with the inhaled steroids BDP and betamethasone valerate in 75 patients with mild to moderate asthma, with a 24-week treatment period. Prednisolone was started at a dose of 20 mg daily, reducing by 5 mg weekly until asthma control was lost, while inhaled corticosteroids were given initially at 800 µg daily, reducing in a similar fashion by 200 µg weekly. Upon loss of asthma symptom control, treatment was increased again until a dose that lead to satisfactory control was achieved. Prednisolone 7.5 mg daily achieved equivalent asthma control to 400 µg of inhaled corticosteroid in the form of number of "failure days" (defined as a day on which regular treatment needed to be increased or <4 puffs of rescue bronchodilator was needed), mean monthly PEF, and percentage of patients requiring an increase in treatment or rescue oral prednisolone. Around 30% of patients receiving systemic treatment reported steroid-related side effects (e.g., weight gain, edema, and dyspepsia) compared to none receiving inhaled treatment. A number of other, smaller studies of shorter (two to four weeks) duration have reported similar findings suggesting that oral prednisolone 7.5–12 mg/day appear to be as effective as 300–2000 µg/day of inhaled beclomethasone or equivalent (74–77). These studies have been the subject of a Cochrane review (78), although differences in study design have precluded a formal meta-analysis.

It has been suggested that where maintenance systemic corticosteroids are required an alternate-day regime may provide sufficient therapeutic benefit while minimizing adverse effects (79). This recommendation appears to be based on an early study by Harter et al., which assessed various oral corticosteroid dosing schedules and concluded that single doses given at 48-hour intervals resulted in adequate asthma control with minimal side effects (80). This study predated the widespread introduction of inhaled corticosteroids, however, and it has subsequently been reported that inhaled corticosteroids appear to be more effective than alternate-day doses of prednisolone up to 60 mg (78,81), in contrast to the findings with daily regimes. Furthermore, there is no evidence to support the suggestion that a significant reduction in side effects is seen with intermittent dosing (82).

A further option for the systemic administration of corticosteroids in chronic asthma is the use of intramuscular triamcinolone acetate. A small number of randomized, controlled trials support its use in this setting. McLeod et al. (83) performed a double-blind, cross-over study in 17 patients with chronic severe asthma comparing triamcinolone 80 mg IM with prednisolone 10 mg daily, each drug given for 24 weeks. Asthma symptom scores, lung function, need for rescue prednisolone, and weight gain were all significantly better in the triamcinolone-treated group, although side effects, particularly adrenal suppression, bruising, and hirsuitism, were reported more commonly. Similar findings were reported by Willey et al. (84). Higher doses of triamcinolone were used in the study of Ogirala et al. (85) Here 12 patients with chronic oral corticosteroid–dependent asthma undertook a randomized, double-blind, cross-over study comparing triamcinolone 120 mg daily for three days with oral prednisolone at a median dose of 12.5 mg daily. Treatment with triamcinolone resulted in significant improvements in peak expiratory flow, emergency room visits, and hospitalizations than oral prednisolone, although side effects again tended to be more common. The results of this study have been criticized, however, since the use of inhaled corticosteroids was not reported, and since patients were encouraged to taper their treatment, including the trial tablets, when they felt that their symptoms were well controlled. This has raised the question that patients may have been under-treated during the oral corticosteroid treatment period, although one could argue that the tapering of treatment during a period of apparent stability reflects the behavior of many patients in routine clinical practice. The available data, along with the clear anti-inflammatory effects of intramuscular triamcinolone (40), do support a role for its use in a small number of patients who are for some reason unable to tolerate or absorb oral corticosteroids or who fail to comply with prescribed regimes, although the risk of side effects must be carefully considered. Further prospective studies in this area are required.

V. Safety

A. Adverse Effects

As in other chronic inflammatory diseases the major limitation for the use of systemic corticosteroids in asthma is their propensity for potentially serious adverse effects. Since all nucleated cells have glucocorticoid receptors, a wide range of complications affecting most organ systems can occur. The frequency of such complications in asthma is difficult to determine due to a lack of reliable studies, and there is little evidence to suggest that the profile of adverse effects in asthma differs from that seen in other corticosteroid-dependent diseases. Those that are a frequent cause of morbidity in patients with asthma requiring systemic corticosteroids are discussed below, and a more comprehensive list of potential adverse effects is given in Table 3.

Osteoporosis

The frequency of osteoporosis in chronic systemic corticosteroid use is thought to be similar to that seen in Cushing's disease at around 30% to 50% (86). The effects appear to depend on both the cumulative dose and duration of use, with highest rates of bone loss within the first six months of treatment (87). Fracture risk declines rapidly on stopping treatment but may not return to baseline. Alternate-dose regimens have been advocated but do not prevent accelerated bone loss (88). It has been suggested that doses of < 7.5 mg prednisone or equivalent may be safe (86), but this is controversial since accelerated rates of bone loss have been described in patients with additional risk factors (such as postmenopausal status) taking lower oral doses (89) and with inhaled corticosteroids (90). It has been suggested that corticoste roids contribute to an increased fracture risk over and above their effects on bone mineral density with higher risks of fracture than are seen in postmenopausal osteoporosis (91). A retrospective cohort study comparing almost a quarter of a million oral corticosteroid users in the United Kingdom with age- and sex-matched controls calculated relative risks for vertebral fractures in patients taking oral corticosteroids at a daily dose of < 2.5 mg prednisolone of 1.55 (95% CI 1.20–2.01) rising to 5.18 (CI 4.25–6.31) at doses of 7.5 mg or greater (92).

Corticosteroids predispose to osteoporosis via a range of mechanisms on calcium and bone metabolism. Gastrointestinal absorption of calcium is impaired and renal calcium excretion increased leading to secondary hyperparathyroidism and subsequent bone resorption. Further effects occur via the suppression of pituitary and anabolic sex hormones. Additionally, corticosteroids directly reduce bone formation by inhibition of osteoblast proliferation and synthesis of Type I collagen and other proteins (93). In adults these mechanisms preferentially result in loss of trabecular bone, predisposing them to spinal and rib fractures.

All patients requiring long-term systemic corticosteroids should be given general advice to reduce bone loss, including good nutrition, adequate dietary calcium, appropriate physical activity, and minimization of tobacco use and alcohol abuse (87). Supplementation with calcium and vitamin D should be considered for all patients receiving long-term corticosteroids since several randomized, controlled trials have shown that this strategy

Table 3 Potential Adverse Effects Associated with Systemic Corticosteroid Treatment

Metabolic
Hyperglycaemia
Weight gain
Hyperlipidaemia
Hypokalaemia

Endocrine
Suppression of growth in children
Adrenal suppression
Cushingoid habitus
Amenorrhoea

Musculoskeletal
Osteoporosis
Myopathy
Aseptic necrosis of bone

Ophthalmological
Cataracts
Glaucoma

Psychological and central nervous system
Altered mood
Insomnia
Psychosis
Pseudotumor cerebri

Immunological
Reduction of circulating immunoglobulins
Reactivation of previous infection including latent tuberculosis

Cardiovascular
Hypertension
Edema

Gastrointestinal
Gastric ulceration and hemorrhage
Pancreatitis

Dermatological
Acne
Increased skin fragility
Subcutaneous tissue atrophy
Impaired wound healing

can significantly reduce and even reverse bone loss (94–96). Calcium alone does not have a similar protective effect (96). Measurements of bone mass using dual X-ray absorpiometry (DEXA) should be considered to assess fracture risk and is recommended by some groups (97). Bone-protective therapy should then be offered to all patients shown to have low-bone mineral density and bone mineral density measurements repeated on an approximately annual basis. The use of bone-protective therapy for all patients at high-fracture risk (e.g., aged over 65 years or with past history of fragility fracture) regardless of baseline bone densitometry is an alternative approach (87). Studies have suggested that in postmenopausal women, hormone replacement therapy (HRT) prevents bone loss in those receiving low to moderate doses of systemic corticosteroids (98). No studies, however, have demonstrated similar efficacy in those requiring higher dose treatment or have evaluated the role of HRT in preventing bone loss at the initiation of corticosteroid treatment. Furthermore, there have been recent concerns over the association between HRT and increased rates of breast cancer and other diseases (99,100). Several large randomized, controlled trials have shown that the bisphosphonates etidronate, alendronate, and risedronate are effective in both the prevention and treatment of corticosteoid-induced osteoporosis (101–103). While fracture prevention was not a primary end point of any of these trials, post hoc and safety analyses have suggested that each of these agents leads to a reduction in vertebral fracture (95,102,104). The data for pamidronate and clodronate are less consistent (105,106). Calcitonin has been suggested as an alternative bone-sparing agent but needs to be given via the intranasal and subcutaneous route and studies of its effect have been inconsistent (107,108). Bisphosphonates used in conjunction with calcium and vitamin D supplements are therefore probably the treatment of choice for the prevention and treatment of osteoporosis in the majority of patients requiring long-term systemic corticosteroids.

Myopathy

Prolonged treatment with moderately high doses of systemic corticosteroids is associated with the development of a chronic myopathy, predominantly affecting the proximal limb muscles. The weakness tends to develop gradually and may be accompanied by reduced respiratory muscle force. The incidence of this complication has not been clearly evaluated but in one study a degree of muscle weakness was observed in over 60% of patients with asthma taking at least 40 mg of prednisone per day, but was almost never seen in patients taking less than 30 mg a day (56). No correlation between the degree of muscle weakness and biochemical markers, including muscle enzymes and urinary creatinine excretion, was seen in these patients, and there is currently no reliable biochemical test to confirm the diagnosis. A number of case reports have described the development of an acute-onset severe generalized myopathy in patients admitted to the hospital with acute severe exacerbations of asthma (109,110). The majority of patients developing this complication had been intubated for a near fatal attack and had received both parenteral corticosteroids and muscle relaxants. Recent cohort studies have estimated that of patients undergoing mechanical ventilation for severe asthma, around 30% of those treated with both corticosteroids and a neuromuscular blocking agent develop acute myopathy compared to between 0% and 10% in those who receive corticosteroids alone (111,112). Very high levels of skeletal muscle enzymes associated with diffuse skeletal muscle necrosis may be seen, although the exact mechanism is unclear (109). Patients may require extensive rehabilitation over several months before fully regaining muscle function.

Adrenal Suppression

It is well recognized that systemic oral corticosteroids lead to suppression of the adrenal cortex, with a significant dose-related reduction in morning cortisol (77,113). This may lead to isolated central adrenal insufficiency with prolonged suppression of the hypothalamic–pituitary axis but normal adrenal function or, in more severe cases, complete suppression of the hypothalamic–pituitary–adrenal axis (114). Patients tend to present in a nonspecific manner and adrenal insufficiency should therefore be considered in all patients receiving at least 5 mg of prednisone or equivalent per day. Confirmation of the diagnosis requires the demonstration of subnormal cortisol levels that remain low despite adrenal stimulation and should be treated with adequate glucocorticoid replacement therapy. The risk of adrenal suppression increases with increased steroid potency, and there is some evidence to suggest that taking corticosteroids only on alternate days may reduce the risk of adrenal suppression (115).

All patients requiring long-term systemic corticosteroid therapy should be considered at risk of adrenal insufficiency and advised to increase their usual maintenance dose to cover intercurrent illnesses or surgery (116). Recent evidence suggests that relatively low doses of additional corticosteroid will prevent adrenal crises (117), and even that simply continuing the maintenance dose on the day of surgery is sufficient (118). The risk of adrenal insufficiency persists up to 12 months after cessation of systemic corticosteroids (119). It is thought that a protocol of slow tapering of the corticosteroid dose minimizes the risk of adrenal crisis, but controlled trials comparing this approach to abrupt steroid cessation following prolonged steroid use have not been done.

Cataracts

Prolonged use of systemic corticosteroids is an important risk factor for the development of posterior subcapsular cataracts (120). Cataracts were reported in 18% of respiratory patients requiring long-term corticosteroids compared to 8% of matched controls in one recent study (121). It is not clear whether the risk of cataracts is dose dependent (122), and it has been suggested that a subset of patients may be particularly susceptible (123).

The mechanism by which corticosteroids predispose to cataract formation is unknown and treatment requires surgical removal of the lens.

B. Interaction with Other Drugs

A number of other drugs may affect the pharmacokinetics of corticosteroids, increasing the potential for adverse effects and in some circumstances reducing the therapeutic response. Common drug interactions are given in Table 3.

C. Special Situations

Children

The main concern when using systemic corticosteroids in children is the risk of suppression of linear growth. Even small daily doses of 2.5–5 mg of prednisolone per day given to children with mild asthma over periods as short as two weeks have been associated with growth suppression in children with asthma (124). Systemic corticosteroid naïve children with asthma are also at risk of growth retardation. Chang et al. (125) studied over 230 asthmatic children and found that those who had never received oral corticosteroids or who had been given only occasional rescue courses had an average height of around one standard deviation lower than their age- and sex-specific predicted means. Children treated with oral corticosteroids for two years or more had a mean height of two standard deviations lower than predicted (125). No difference was seen between children treated with an alternate day or daily corticosteroid regime, although other studies have suggested that inhibition of growth may be less with an alternate-day regime (126,127). The mechanisms of linear growth suppression are poorly understood but may be analogous to those leading to osteoporosis in corticosteroid-treated adults. Aside from growth delay, children may be particularly susceptible to the other corticosteroid-related side effects outlined earlier. Adrenal suppression, for example, has been observed in 20% of children receiving four or more short-rescue courses of oral corticosteroids per year for asthma exacerbations (128). Children are particularly vulnerable to the development of posterior subcapsular cataracts, which occur at lower corticosteroid doses than in adults (129) and have been seen after only six months of systemic treatment (122). As in adults, prolonged treatment with systemic corticosteroids should be recommended only where absolutely necessary and where a clear clinical benefit can be demonstrated (see recommendations).

Pregnancy and Breastfeeding

Approximately 10% to 15% of pregnant women with asthma experience at least one acute exacerbation requiring emergency treatment (130). Concern over the safety of oral corticosteroids in pregnancy has at times resulted in a reluctance to prescribe oral steroids in this setting (131). Numerous studies, however, including a large case–control study of over 20,000 subjects, have shown no association between the use of systemic corticosteroids in pregnancy and adverse fetal events, including congenital malformation (132,133). Findings of an early animal study that raised questions over the development of cleft palate (134) have not been confirmed in humans (132). The results of one case–control study, which did report a possible link between oral corticosteroid use and cleft lip, are seriously limited by flaws in study design (135) and an alternative analysis of the data does not support a positive association (136). Both severe asthma and systemic corticosteroids have been associated with an increased risk of maternal pre-eclampsia (137,138). Finally, a recent multicenter, prospective study of over 2000 patients with asthma found that the use of oral steroids during pregnancy was associated with both preterm delivery [odds ratio (OR) 1.54, 95% CI 1.02–2.33] and low birth weight $< 2500\,g$ (OR 1.8, 95% CI 1.13–2.88), even controlling for asthma severity (139). Despite this, the major risk to both mother and fetus during pregnancy comes from inadequate treatment of severe asthma, and pregnancy should never be a contraindication to the use of systemic corticosteroids in asthma (82).

There is no evidence to support the theory that maternal systemic corticosteroid use leads to adrenal suppression in the fetus (140). Similarly, the incidence of maternal adrenal suppression is unknown, although guidelines suggest that intravenous hydrocortisone should be administered during labor to women receiving prednisolone of more than 7.5 mg daily for more than two weeks in view of the theoretical risk (82). Concentrations of corticosteroids in the breast milk of mothers treated with systemic steroids are very low, and there are no clinically important risks to breastfed infants (141).

VI. Recommendations

A. Systemic Corticosteroids in the Management of Acute Severe Asthma

Systemic corticosteroids are essential in the management of asthma exacerbations. Current guidelines recommend that they be given in all but the mildest of exacerbations (defined as a prompt response to inhaled β_2-agonists resulting in a PEF of $> 80\%$ of predicted or best after one hour) (142). Unless there are problems of absorption or recurrent vomiting, oral administration is as effective as the intravenous route, although intramuscular injections may be considered where compliance is in doubt yet hospital admission is not required (141,143). Daily doses of 40–50 mg of prednisolone, 60–80 mg of methylprednisolone, or 400 mg of hydrocortisone (100 mg every six hours) are recommended for adults and 1 mg/kg/day for children (82,141). Systemic corticosteroids should be continued until recovery and, therefore, the optimum duration of treatment should be tailored to the individual, although at least five days is usually needed (82). Providing inhaled corticosteroids are given, abrupt cessation of treatment is appropriate except in the few patients receiving prolonged courses of oral corticosteroids (82).

B. The Management of Chronic Oral Corticosteroid-Dependent Asthma

Where adequate control of symptoms, airflow obstruction, and/or recurrent exacerbations cannot be achieved with inhaled corticosteroids and bronchodilators, maintenance doses of oral corticosteroids may be considered. Given the narrow therapeutic window and potential severity of adverse effects we suggest that a number of steps be made before systemic corticosteroids are recommended in this way. First, failure to respond to conventional treatment, including inhaled corticosteroids, should always prompt a review of the accuracy of the asthma diagnosis. Objective confirmation of a diagnosis of asthma may be particularly difficult in this group since it is often difficult to withdraw treatment such as high-dose bronchodilators, the presence of which may limit the interpretation of physiological tests. Nevertheless, stringent attempts at demonstrating variable airflow obstruction should be made using peak expiratory flow monitoring, spirometry before and after bronchodilators and/or oral corticosteroids, and measurements of AHR to methacholine, histamine, or exercise (141). The demonstration of airway inflammation using induced sputum and/or exhaled nitric oxide (NO) may also be helpful, although no test is specific to asthma. Alternative diagnoses should be rigorously excluded in patients with a lack of objective evidence of asthma coupled with a poor response to inhaled treatment.

Second, even where objective confirmation of asthma is obtained, consideration of additional comorbidities should be given since current symptoms may not be due to asthma. Thus, the presence of dysfunctional breathlessness, gastroesophageal reflux, rhinosinusitis, nasal polyposis, bronchiectasis, and other additional pathologies should be identified and appropriately treated. Inhaled corticosteroids are less effective in cigarette smokers (144) and smoking cessation advice should be given. Third, non-concordance to inhaled treatment should be considered, although this may be difficult to identify. This may arise for a number of reasons, including poor technique with the prescribed device, a lack of understanding of the rationale of treatment, concern over potential side effects, or because the patient's perception of the goals of treatment differs from that of their health professional. Successful strategies for managing non-concordance remain unclear, although patient education, including the provision of written material, may help (145).

Having addressed these areas consideration should be given to the nature and extent of the underlying pathophysiology, since this may provide important information about the likelihood of systemic corticosteroid response. The identification of persistent eosinophilic airway inflammation, for example, appears to be a marker not only of recurrent severe exacerbations but also of a potential for improvement with additional anti-inflammatory treatment (36,43). Conversely, neutrophilic airway inflammation has been associated with a poor response to corticosteroids (146,147). Additionally, patients who achieve significant improvements in symptoms and airflow obstruction following short treatment trials may be more likely to benefit from systemic corticosteroids in the longer term.

Once a decision to treat with systemic corticosteroids has been made priority should be given to the prevention of adverse effects. The lowest possible dose to control symptoms, airflow obstruction, and exacerbations should be given and the addition of steroid-sparing agents should be considered. High doses of inhaled corticosteroids have been shown to be the most effective of these (148) and should always be continued. Additional options include methotrexate, gold, and cyclopsorin, although the response to these agents is unpredictable (82). The use of alternate-day dosing regimes is controversial, being recommended by some guidelines (141) but not others (82). Oral corticosteroids have a preferable side-effect profile, although intramuscular triamcinolone is a useful alternative, particularly where non-concordance is an issue. Patients and clinicians should be aware of the range of potential side effects and, in particular, strategies for the prevention of osteoporosis should be applied as already discussed. Finally, patients receiving chronic systemic corticosteroid treatment should remain under specialist care and the continuing need for this treatment should be reassessed at every opportunity.

References

1. American Thoracic Society. Proceedings of the ATS workshop on refractory asthma: current understanding, recommendations, and unanswered questions. American Thoracic Society. Am J Respir Crit Care Med 2000; 162(6): 2341–2351.
2. Frey BM, Frey FJ. Clinical pharmacokinetics of prednisone and prednisolone. Clin Pharmacokinet 1990; 19(2):126–146.
3. Mortimer O, Grettve L, Lindstrom B, Lonnerholm G, Zetterstrom O. Bioavailability of prednisolone in asthmatic patients with a poor response to steroid treatment. Eur J Respir Dis 1987; 71(5):372–379.
4. West HF. Prevention of peptic ulceration during corticosteroid therapy. Br Med J 1959; 5153:680.
5. Adair CG, McCallion O, McElnay JC, Scott MG, Hamilton BA, McCann JP, Stanford CF, Nicholls DP. A pharmacokinetic and pharmacodynamic compar-

ison of plain and enteric-coated prednisolone tablets. Br J Clin Pharmacol 1992; 33(5):495–499.

6. Al Habet S, Rogers HJ. Pharmacokinetics of intravenous and oral prednisolone. Br J Clin Pharmacol 1980; 10(5):503–508.

7. Al Habet SM, Rogers HJ. Effect of food on the absorption and pharmacokinetics of prednisolone from enteric-coated tablets. Eur J Clin Pharmacol 1989; 37(4):423–426.

8. Szefler SJ, Ebling WF, Georgitis JW, Jusko WJ. Methylprednisolone versus prednisolone pharmacokinetics in relation to dose in adults. Eur J Clin Pharmacol 1986; 30(3):323–329.

9. Frey FJ, Amend WJ, Lozada F, Frey BM, Holford NH, Benet LZ. Pharmacokinetics of prednisolone and endogenous hydrocortisone levels in cushingoid and non-cushingoid patients. Eur J Clin Pharmacol 1981; 21(3):235–242.

10. McAllister WA, Winfield CR, Collins JV. Pharmacokinetics of prednisolone in normal and asthmatic subjects in relation to dose. Eur J Clin Pharmacol 1981; 20(2):141–145.

11. Ellul-Micallef R, Borthwick RC, McHardy GJ. The time-course of response to prednisolone in chronic bronchial asthma. Clin Sci Mol Med 1974; 47(2):105–117.

12. Nichols AI, Boudinot FD, Jusko WJ. Second generation model for prednisolone pharmacodynamics in the rat. J Pharmacokinet Biopharm 1989; 17(2):209–227.

13. Reiss WG, Slaughter RL, Ludwig BA, Middleton E Jr, Jusko WJ. Steroid dose sparing: phannacodynamic responses to single versus divided doses of methylprednisolone in man. J Allergy Clin Immunol 1990; 85(6):1058–1066.

14. Rose JQ, Nickelsen JA, Middleton E Jr, Yurchak AM, Park BH, Jusko WJ. Prednisolone disposition in steroid-dependent asthmatics. J Allergy Clin Immunol 1980; 66(5):366–373.

15. Hill MR, Szefler SJ, Ball BD, Bartoszek M, Brenner AM. Monitoring glucocorticoid therapy: a pharmacokinetic approach. Clin Pharmacol Ther 1990; 48(4):390–398.

16. Reichardt HM, Kaestner KH, Tuckermann J, Kretz O, Wessely O, Bock R, Gass P, Schmid W, Herrlich P, Aangel P, Schutz G. DNA binding of the glucocorticoid receptor is not essential for survival. Cell 1998; 93(4):531–541.

17. Barnes PJ, Adcock IM. How do corticosteroids work in asthma? Ann Intern Med 2003; 139(5 Pt l):359–370.

18. Ito K, Barnes PJ, Adcock IM. Glucocorticoid receptor recruitment of histone deacetylase 2 inhibits interleukin-1beta-induced histone H4 acetylation on lysines 8 and 12. Mol Cell Biol 2000; 20(18):6891–6903.

19. Leckie MJ, ten Brinke A, Khan J, Diamant Z, O'connor BJ, Walls CM, Mathur AK, Cowley HC, Chung KF, Djukanovic R, Hansel TT, Holgate ST, Sterk PJ, Barnes PJ. Effects of an interleukin-5 blocking monoclonal antibody on eosinophils, airway hyper-responsiveness, and the late asthmatic response. Lancet 2000; 356(9248): 2144–2148.

20. Lamas AM, Leon OG, Schleimer RP. Glucocorticoids inhibit eosinophil responses to granulocyte-macrophage colony-stimulating factor. J Immunol 1991; 147(l):254–259.

21. Gillis S, Crabtree GR, Smith KA. Glucocorticoid-induced inhibition of T-cell growth factor production. I. The effect on mitogen-induced lymphocyte proliferation. J Immunol 1979; 123(4):1624–1631.
22. Reed JC, Abidi AH, Alpers JD, Hoover RG, Robb RJ, Nowell PC. Effect of cyclosporin A and dexamethasone on interleukin 2 receptor gene expression. J Immunol 1986; 137(1):150–154.
23. Cox G. Glucocorticoid treatment inhibits apoptosis in human neutrophils. Separation of survival and activation outcomes. J Immunol 1995; 154(9): 4719–4725.
24. Schwiebert LM, Stellato C, Schleimer RP. The epithelium as a target of glucocorticoid action in the treatment of asthma. Am J Respir Crit Care Med 1996; 154(2 Pt 2):S16–S19.
25. Boschetto P, Rogers DF, Fabbri LM, Barnes PJ. Corticosteroid inhibition of airway microvascular leakage. Am Rev Respir Dis 1991; 143(3):605–609.
26. Marom Z, Shelhamer J, Alling D, Kaliner M. The effects of corticosteroids on mucous glycoprotein secretion from human airways in vitro. Am Rev Respir Dis 1984; 129(l):62–65.
27. Holgate ST, Baldwin CJ, Tattersfield AE. Beta-adrenergic agonist resistance in normal human airways. Lancet 1977; 2(8034):375–377.
28. Hui KK, Conolly ME, Tashkin DP. Reversal of human lymphocyte beta-adrenoceptor desensitization by glucocorticoids. Clin Pharmacol Ther 1982; 32(5):566–571.
29. Djukanovic R, Homeyard S, Gratziou C, Madden J, Walls A, Montefort S, Peroni D, Polosa R, Holgate S, Howarth P. The effect of treatment with oral corticosteroids on asthma symptoms and airway inflammation. Am J Respir Crit Care Med 1997; 155(3):826–832.
30. Robinson D, Hamid Q, Ying S, Bentley A, Assoufi B, Durham S, Kay AB. Prednisolone treatment in asthma is associated with modulation of bronchoalveolar lavage cell interleukin-4, interleukin-5, and interferon-gamma cytokine gene expression. Am Rev Respir Dis 1993; 148(2):401–406.
31. Bentley AM, Hamid Q, Robinson DS, Schotman E, Meng Q, Assoufi B, Kay AB, Durham SR. Prednisolone treatment in asthma. Reduction in the numbers of eosinophils, T cells, tryptase-only positive mast cells, and modulation of IL-4, IL-5, and interferon-gamma cytokine gene expression within the bronchial mucosa. Am J Respir Crit Care Med 1996; 153(2):551–556.
32. Claman DM, Boushey HA, Liu J, Wong H, Fahy JV. Analysis of induced sputum to examine the effects of prednisone on airway inflammation in asthmatic subjects. J Allergy Clin Immunol 1994; 94(5):861–869.
33. Meijer RJ, Kerstjens HA, Arends LR, Kauffman HF, Koeter GH, Postma DS. Effects of inhaled fluticasone and oral prednisolone on clinical and inflammatory parameters in patients with asthma. Thorax 1999; 54(10):894–899.
34. Keatings VM, Jatakanon A, Worsdell YM, Barnes PJ. Effects of inhaled and oral glucocorticoids on inflammatory indices in asthma and COPD. Am J Respir Crit Care Med 1997; 155(2):542–548.
35. Pizzichini MM, Pizzichini E, Clelland L, Efthimiadis A, Mahony J, Dolovich J, Hargreave FE. Sputum in severe exacerbations of asthma: kinetics of inflam-

matory indices after prednisone treatment. Am J Respir Crit Care Med 1997; 155(5):1501–1508.

36. Little SA, Chalmers GW, MacLeod KJ, McSharry C, Thomson NC. Non-invasive markers of airway inflammation as predictors of oral steroid responsiveness in asthma. Thorax 2000; 55(3):232–234.

37. Zanconato S, Scollo M, Zaramella C, Landi L, Zacchello F, Baraldi E. Exhaled carbon monoxide levels after a course of oral prednisone in children with asthma exacerbation. J Allergy Clin Immunol 2002; 109(3):440–445.

38. Payne DN, Wilson NM, James A, Hablas H, Agrafioti C, Bush A. Evidence for different subgroups of difficult asthma in children. Thorax 2001; 56(5): 345–350.

39. Stirling RG, Kharitonov SA, Campbell D, Robinson DS, Durham SR, Chung KF, Barnes PJ. Increase in exhaled nitric oxide levels in patients with difficult asthma and correlation with symptoms and disease severity despite treatment with oral and inhaled corticosteroids. Asthma and Allergy Group. Thorax 1998; 53(12): 1030–1034.

40. ten Brinke A, Zwinderman AH, Sterk PJ, Rabe KF, Bel EH. 'Refractory' eosinophilic airway inflammation in severe asthma: effect of parenteral corticosteroids. Am J Respir Crit Care Med 2004.

41. Pavord ID, Brightling CE, Woltmann G, Wardlaw AJ. Non-eosinophilic corticosteroid unresponsive asthma [letter]. Lancet 1999; 353(9171):2213–2214.

42. Brightling CE, Monteiro W, Ward R, Parker D, Morgan MD, Wardlaw AJ, Pavord ID. Sputum eosinophilia and short-term response to prednisolone in chronic obstructive pulmonary disease: a randomised controlled trial. Lancet 2000; 356(9240):1480–1485.

43. Green RH, Brightling CE, McKenna S, Hargadon B, Parker D, Bradding P, Wardlaw AJ, Pavord ID. Asthma exacerbations and sputum eosinophil counts: a randomised controlled trial. Lancet 2002; 360:1715–1721.

44. Gibson PG, Hargreave FE, Girgis-Gabardo A, Morris M, Denburg JA, Dolovich J. Chronic cough with eosinophilic bronchitis: examination for variable airflow obstruction and response to corticosteroid. Clin Exp Allergy 1995; 25(2):127–132.

45. Brightling CE, Bradding P, Symon FA, Holgate ST, Wardlaw AJ, Pavord ID. Mast-cell infiltration of airway smooth muscle in asthma. N Engl J Med 2002; 346(22):1699–1705.

46. Bhagat RG, Grunstein MM. Effect of corticosteroids on bronchial responsiveness to methacholine in asthmatic children. Am Rev Respir Dis 1985; 131(6):902–906.

47. Mattoli S, Rosati G, Mormile F, Ciappi G. The immediate and short-term effects of corticosteroids on cholinergic hyperreactivity and pulmonary function in subjects with well-controlled asthma. J Allergy Clin Immunol 1985; 76(2 Pt 1):214–222.

48. Jenkins CR, Woolcock AJ. Effect of prednisone and beclomethasone dipropionate on airway responsiveness in asthma: a comparative study. Thorax 1988; 43(5):378–384.

49. van den Berge M, Kerstjens HA, Meijer RJ, de Reus DM, Koeter GH, Kauffman HF, Postma DS. Corticosteroid-induced improvement in the

PC20 of adenosine monophosphate is more closely associated with reduction in airway inflammation than improvement in the PC20 of methacholine. Am J Respir Crit Care Med 2001; 164(7):1127–1132.

50. Bucknall CE, Slack R, Godley CC, Mackay TW, Wright SC. Scottish Confidential Inquiry into Asthma Deaths (SCIAD), 1994–1996. Thorax 1999; 54(11):978–984.

51. Controlled trial of effects of cortisone acetate in status asthmaticus; report to the Medical Research Council by the subcommittee on clinical trials in asthma. Lancet 1956; 271(6947):803–806.

52. Loren ML, Chai H, Leung P, Rohr C, Brenner AM. Corticosteroids in the treatment of acute exacerbations of asthma. Ann Allergy 1980; 45(2):67–71.

53. Fanta CH, Rossing TH, McFadden ER Jr. Glucocorticoids in acute asthma. A critical controlled trial. Am J Med 1983; 74(5):845–851.

54. Littenberg B, Gluck EH. A controlled trial of methylprednisolone in the emergency treatment of acute asthma. N Engl J Med 1986; 314(3):150–152.

55. Stein LM, Cole RP. Early administration of corticosteroids in emergency room treatment of acute asthma. Ann Intern Med 1990; 112(11):822–827.

56. Bowyer SL, LaMothe MP, Hollister JR. Steroid myopathy: incidence and detection in a population with asthma. J Allergy Clin Immunol 1985; 76(2 Pt 1):234–242.

57. Haskell RJ, Wong BM, Hansen JE. A double-blind, randomized clinical trial of methylprednisolone in status asthmaticus. Arch Intern Med 1983; 143(7): 1324–1327.

58. Bowler SD, Mitchell CA, Armstrong JG. Corticosteroids in acute severe asthma: effectiveness of low doses. Thorax 1992; 47(8):584–587.

59. Marquette CH, Stach B, Cardot E, Bervar JF, Saulnier F, Lafitte JJ, et al. High-dose and low-dose systemic corticosteroids are equally efficient in acute severe asthma. Eur Respir J 1995; 8(1):22–27.

60. Morell F, Orriols R, de Gracia J, Curull V, Pujol A. Controlled trial of intravenous corticosteroids in severe acute asthma. Thorax 1992; 47(8):588–591.

61. Manser R, Reid D, Abramson M. Corticosteroids for acute severe asthma in hospitalised patients. Cochrane Database Syst Rev 2001; (1):CD001740.

62. Ratto D, Alfaro C, Sipsey J, Glovsky MM, Sharma OP. Are intravenous corticosteroids required in status asthmaticus? JAMA 1988; 260(4):527–529.

63. McCarren M, McDermott MF, Zalenski RJ, Jovanovic B, Marder D, Murphy DG, Kampe LM, Misiewicz VM, Rydman RJ. Prediction of relapse within eight weeks after an acute asthma exacerbation in adults. J Clin Epidemiol 1998; 51(2):107–118.

64. Chapman KR, Verbeek PR, White JG, Rebuck AS. Effect of a short course of prednisone in the prevention of early relapse after the emergency room treatment of acute asthma. N Engl J Med 1991; 324(12):788–794.

65. Fiel SB, Swartz MA, Glanz K, Francis ME. Efficacy of short-term corticosteroid therapy in outpatient treatment of acute bronchial asthma. Am J Med 1983; 75(2):259–262.

66. Shapiro GG, Furukawa CT, Pierson WE, Gardinier R, Bierman CW. Double-blind evaluation of methylprednisolone versus placebo for acute asthma episodes. Pediatrics 1983; 71(4):510–514.

67. McNamara RM, Rubin JM. Intramuscular methylprednisolone acetate for the prevention of relapse in acute asthma. Ann Emerg Med 1993; 22(12):1829–1835.

68. Rowe BH, Spooner CH, Ducharme FM, Bretzlaff JA, Bota GW. Corticosteroids for preventing relapse following acute exacerbations of asthma. Cochrane Database Syst Rev 2001; (1):CD000195.

69. O'Driscoll BR, Kalra S, Wilson M, Pickering CA, Carroll KB, Woodcock AA. Double-blind trial of steroid tapering in acute asthma. Lancet 1993; 341(8841): 324–327.

70. Lederle FA, Pluhar RE, Joseph AM, Niewoehner DE. Tapering of corticosteroid therapy following exacerbation of asthma. A randomized, double-blind, placebo-controlled trial. Arch Intern Med 1987; 147(12):2201–2203.

71. Cameron SJ, Cooper EJ, Crompton GK, Hoare MV, Grant IW. Substitution of beclomethasone aerosol for oral prednisolone in the treatment of chronic asthma. Br Med J 1973; 4(5886):205–207.

72. A controlled trial of inhaled corticosteroids in patients receiving Prednisone tablets for asthma. Br J Dis Chest 1976; 70(2):95–103.

73. Bosman HG, van Uffelen R, Tamminga JJ, Paanakker LR. Comparison of inhaled beclomethasone dipropionate 1000 micrograms twice daily and oral prednisone 10 mg once daily in asthmatic patients. Thorax 1994; 49(1):37–40.

74. Eriksson NE, Lindgren S, Lindholm N. A double-blind comparison of beclomethasone dipropionate aerosol and prednisolone in asthmatic patients. Postgrad Med J 1975; 51(suppl 4):67–70.

75. Namsirikul P, Chaisupamongkollarp S, Chantadisai N, Bamberg P. Comparison of inhaled budesonide with oral prednisolone at two dose-levels commonly used for the treatment of moderate asthma. Eur Respir J 1989; 2(4):317–324.

76. Toogood JH, Baskerville J, Jennings B, Lefcoe NM, Johansson SA. Bioequivalent doses of budesonide and prednisone in moderate and severe asthma. J Allerg Clin Immunol 1989; 84(5 Pt 1):688–700.

77. Mash B, Bheekie A, Jones PW. Inhaled vs oral steroids for adults with chronic asthma. Cochrane Database Syst Rev 2001; (1):CD002160.

78. Dunlap NE, Fulmer JD. Corticosteroid therapy in asthma. Clin Chest Med 1984; 5(4):669–683.

79. Harter JG, Reddy WJ, Thorn GW. Studies on an intermittent corticosteroid dosage regimen. N Engl J Med 1963; 269:591–596.

80. Toogood JH. Efficiency of inhaled versus oral steroid treatment of chronic asthma. N Engl Reg Allerg Proc 1987; 8(2):98–103.

81. British Thoracic Society, Scottish Intercollegiate Network. British guideline on the management of asthma. Thorax 2003; 58(suppl l):i1–i94.

82. McLeod DT, Capewell SJ, Law J, MacLaren W, Seaton A. Intramuscular triamcinolone acetonide in chronic severe asthma. Thorax 1985; 40(11):840–845.

83. Willey RF, Fergusson RJ, Godden DJ, Crompton GK, Grant IW. Comparison of oral prednisolone and intramuscular depot triamcinolone in patients with severe chronic asthma. Thorax 1984; 39(5):340–344.

84. Ogirala RG, Aldrich TK, Prezant DJ, Sinnett MJ, Enden JB, Williams MH Jr. High-dose intramuscular triamcinolone in severe, chronic, life-threatening asthma. N Engl J Med 1991; 324(9):585–589.

85. Lukert BP, Raisz LG. Glucocorticoid-induced osteoporosis: pathogenesis and management. Ann Intern Med 1990; 112(5):352–364.

86. Compston J (chairman). Glucocorticoid-induced osteoporosis—Guidelines for prevention and treatment. National Osteoporosis Society 2002. http://www.nos.org/glucocorticoid.asp (accessed June 2004).

87. Gluck OS, Murphy WA, Hahn TJ, Hahn B. Bone loss in adults receiving alternate day glucocorticoid therapy. A comparison with daily therapy. Arthritis Rheum 1981; 24(7):892–898.

88. Buckley LM, Leib ES, Cartularo KS, Vacek PM, Cooper SM. Effects of low dose corticosteroids on the bone mineral density of patients with rheumatoid arthritis. J Rheumatol 1995; 22(6):1055–1059.

89. Wong CA, Walsh LJ, Smith CJ, Wisniewski AF, Lewis SA, Hubbard R, Cawte S, Green DJ, Pringle M, Tattersfield AE. Inhaled corticosteroid use and bone-mineral density in patients with asthma. Lancet 2000; 355(9213):1399–1403.

90. Luengo M, Picado C, Del Rio L, Guanabens N, Montserrat JM, Setoain J. Vertebral fractures in steroid dependent asthma and involutional osteoporosis: a comparative study. Thorax 1991; 46(11):803–806.

91. van Staa TP, Leufkens HG, Abenhaim L, Zhang B, Cooper C. Use of oral corticosteroids and risk of fractures. J Bone Miner Res 2000; 15(6):993–1000.

92. Canalis E. Clinical review 83: mechanisms of glucocorticoid action in bone: implications to glucocorticoid-induced osteoporosis. J Clin Endocrinol Metab 1996; 81(10):3441–3447.

93. Buckley LM, Leib ES, Cartularo KS, Vacek PM, Cooper SM. Calcium and vitamin D3 supplementation prevents bone loss in the spine secondary to low-dose corticosteroids in patients with rheumatoid arthritis. A randomized, double-blind, placebo-controlled trial. Ann Intern Med 1996; 125(12):961–968.

94. Reid DM, Hughes RA, Laan RF, Sacco-Gibson NA, Wenderoth DH, Adami S, Eusebio RA, Devogelaer JP. Efficacy and safety of daily risedronate in the treatment of corticosteroid-induced osteoporosis in men and women: a randomized trial. European Corticosteroid-Induced Osteoporosis Treatment Study. J Bone Miner Res 2000; 15(6):1006–1013.

95. Sambrook P, Birmingham J, Kelly P, Kempler S, Nguyen T, Pocock N, Eisman J. Prevention of corticosteroid osteoporosis. A comparison of calcium, calcitriol, and calcitonin. N Engl J Med 1993; 328(24):1747–1752.

96. Recommendations for the prevention and treatment of glucocorticoid-induced osteoporosis: 2001 update. American College of Rheumatology Ad Hoc Committee on Glucocoritcoid-Induced Osteoporosis. Arthritis Rheum 2001; 44(7):1496–1503.

97. Hall GM, Daniels M, Doyle DV, Spector TD. Effect of hormone replacement therapy on bone mass in rheumatoid arthritis patients treated with and without steroids. Arthritis Rheum 1994; 37(10):1499–1505.

98. Beral V. Breast cancer and hormone-replacement therapy in the Million Women Study. Lancet 2003; 362(9382):419–427.

99. Beral V, Banks E, Reeves G. Evidence from randomised trials on the long-term effects of hormone replacement therapy. Lancet 2002; 360(9337):942–944.

100. Adachi JD, Bensen WG, Brown J, Hanley D, Hodsman A, Josse R, et al. Intermittent etidronate therapy to prevent corticosteroid-induced osteoporosis. N Engl J Med 1997; 337(6):382–387.

101. Saag KG, Emkey R, Schnitzer TJ, Brown JP, Hawkins F, Goemaere S, et al. Alendronate for the prevention and treatment of glucocorticoid-induced

osteoporosis. Glucocorticoid-Induced Osteoporosis Intervention Study Group. N Engl J Med 1998; 339(5):292–299.

102. Cohen S, Levy RM, Keller M, Boling E, Emkey RD, Greenwald M, et al. Risedronate therapy prevents corticosteroid-induced bone loss: a twelve-month, multicenter, randomized, double-blind, placebo-controlled, parallel-group study. Arthritis Rheum 1999; 42(11):2309–2318.

103. Disla E, Tamayo B, Fahmy A. Intermittent etidronate and corticosteroid-induced osteoporosis. N Engl J Med 1997; 337(26):1921.

104. Aris RM, Lester GE, Renner JB, Winders A, Denene Blackwood A, Lark RK, Ontjes DA. Efficacy of pamidronate for osteoporosis in patients with cystic fibrosis following lung transplantation. Am J Respir Crit Care Med 2000; 162(3 Pt 1):941–946.

105. Grotz WH, Rump LC, Niessen A, Schmidt-Gayk H, Reichelt A, Kirste G, Olschewski M, Schollmeyer PJ. Treatment of osteopenia and osteoporosis after kidney transplantation. Transplantation 1998; 66(8):1004–1008.

106. Luengo M, Picado C, Del Rio L, Guanabens N, Montserrat JM, Setoain J. Treatment of steroid-induced osteopenia with calcitonin in corticosteroid-dependent asthma. A one-year follow-up study. Am Rev Respir Dis 1990; 142(1):104–107.

107. Kotaniemi A, Piirainen H, Paimela L, Leirisalo-Repo M, Uoti-Reilama K, Lahdentausta P, Ruotsalainen P, Kataja M, Vaisanen E, Kurki P. Is continuous intranasal salmon calcitonin effective in treating axial bone loss in patients with active rheumatoid arthritis receiving low dose glucocorticoid therapy?. J Rheumatol 1996; 23(11):1875–1879.

108. Douglass JA, Tuxen DV, Horne M, Scheinkestel CD, Weinmann M, Czarny D, Bowes G. Myopathy in severe asthma. Am Rev Respir Dis 1992; 146(2):517–519.

109. Knox AJ, Mascie-Taylor BH, Muers MF. Acute hydrocortisone myopathy in acute severe asthma. Thorax 1986; 41(5):411–412.

110. Leatherman JW, Fluegel WL, David WS, Davies SF, Iber C. Muscle weakness in mechanically ventilated patients with severe asthma. Am J Respir Crit Care Med 1996; 153(5):1686–1690.

111. Behbehani NA, Al Mane F, D'yachkova Y, Pare P, FitzGerald JM. Myopathy following mechanical ventilation for acute severe asthma: the role of muscle relaxants and corticosteroids. Chest 1999; 115(6):1627–1631.

112. Wilson AM, McFarlane LC, Lipworth BJ. Systemic bioactivity profiles of oral prednisolone and nebulized budesonide in adult asthmatics. Chest 1998; 114(4):1022–1027.

113. Jasani MK, Boyle JA, Greig WR, Dalakos TG, Browning MC, Thompson A, Buchanan WW. Corticosteroid-induced suppression of the hypothalamo-pituitary-adrenal axis: observations on patients given oral corticosteroids for rheumatoid arthritis. Q J Med 1967; 36(143):261–276.

114. Ackerman GL, Nolsn CM. Adrenocortical responsiveness after alternate-day corticosteroid therapy. N Engl J Med 1968; 278(8):405–409.

115. Krasner AS. Glucocorticoid-induced adrenal insufficiency. JAMA 1999; 282(7):671–676.

116. Salem M, Tainsh RE Jr, Bromberg J, Loriaux DL, Chernow B. Perioperative glucocorticoid coverage. A reassessment 42 years after emergence of a problem. Ann Surg 1994; 219(4):416–425.

117. Glowniak JV, Loriaux DL. A double-blind study of perioperative steroid requirements in secondary adrenal insufficiency. Surgery 1997; 121(2):123–129.

118. Graber AL, Ney RL, Nicholson WE, Island DP, Liddle GW. Natural history of pituitary-adrenal recovery following long-term suppression with corticosteroids. J Clin Endocrinol Metab 1965; 25:11–16.

119. Delcourt C, Cristol JP, Tessier F, Leger CL, Michel F, Papoz L. Risk factors for cortical, nuclear, and posterior subcapsular cataracts: the POLA study. Pathologies Oculaires Liees a l'Age. Am J Epidemiol 2000; 151(5):497–504.

120. Walsh LJ, Wong CA, Oborne J, Cooper S, Lewis SA, Pringle M, et al. Adverse effects of oral corticosteroids in relation to dose in patients with lung disease. Thorax 2001; 56(4):279–284.

121. Jobling AI, Augusteyn RC. What causes steroid cataracts? A review of steroid-induced posterior subcapsular cataracts. Clin Exp Optom 2002; 85(2):61–75.

122. Limaye SR, Pillai S, Tina LU. Relationship of steroid dose to degree of posterior subcapsular cataracts in nephrotic syndrome. Ann Ophthalmol 1988; 20(6):225–227.

123. Wolthers OD, Pedersen S. Short term linear growth in asthmatic children during treatment with prednisolone. BMJ 1990; 301(6744):145–148.

124. Chang KC, Miklich DR, Barwise G, Chai H, Miles-Lawrence R. Linear growth of chronic asthmatic children: the effects of the disease and various forms of steroid therapy. Clin Allerg 1982; 12(4):369–378.

125. Nassif E, Weinberger M, Sherman B, Brown K. Extrapulmonary effects of maintenance corticosteroid therapy with alternate-day prednisone and inhaled beclomethasone in children with chronic asthma. J Allerg Clin Immunol 1987; 80(4):518–529.

126. Reimer LG, Morris HG, Ellis EF. Growth of asthmatic children during treatment with alternate-day steriods. J Allerg Clin Immunol 1975; 55(4):224–231.

127. Dolan LM, Kesarwala HH, Holroyde JC, Fischer TJ. Short-term, high-dose, systemic steroids in children with asthma: the effect on the hypothalamic-pituitary-adrenal axis. J Allerg Clin Immunol 1987; 80(1):81–87.

128. Bihari M, Grossman BJ. Posterior subcapsular cataracts. Related to long-term corticosteroid treatment in children. Am J Dis Child 1968; 116(6):604–608.

129. Wendel PJ, Ramin SM, Barnett-Hamm C, Rowe TF, Cunningham FG. Asthma treatment in pregnancy: a randomized controlled study. Am J Obstet Gynecol 1996; 175(1):150–154.

130. Cydulka RK, Emerman CL, Schreiber D, Molander KH, Woodruff PG, Camargo CA Jr. Acute asthma among pregnant women presenting to the emergency department. Am J Respir Crit Care Med 1999; 160(3):887–892.

131. Czeizel AE, Rockenbauer M. Population-based case-control study of teratogenic potential of corticosteroids. Teratology 1997; 56(5):335–340.

132. Fitzsimons R, Greenberger PA, Patterson R. Outcome of pregnancy in women requiring corticosteroids for severe asthma. J Allerg Clin Immunol 1986; 78(2):349–353.

133. Fainstat T. Cortisone-induced congenital cleft palate in rabbits. Endocrinology 1954; 55(4):502–508.

134. Rodriguez-Pinilla E, Martinez-Frias ML. Corticosteroids during pregnancy and oral clefts: a case-control study. Teratology 1998; 58(1):2–5.

135. Nelson-Piercy C. Asthma in pregnancy. Thorax 2001; 56(4):325–328.

136. Stenius-Aarniala B, Piirila P, Teramo K. Asthma and pregnancy: a prospective study of 198 pregnancies. Thorax 1988; 43(1):12–18.

137. Schatz M, Zeiger RS, Harden K, Hoffman CC, Chilingar L, Petitti D. The safety of asthma and allergy medications during pregnancy. J Allerg Clin Immunol 1997; 100(3):301–306.

138. Arad I, Landau H. Adrenocortical reserve of neonates born of long-term, steroid-treated mothers. Eur J Pediatr 1984; 142(4):279–280.

139. Schatz M, Dombrowski MP, Wise R, Momirova V, Landon M, Mabie W, Newman RB, Hauth JC, Lindheimer M, Caritis SN, Leveno KJ, Meis P, Miodovnik M, Wapner RJ, Paul RH, Varner MW, O'Sullivan MJ, Thurnau GR, Conway DL. Maternal-Fetal Medicine Units Network, The National Institute of Child Health and Development; The National Heart, Lung and Blood Institute. The reiationship of asthma medication use to perinatal outcomes. J Allergy Clin Immunol 2004 Jun; 113(6):1040–1045.

140. Ost L, Wettrell G, Bjorkhem I, Rane A. Prednisolone excretion in human milk. J Pediatr 1985; 106(6):1008–1011.

141. Global Initiative for Asthma. Global strategy for asthma management and prevention. National Heart, Lung and Blood Institute . (Updated November 2003). http://www.ginasthma.com (accessed June 2004).

142. Chan JS, Cowie RL, Lazarenko GC, Little C, Scott S, Ford GT. Comparison of intramuscular betamethasone and oral prednisone in the prevention of relapse of acute asthma. Can Respir J 2001; 8(3):147–152.

143. Chalmers GW, MacLeod KJ, Little SA, Thomson LJ, McSharry CP, Thomson NC. Influence of cigarette smoking on inhaled corticosteroid treatment in mild asthma. Thorax 2002; 57(3):226–230.

144. Haynes RB, McDonald H, Garg AX, Montague P. Interventions for helping patients to follow prescriptions for medications. Cochrane Database Syst Rev 2002;(2):CD000011.

145. Green RH, Brightling CE, Woltmann G, Parker D, Wardlaw AJ, Pavord ID. Analysis of induced sputum in adults with asthma: identification of subgroup with isolated sputum neutrophilia and poor response to inlialed corticosteroids. Thorax 2002; 57(10):875–879.

146. Wenzel SE, Schwartz LB, Langmack EL, Halliday JL, Trudeau JB, Gibbs RL, et al. Evidence that severe asthma can be divided pathologically into two inflammatory subtypes with distinct physiologic and clinical characteristics. Am JRespir Crit Care Med 1999; 160(3):1001–1008.

147. Adams N, Bestall J, Jones PW. Inhaled fluticasone proprionate for chronic asthma (Cochrane Review). Cochrane Database Syst Rev 2001; 3:CD003135.

9

Anti-IgE Therapy for Asthma

S. G. O. JOHANSSON

Department of Medicine, Unit of Clinical
    Immunology and Allergy,
    Karolinska University Hospital
Stockholm, Sweden

ROLAND BUHL

Pulmonary Department, Mainz University
    Hospital
Mainz, Germany

I. Introduction

Allergic diseases, such as allergic asthma, are hypersensitivity reactions
initiated by immunological mechanisms (1,2). They are usually mediated
by IgE antibodies, triggering an inflammation characterized by an increase
in production of Th2-type cytokines at a mucosal surface, the interface
between the external and the internal environments. Allergic diseases usually
occur in atopic individuals who are genetically predisposed to producing IgE
antibodies in response to low doses of general environmental allergens, e.g.,
pollens, mites, and danders. Although allergies mediated by other immunoglobulins (e.g., IgG-immune complexes that can activate complement) or
lymphocytes (e.g., allergic contact dermatitis to chromium and nickel) also
exist, the major part, if not all, of allergic asthma is IgE mediated. The
cross-linking of mast cell/basophil membrane cell-bound IgE antibodies by
allergen results in the release of inflammatory mediators that are responsible
for the signs and symptoms of allergy. IgE sensitization to an allergen can
develop in childhood or throughout life, and subsequent allergen contact,
which may occur years later, can initiate a severe attack of allergic asthma.

An anti-IgE antibody, omalizumab (Xolair®), was approved in the United States in July 2003 for the treatment of moderate to severe allergic asthma in adults and adolescents. Omalizumab is licensed for use in allergic asthma in Australia and is under evaluation for use in patients with uncontrolled severe persistent allergic asthma in Europe. In this chapter, we will describe the role of IgE in allergic asthma and the rationale for anti-IgE therapy. We will present clinical data illustrating proof of the anti-IgE concept and results from the pivotal phase-III clinical studies showing efficacy of omalizumab in adult and pediatric asthma patients. Consideration will be given to the anti-inflammatory effects of anti-IgE treatment with omalizumab and which patients are most likely to benefit from anti-IgE therapy.

II. What Is IgE?

The discovery of IgE in 1968 represented a major breakthrough in our understanding of allergic disease (3). Although allergy had been recognized for centuries, and the possible existence of the "reagins" responsible had been reported in the early 20th century, allergology had been regarded with suspicion until this new immunoglobulin was declared.

IgE has a molecular weight of 190 kDa. Its structure is shown in Figure 1. The heavy chain includes four constant regions, Cε1–4, of which

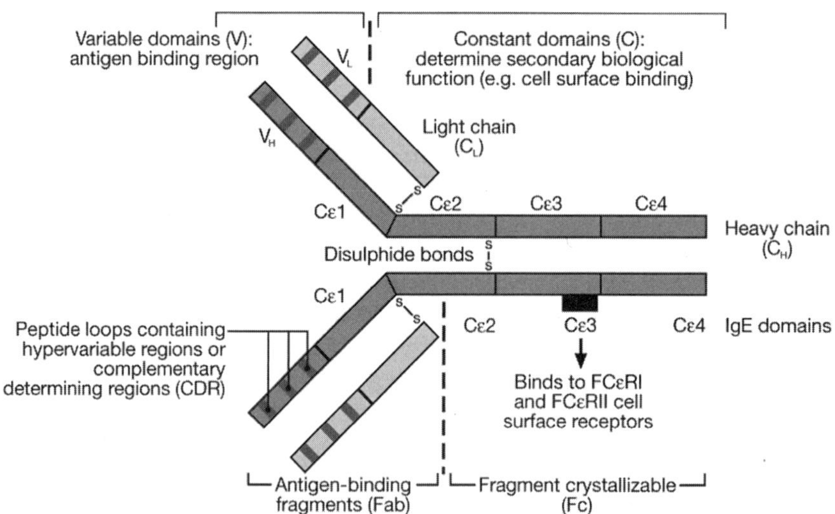

Figure 1   The primary structure of IgE. Variable domains bind antigen, while constant domains determine secondary biological function (e.g., cell surface binding). *Abbreviations*: V$_L$, variable domain of the light chain; V$_H$, variable domain of the heavy chain; C$_L$, constant domain of the light chain; Cε1–4, constant domains of the heavy chain; Fab, antigen binding fragments; Fc, crystallizable fragments.

Cε2–4 constitute the Fc fragment. As in other antibodies, the antigen-binding site is contained in the Fab fragment (at the VL/VH domains). The Cε3 domains of Fc bind either of the two IgE receptors, the high-affinity receptor FcεRI [$K_D = (1-2) \times 10^{-9}$ M], or the low-affinity receptor FcεRII ($K_D = 1 \times 10^{-6}$ M). Monomeric IgE, free in circulation, has been reported to have a half-life of two to three days but recent studies of transfused IgE antibodies showed a half-life as short as 1.13 days (4). However, once IgE binds to receptors it can remain stable for weeks. Its concentration in the serum is highly dependent on age and sex (decreasing from the age of 20 years) and is very low. The range is approximately 1–100 μg/L, which corresponds to 20–40 IU/mL using the NIBSC/WHO reference 75/502 (5–7), which is considerably lower than that of any other immunoglobulin, e.g., 1/100,000 of IgG. Levels are typically higher in allergic populations, e.g., allergic asthma (10–1000 μg/L) (8), and highest in comorbid patients with more than one allergic disorder, e.g., in patients with asthma and "atopic dermatitis" (9,10). However, high serum IgE levels, without any related IgE antibodies, have been reported in viral infections (11), in response to air pollution like cigarette smoke (12), and also in immunological interactions like graft-versus-host disease after bone marrow transplantation (13).

A. The Role of IgE in Asthma

The role of IgE in the initiation of the allergic cascade is well established (14). The IgE-mediated allergic cascade involves a biphasic response with an immediate or early allergic response (EAR) and a late allergic response (LAR) (15). EAR is an acute response that occurs within one hour of exposure to allergen. It is characterized by constriction of the bronchi and bronchioles, contraction of smooth muscle and vasodilation of capillaries, and overstimulation of mucous glands and nerve endings. LAR occurs 4 to 24 hours after initial allergen challenge. It is characterized by chronic infiltration of the airways by immune cells, resulting in prolonged airflow obstruction and determining the severity of bronchial hyper-responsiveness. After 24 to 48 hours, infiltrating Th2 cells stimulate the release of proinflammatory cytokines. IgE plays a critical role in both the EAR and the LAR via interaction with the FcεRI and FcεRII receptors. In addition, IgE enhances the efficiency of antigen presentation to T cells via interaction with FcεRI receptors on antigen-presenting cells (16).

The complete form of FcεRI is a tetramer ($\alpha\beta\gamma_2$) and is expressed on a variety of cell types, predominantly on mast cells and basophils. FcεRI is expressed as a trimer ($\alpha\gamma_2$) on antigen-presenting cells (16), such as monocytes (17), epidermal Langerhans cells (18), and peripheral blood dendritic cells (19) (but is not expressed on their progenitors). It is also expressed on epithelial cells (20), platelets (21), and, at a low level, on eosinophils (22). The IgE–FcεRI interaction has 1:1 stoichiometry (23).

FcεRII (also called CD23) is expressed on B cells, eosinophils, platelets, natural killer cells, Th2 cells, follicular dendritic cells, Langerhans cells, and epithelial cells (24). FcεRII exists in two forms (FcεRIIa and FcεRIIb). FcεRIIa mediates endocytosis by B cells, and FcεRIIb, the sequence of which differs only in a few amino acids, plays a role in IgE-mediated phagocytosis by diverse cells (25). Eosinophils express both forms (26). The IgE–FcεRII interaction has 2:1 stoichiometry.

EAR results from IgE-mediated mast-cell degranulation. Mast cells are major players in the allergic response (27). When IgE antibodies on mast cells or basophils are cross-linked by allergen, the cells become activated. Interaction of receptor-bound IgE antibodies with soluble multivalent allergen leads to receptor aggregation. By signal transduction, a complex series of events ensues, including recruitment of intracellular protein kinases, phospholipases, influx of Ca^{2+} ions, and synthesis of proinflammatory mediators. This culminates in rapid (i.e., within minutes) degranulation, the release of the stored contents of cytoplasmic granules and of newly formed mediators by exocytosis (Fig. 2A). A plethora of mediators is released, including histamine, leukotrienes, the anticoagulant heparin, neutral proteases (such as tryptase and chymase, which constitute approximately 30% of the total granule protein), complex-carbohydrate-cleaving enzymes, platelet activating factor, chemokines, prostaglandins, and an array of cytokines [IL-3, IL-4, IL-5, IL-6, IL-10 and IL-13, tumor necrosis factor (TNF)-α, GM-CSF, and others] (28). Acute allergic symptoms are generated by interaction of these preformed and newly formed mediators with specific receptors on the target tissues. Unlike basophils, mast cells do not circulate, although they can migrate through the tissues in which they are localized, and are usually present in perivascular connective tissue, epithelia, and lymph nodes. In patients with allergic asthma, mast cells localize in the bronchial smooth muscle bundles. Asthma severity increases with smooth-muscle mast-cell density, because mast cell migration to airway mucus glands and degranulation increase bronchial hyper-responsiveness and mucous secretion (27).

The cause and significance of the LAR is less understood. A number of studies have shown that eosinophils play a major role. Eosinophilic inflammation has been shown to be related to asthma severity (29) and asthma exacerbations (30). However, long-term suppression of circulating eosinophils by an antibody to IL-5 did not protect against the LAR, indicating that eosinophils are not solely responsible for the effect (31). Eosinophils are selectively recruited to the site of inflammation from the microcirculation (Fig. 2B). Their cytoplasmic granules have a crystalloid core of major basic protein and a matrix of eosinophil cationic protein, eosinophil-derived neurotoxin, and eosinophil peroxidase. These unique toxic inflammatory mediators and a variety of cytokines and lipid mediators are both synthesized and released by degranulation in response to

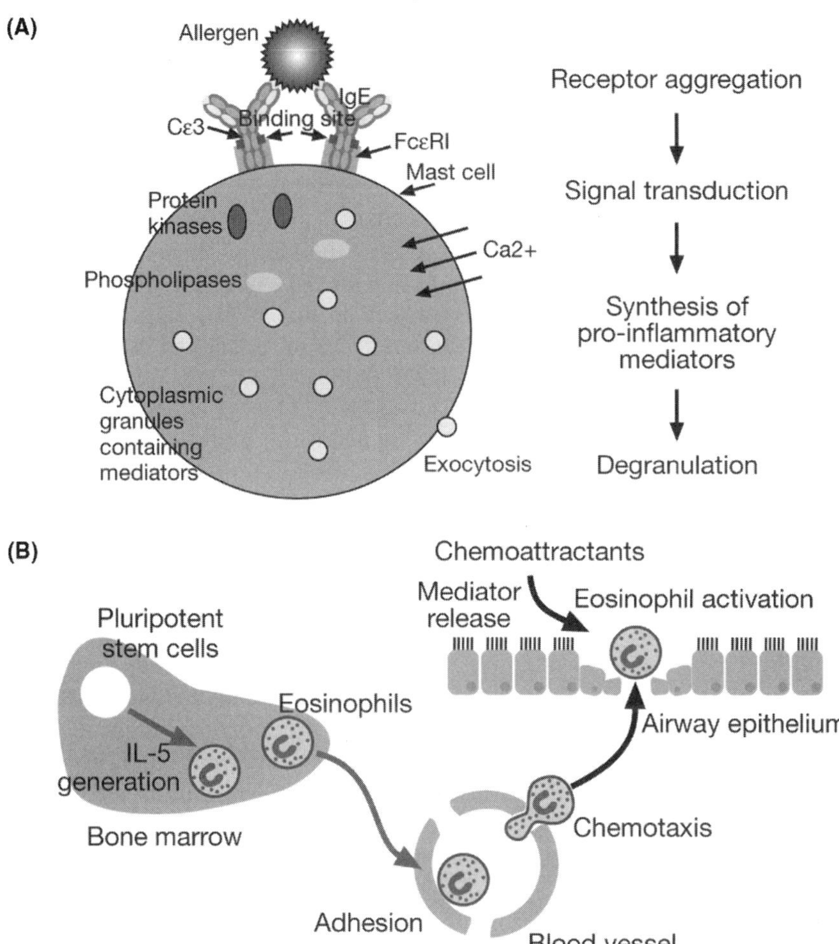

Figure 2 Early and late asthmatic responses. (**A**) Sequence of events following mast-cell sensitization by IgE (activation and degranulation), the early allergenic response. (**B**) Role of eosinophils in the late allergenic response.

IgE binding to the FcεRI receptor. However, whether this is the major pathway of the LAR is uncertain, due to the low level of FcεRI expression on eosinophils (32). Major basic protein and eosinophil cationic protein have profound cytotoxic effects on the airway epithelium (33), and for this reason, eosinophils are often regarded as the primary effector cells in asthma.

Interaction of IgE with the FcεRII receptor has been implicated in allergy, although its role has not yet been fully elucidated. FcεRII is multifunctional and its roles include the induction of IgE synthesis (34–36) and the maintenance and modulation of the IgE response (35). IgE binding to the FcεRII receptor has been shown to be responsible for rapid and specific transepithelial antigen transport in allergic rats (36). As asthmatic airway smooth muscle expresses surface FcεRII, and expression is upregulated by IgE–FcεRII binding (37), it is possible that FcεRII is involved in a similar transepithelial migration pathway in humans, acting like an adhesion molecule to facilitate the phagocytosis of IgE-bound antigen. FcεRI has also been implicated in the IgE-mediated presentation of allergen on antigen-presenting cells (38). In addition, although not as predominant as its role in binding IgE, membrane-bound FcεRII (and the soluble form) has functions in the allergic response that do not involve interaction with IgE, such as in cell–cell interaction, acting as an adhesion molecule that binds β integrins, and in cytokine-like activities (39).

Allergen presentation to T cells is enhanced by IgE–FcεRI complexes on antigen-presenting cells (16), including dendritic cells (40), macrophages (41), and Langerhans cells (42). Allergen presentation leads to Th2-cell-mediated allergic reactions and their associated clinical symptoms. Circulating myeloid dendritic cells are rapidly recruited to the airway epithelia following allergen inhalation (43,44), and numbers of dendritic cells are significantly higher in the airways of patients with asthma compared with control individuals ($p < 0.02$) (45). Dendritic cells express FcεRIα, but not FcεRIβ (46,47), and expression of FcεRIα is significantly increased in patients with asthma compared with control individuals ($p < 0.003$) (45). Allergens can thus be internalized and presented by dendritic cells by cross-linking of allergen-IgE antibodies bound to the α chain of FcεRI (48). However, the β chain is necessary for signal transduction (48).

These roles of T cells, B cells, mast cells, and eosinophils in the early and late asthmatic reactions are summarized in Figure 3.

III. Anti-IgE as a Therapeutic Strategy

The majority of asthma is allergic in nature and initiated by IgE antibody (49). Targeting of factors involved in the allergic response, such as IgE, represents a novel strategy for the development of new therapeutic agents for allergic diseases. The importance of FcεRI-mediated mast-cell degranulation and FcεRI and FcεRII-mediated enhancement of antigen presentation in the development of an allergic reaction make these two processes particularly suitable for therapeutic intervention. IgE binding to its Fc receptors mediates both processes and therefore represents an ideal target for therapeutic attenuation of the allergic cascade. This IgE-receptor-binding step might be blocked by inhibitory peptides with structures based on the receptor. However, such receptor-derived peptides may elicit an anti-peptide immune response and anaphylaxis through receptor cross-linking. A preferable strategy is to use a monoclonal anti-IgE antibody that binds

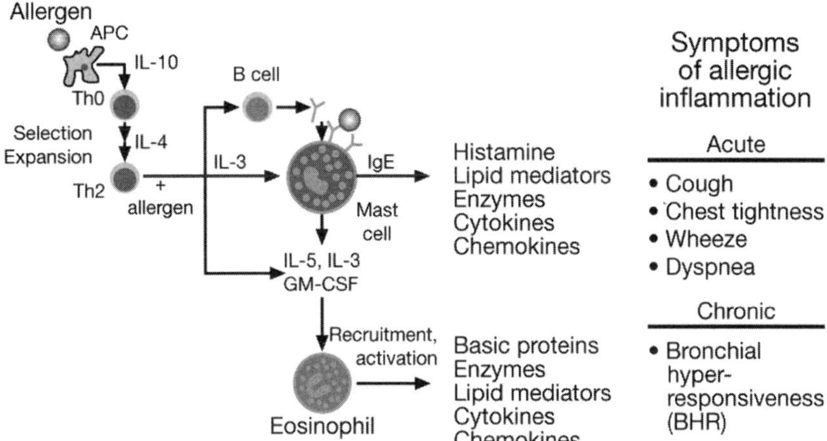

Figure 3   The interactions between mast cells, B cells, antigen-presenting cells, eosinophils, and airway tissues that are mediated by IgE during chronic asthma. *Source*: From Ref. 49.

free, but not receptor-bound, IgE and thereby inhibits initiation of the allergic cascade by preventing IgE binding to receptors.

As IgE-receptor binding directs immune responses through the multiple cell types on which Fc receptors are expressed, the effects of blocking it could be expected to be manifold (Fig. 3). Blocking IgE binding to FcɛRI receptors on dendritic cells could reduce the efficiency of antigen presentation to T cells (16), while blocking binding to FcɛRI receptors on mast cells and basophils could prevent allergen-induced degranulation and avoid the effects following the release of inflammatory mediators (27). In addition, blocking IgE binding to FcɛRII receptors on monocytes and eosinophils could prevent IgE-mediated phagocytosis (25).

For reasons of tolerability, a therapeutic anti-IgE antibody must be non-immunogenic and non-anaphylactogenic. In addition, the binding affinity between IgE and the antibody should favor the formation of immune complexes small enough to result in a reasonable rate of clearance without immune-complex-mediated adverse reactions. To achieve therapeutic efficacy, a dose of anti-IgE capable of nearly completely removing free IgE might be necessary, as FcɛRI receptor density on effector cells is high (10^4–10^6 per cell) and only 2000 IgE molecules are required for half-maximal histamine release from basophils exposed to allergen (50).

IV.   Anti-IgE Therapy with Omalizumab—Proof of Concept

A monoclonal humanized recombinant anti-IgE antibody (omalizumab) has been generated from a human IgG_1 framework onto which is grafted the complementarity-determining region from a murine anti-IgE antibody (51). This was designed for optimal safety. As the entire molecule contains fewer than 5% murine residues, it has a low potential for immunogenicity (51). Omalizumab recognizes the Cε3 domain of free human IgE (Figs. 1 and 4). As this is the same site that binds the FcεRIα and FcεRII receptors, omalizumab cannot bind receptor-bound IgE and is thereby prevented from inducing mast-cell or basophil degranulation and anaphylaxis (51). This has been demonstrated by in vitro and in vivo studies (52) and clinical studies in 2845 patients. Analytical ultracentrifugation and size-exclusion chromatography revealed that omalizumab-IgE complexes are generally small, the largest consisting of a cyclic or near-cyclic heterohexamer of three IgE and three anti-IgE molecules ($\leq 10^3$ kDa) (53). While this species formed at a molar ratio of 1:1, a heterotrimer of two IgE molecules and one anti-IgE was the dominant species formed at the more physiological molar ratio of 10:1 (IgE to anti-IgE), and a heterotrimer of one IgE and two anti-IgE molecules was dominant at a 1:10 molar ratio.

The therapeutic potential of omalizumab was confirmed in a multicenter, double-blind, placebo-controlled trial enrolling 240 patients, which found omalizumab to considerably reduce serum free IgE (54). In some patients, concentrations of serum free IgE decreased by $\geq 90\%$ over 12 weeks of omalizumab administration (from 160 IU/mL to below the detection limit of 10 IU/mL, 24 ng/mL), and a dose of 0.005 mg/kg/week omalizumab for each IU/mL of free IgE in serum at baseline was effective in reducing serum levels of free IgE to the lowest detectable level at steady state. Another study, which found omalizumab to reduce serum levels of free IgE to 1% of pretreatment levels, also reported a marked reduction of FcεRI on basophils: the pretreatment median receptor density was 220,000 per basophil, reducing to a median of 8300 after three months of omalizumab therapy (55). This reduction in receptor density was accompanied

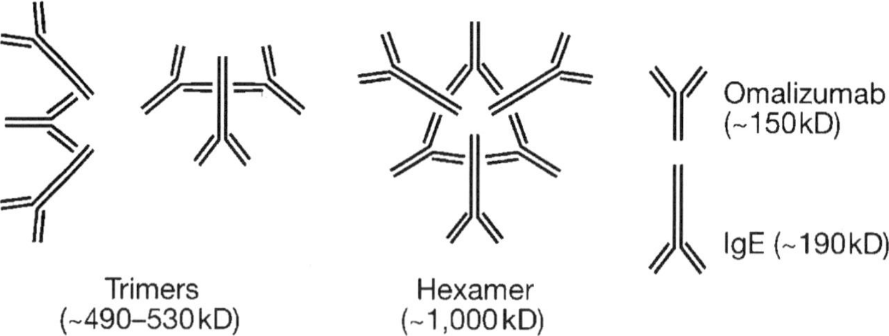

Figure 4 Structures of the complexes formed by interaction of the antigen-recognition site of omalizumab with the Cε3 site of IgE. The heterotrimer is formed at molar ratios of 1:10 and 10:1, and the heterohexamer at a molar ratio of 1:1.

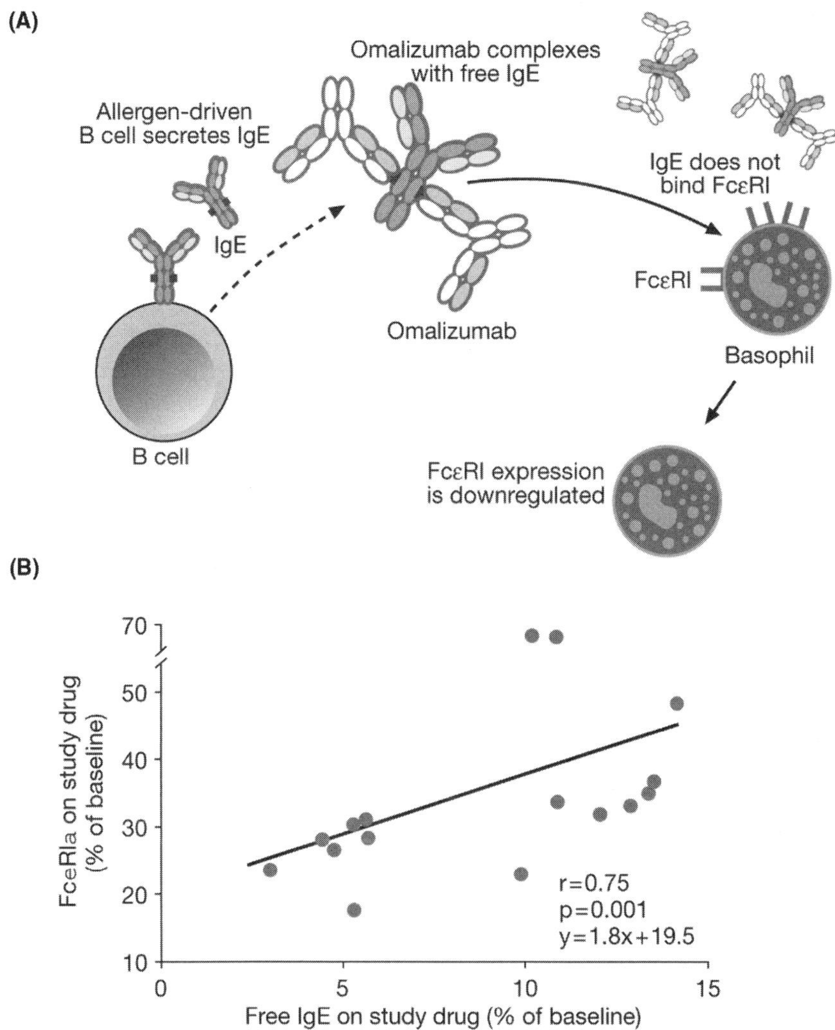

Figure 5 The reduction in serum free IgE by omalizumab binding is associated with downregulation of the high affinity FcεRI receptor. (**A**) Schematic showing receptor downregulation by IgE. Likewise, an increase in serum free IgE is associated with an increase in FcεRI-receptor expression. This process is believed to occur in both basophils and mast cells. (**B**) Correlation between basophil FcεRI expression and serum levels of free IgE in patients receiving omalizumab. *Source*: From Ref. 56.

by a reduction in responsiveness of basophils to stimulation by allergen of approximately 90%, suggesting that FcεRI density on basophils is regulated by serum levels of free IgE (Fig. 5A,B) (56). The mast-cell response, as measured by skin tests, was also markedly reduced (55), and it is likely that similar FcεRI down-regulation occurs in mast cells, which are morphologically very similar to basophils. This suggests that FcεRI-receptor density is regulated by circulating levels of free IgE, and that moderately reducing free IgE with omalizumab is very effective in reducing FcεRI expression.

Two preliminary studies further support the therapeutic use of omalizumab in patients. In patients with allergic asthma, nine weeks' omalizumab therapy (57) reduced serum free IgE to levels below or approaching the detection limit and increased the dose of allergen required to provoke an allergic response (for bronchoconstriction, increased from 1:870 to 1:459; for cutaneous reaction, increased from 1:10,000 to 1:2000). In addition, it attenuated both the EAR [mean maximum fall in forced expiratory volume in one second (FEV_1) during which EAR decreased from 30% to 18.8%, $p = 0.01$ vs. placebo], and the LAR (mean maximum fall in FEV_1 during which EAR decreased from 24% to 9%, $p = 0.047$; induced sputum eosinophil count reduced 11-fold; methacholine responsiveness PC_{20} improved). Similarly, 11 weeks' omalizumab therapy (58) reduced serum free IgE by 89%, and attenuated the EAR [scored as improvements in methacholine responsiveness (PC_{20}, $p < 0.05$, final measurement) and allergen responsiveness (PC_{15}, $p \leq 0.002$, throughout)].

Clinical benefit with omalizumab is observed when free IgE levels in serum are reduced to 50 ng/mL (20.8 IU/mL) or less [target 25 ng/mL (10.4 IU/mL)]. The ability of omalizumab to reduce free IgE levels to this extent depends on dose and the patient's weight and baseline IgE level. To simplify dosing and ensure that free IgE reduction is achieved, an individualized tiered dosing table was developed. According to this table, patients receive omalizumab, 150–375 mg, by subcutaneous injection for every two or four weeks, depending on weight and starting IgE level (Fig. 6) (59).

Body weight (kg)	30–60	>60–70	>70–80	>80–90	>90–150	
Baseline IgE (IU/mL)			Mg/dose			**Frequency of dosing**
≥30–100	150	150	150	150	300	Q4wk
>100–200	300	300	300	300	225	Q2wk
>200–300	300	225	225	225	300	
>300–400	225	225	300	300		
>400–500	300	300	375	375		Not dosed
>500–600	300	375				
>600–700	375					

Figure 6 Omalizumab subcutaneous doses for adolescents and adults with allergic asthma. *Source*: From Ref. 59.

V. Pivotal Studies in Asthma

Pivotal in the clinical evaluation of omalizumab were three large, multicenter, randomized, double-blind, placebo-controlled, phase III studies conducted in a total of 1405 children, adolescents, and adults (aged 6 to 76 years) with moderate to severe allergic asthma. Patients had a positive skin prick test to one or more common allergens to which they were exposed, and serum total IgE levels 30 to 700 (or an upper limit of 1200 in children) IU/mL (60–62). These three studies had a similar design (Fig. 7): a four- to six-week run-in phase prior to randomization; a 16-week "steroid-stable" phase, where placebo or active treatment was given in addition to stable inhaled corticosteroid (ICS) treatment [beclomethasone dipropionate (BDP)]; and a 12-week "steroid-reduction" phase, in which ICS therapy was gradually reduced to the optimal lowest dose required for an acceptable level of asthma control, ending with four weeks at a constant, minimal ICS dose. Subcutaneous injections of 150–750 mg omalizumab were given every four or two weeks (doses above 225 mg were divided into two and given every two weeks). The dose was calculated from patient baseline IgE and body weight to provide at least 0.016 mg/kg per IU/mL of IgE per four weeks. Baseline characteristics of the patients enrolled are shown in Table 1. The primary endpoint for the studies in adults was reduction in asthma exacerbations during the steroid-stable or steroid-reduction phases. Exacerbations were defined as a worsening of asthma requiring treatment with oral or intravenous corticosteroids or doubling of baseline ICS dose.

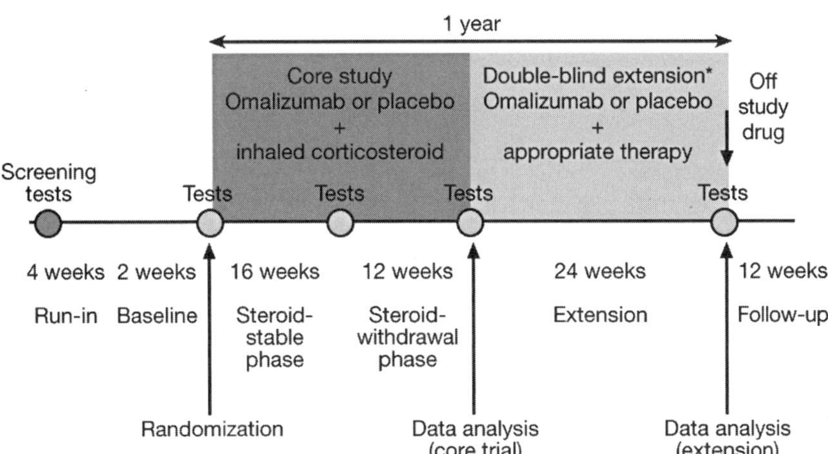

Figure 7 Phase III study design.

Table 1 Phase III Trials: Baseline Characteristics

	Busse et al. (60)		Solér et al. (61)		Milgrom et al. (62)	
	Omalizumab	Placebo	Omalizumab	Placebo	Omalizumab	Placebo
n	268	257	274	272	225	109
Mean age	39	39	40	39	9	10
Mean FEV_1 (% predicted)	68	68	70	70	84	85
Mean BDP dose (μg/day)	679	676	769	772	338	318
Severe asthma (%)	30	31	22	22	9	6

Abbreviations: FEV_1, forced expiratory volume in 1 second; BDP, beclomethasone dipropionate.

These three core studies demonstrated fewer asthma exacerbations in patients treated with omalizumab compared with placebo (percentage of patients experiencing exacerbations vs. placebo, $p < 0.001$) (Fig. 8). In addition, patients receiving omalizumab significantly reduced their requirement for ICS versus placebo ($p \leq 0.001$) (Fig. 9), and significantly more patients on omalizumab than placebo withdrew completely from ICS therapy [$p < 0.005$ (60–62)]. In the adult studies (60,61), improvements in rescue-bronchodilator use, asthma symptoms, and FEV_1 were also observed versus placebo (all $p < 0.05$) and, in the pediatric study (62), rescue-bronchodilator use was reduced versus placebo ($p = 0.004$) and a trend was seen toward improvement in asthma symptoms and FEV_1.

The long-term efficacy of omalizumab in adults was demonstrated in 24-week double-blind extensions to the Busse core study by Lanier et al. (63), and to the Solèr core study, by Buhl et al. (64). Of 525 patients from the Busse core study, 460 entered the Lanier extension, and were randomized either to omalizumab or placebo added on to the lowest sustained dose of BDP as established during the steroid-reduction phase of the core study (63). More patients in the omalizumab group completed the extension without using ICS (27% vs. 10%, $p < 0.001$) and remained exacerbation-free (68.2% vs. 57.2%, $p = 0.015$) than in the placebo group, and omalizumab recipients used less ICS than placebo recipients overall ($p < 0.001$). Of the 546 patients who took part in the Solèr study, 483 continued for 24 weeks on randomized treatment in the Buhl extension (64). Compared with placebo recipients, more omalizumab recipients completed the extension without

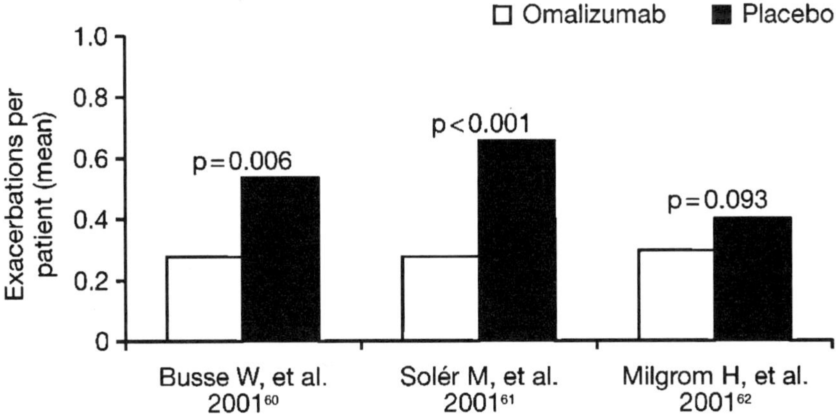

Figure 8 Reduction in asthma exacerbations with omalizumab treatment: pivotal phase III studies (60–62). Patients received either omalizumab (0.016 mg/kg/IU/ mL) or placebo for 16 weeks. Exacerbation was defined as worsening of asthma requiring treatment with oral or I.V. corticosteroids or doubling of baseline beclomethasone dipropionate dose.

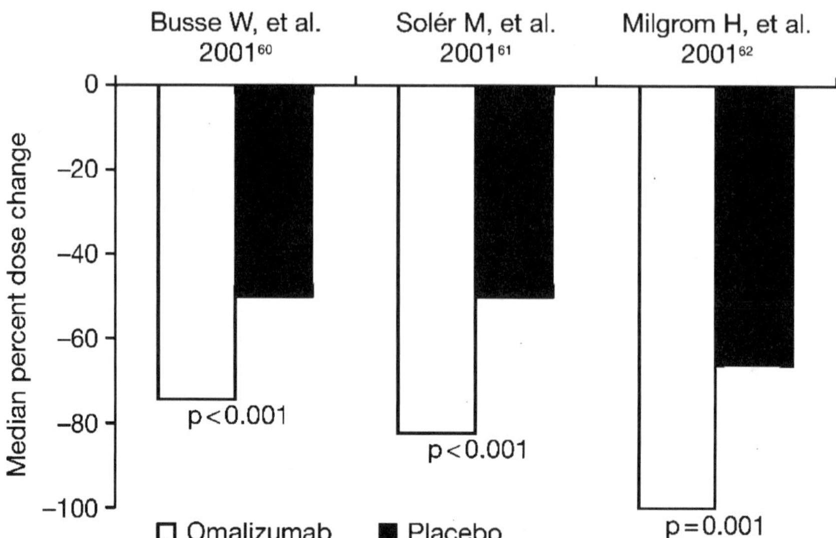

Figure 9   Median (%) change in inhaled corticosteroid dose with omalizumab: pivotal phase III studies (60–62). Patients received either omalizumab (0.016 mg/kg/IU/mL) or placebo for 16 weeks.

using ICS (33.5% vs. 13.5%, $p < 0.001$) and remained exacerbation-free (76% vs. 59.4%, $p < 0.001$), and omalizumab recipients maintained a lower dose of ICS than placebo recipients throughout ($p < 0.001$).

Asthma-related quality of life (QoL) in the three pivotal studies by Busse (60), Solèr (61), and Milgrom (62) was assessed by Finn et al. (65), Buhl et al. (66), and Lemanske et al. (67), respectively. The effect of omalizumab therapy was assessed using the Juniper Asthma Quality of Life Questionnaire (AQLQ) (68) over 52 weeks in adults, and the pediatric AQLQ (PAQLQ) over 28 weeks in children. In adults with moderate to severe asthma (66), progressive improvements throughout the 52 weeks were observed across all four domains of the AQLQ (activities, emotions, symptoms, and exposure) and overall AQLQ, which were significant at the end of each treatment phase versus placebo (all $p < 0.05$). Juniper et al. have determined that improvements in the AQLQ score of $\geq$0.5, 1.0, and 1.5 represented the minimal clinically important difference, a moderate change, and a large change in QoL, respectively (69). The proportion of patients achieving large improvements in AQLQ (increase in overall score $\geq$1.5 points from baseline) was significantly higher in omalizumab recipients than placebo recipients in all domains, except exposure, and overall at the end of the steroid-reduction phase. Results in the Finn assessment (65) were similar, with omalizumab recipients showing significant improvements in AQLQ domain and overall scores at the end of each phase compared to placebo ($p < 0.05$

for all changes, apart from the emotions domain at the end of the extension phase). In addition to the statistical analysis, more omalizumab recipients showed clinically relevant improvements [defined as an increase in AQLQ $\geq$0.5 points from baseline (69)] than placebo recipients in all domains at the end of the steroid-stable and extension phases ($p < 0.05$). In pediatric patients with allergic asthma well controlled by daily ICS (67), at the end of both the 16-week steroid-stable phase and the 12-week steroid-reduction phase, PAQLQ scores improved across all domains, except emotions, and overall in the omalizumab recipients versus placebo recipients at the end of the steroid-reduction phase ($p < 0.05$). Again, the proportion of patients achieving clinically relevant [$\geq$0.5 points (69)] or large [$\geq$1.5 points (69)] improvements was greater in the omalizumab group than in the placebo group, and significantly so in the activities domain and overall at the end of steroid reduction. These studies have shown that the reduction in asthma exacerbations seen with omalizumab treatment correlates with improvements in QoL.

Asthma exacerbations are potentially life-threatening episodes of acute airways inflammation, and hospitalization resulting from exacerbations constitutes the greatest cost to the health care system for asthma. In patients with allergic asthma, exacerbation reduction is one of the most important goals of management (70), particularly for patients with severe asthma. To determine the effect of long-term omalizumab therapy on the rate of serious exacerbations, data from the three phase-III pivotal studies (60–62) were pooled and analyzed (71). The rates of unscheduled, asthma-related outpatient visits (rate ratio 0.60, $p < 0.01$) and emergency room visits (rate ratio 0.47, $p < 0.05$) were lower for omalizumab-treated patients versus patients receiving placebo, and hospitalizations were markedly reduced from 3.42 events per 100 patient years on placebo treatment to 0.26 on omalizumab treatment (rate ratio 0.08, $p < 0.01$).

Following the three pivotal studies in moderate to severe asthma, a study focusing on patients with severe asthma evaluated the efficacy of omalizumab as add-on therapy (72). This multicenter, randomized, double-blind, and placebo-controlled study included 146 patients (aged 12 to 75 years) who required $\geq$1000 µg/day fluticasone to maintain control of their asthma. During a 6- to 10-week run-in, ICS therapies were standardized by switching patients to fluticasone. This was followed by a 32-week double-blind treatment period in which patients received omalizumab [at least 0.016 mg/kg/ IgE (IU/mL) every four weeks; $n = 126$] or placebo ($n = 120$) as add-on therapy, including a 16-week fluticasone-stable period, a 12-week fluticasone-reduction period, and a four-week maintenance period in which patients were maintained on the minimum fluticasone dose for adequate symptom management. Patients receiving omalizumab had a greater reduction in fluticasone dose during the 32-week treatment period than patients receiving placebo (median 60.0% vs. 50.0%, $p = 0.003$), and more patients receiving omalizumab reduced their fluticasone dose by $\geq$50% than patients on placebo (73.8% vs. 50.8%, $p = 0.001$). Despite the reduction in fluticasone dose, there was no loss of control of asthma symptoms with omalizumab. Indeed, patients in the omalizumab group showed improvements in asthma symptom scores (0.9 vs. 1.4) and reduced rescue-medication use (−0.75 vs. 0.1) over placebo at the end of the 32-week steroid-stable period, which were significant at most time points throughout the steroid-stable and steroid-reduction periods ($p < 0.05$). Likewise, more omalizumab than placebo recipients showed improvements in asthma-related QoL [AQLQ (68)] scores throughout the 32-week treatment period that were clinically relevant (≥ 0.5 points; overall score 57.5% vs. 38.6%, $p < 0.001$) and large (≥ 1.5 points; overall score 16.0% vs. 5.9%, $p < 0.05$). The results showed that add-on therapy with omalizumab in patients with severe allergic asthma not only reduced the requirement for ICS, but also improved disease control. This suggests that omalizumab therapy is particularly beneficial for this very severe patient population.

VI. Selecting Patients for Anti-IgE Therapy with Omalizumab

Omalizumab is currently licensed in the United States for the treatment of moderate to severe persistent allergic asthma in patients of 12 years of age or more. Patients are required to have a positive skin test or in vitro IgE reactivity to a perennial aeroallergen and symptoms that are inadequately controlled with inhaled corticosteroids. To help identify the place of omalizumab in therapy, additional analyses of clinical data from asthma studies have been performed to determine which patients are most likely to benefit from omalizumab therapy.

One such analysis investigated whether patients at high risk of exacerbations and hospitalizations would be likely to benefit. This meta-analysis (73) evaluated three randomized, double-blind, placebo-controlled studies (60,61,72), including a total of 1412 adults and adolescents with moderate to severe asthma requiring daily treatment with ICS. A subgroup of 254 patients [69/525 patients from Busse 2001 (60), 73/546 patients from Solèr 2001 (61), and 112/341 patients from Holgate 2001 (72)] was identified as being at high risk of serious asthma-related morbidity or mortality on the basis of baseline asthma history: Patients were identified as high risk if they had ever been intubated before screening, or if they had visited an emergency room, experienced overnight hospitalization, or undergone treatment in an intensive care unit during the year prior to screening. Of the 254 high-risk patients, 135 were treated with omalizumab and 119 received placebo. The primary outcome measure was the annualized rate of significant asthma exacerbation episodes in the 16-week steroid-stable phase. Significant asthma exacerbation episodes were defined as exacerbations that required a doubling of baseline ICS dose (60,61) or use of systemic corticosteroids (in all three studies).

The significant asthma exacerbation rate in the steroid-stable phase was more than halved in the omalizumab group to 0.69 per patient year compared with 1.56 in the placebo group ($p = 0.007$). This translated into prevention of 87 significant asthma exacerbations for every 100 patients treated with omalizumab for one year. In addition, the proportion of patients with at least one significant asthma exacerbation during this phase was reduced to 18% with omalizumab compared with 35% with placebo. Although most patients experiencing significant asthma exacerbations experienced only a single significant asthma exacerbation, fewer patients receiving omalizumab experienced multiple significant asthma exacerbations. Likewise, over the whole 32-week study period, the significant asthma exacerbation rate decreased to 0.92 from 2.04 (omalizumab vs. placebo, $p < 0.001$) and the proportion of patients with at least one significant asthma exacerbation decreased to 44% from 66% (omalizumab vs. placebo). On the basis of these results, it was estimated that omalizumab would prevent significant asthma exacerbations in 17 patients of every 100 treated during stable ICS treatment, and in 22 of every 100 treated in the entire 32-week study. This corresponds to a number needed to treat (NNT) of 5.7 or 4.6 patients to maintain one patient free of significant asthma exacerbations (steroid-stable phase or whole study period, respectively).

Another analysis was used to determine which patient characteristics are associated with a response to omalizumab. This was a pooled exploratory analysis (74) of the two adult pivotal studies (60,61). Among the participants in these two studies were 1070 poorly controlled patients, who were symptomatic despite therapy with moderate to high doses of ICS (mean dose 725 µg/day BDP) or who had a history of emergency asthma treatment in the last year. Of these, 542 received omalizumab and 528 received placebo over a 16-week period. The factor most predictive of best response on treatment with omalizumab was a history of emergency asthma treatment in the preceding year: The response rate in patients with this history was 67% with omalizumab and 42% with placebo, versus 63% and 54%, respectively, in patients without ($p = 0.015$). High dose of ICS (≥ 800µg/day) was also predictive: Response rates were 65% with omalizumab and 40% with placebo in patients receiving high-dose ICS versus 63% and 55%, respectively, in patients receiving lower-dose ICS ($p = 0.037$). Low FEV_1 ($\leq 65\%$ predicted) was suggestive of a response: Response rates were 60% with omalizumab and 40% with placebo in patients with low FEV_1 versus 67% and 53%, respectively, in patients with high FEV_1 ($p = 0.072$). Patients with at least one of these factors showed odds of responding that were 2.25 times higher than placebo (95% CI; 1.68–3.01). These results suggest that omalizumab treatment is most likely to benefit patients with severe, poorly controlled asthma.

The same analysis (74) also evaluated the time taken for patients to respond to omalizumab therapy and how this related to the eventual response at study end (16 weeks). Of the patients who responded at 16 weeks, 61% had responded as early as four weeks after initiation of therapy, while the figure increased to 87% at 12 weeks. These findings support a minimum duration of treatment of 12 weeks as add-on therapy with omalizumab before deciding whether to continue therapy.

The efficacy of add-on therapy with omalizumab in a poorly controlled subpopulation of patients has since been confirmed in a "real-life" clinical setting by Ayres et al. (75). Patients enrolled in this randomized, open-label, multicenter, parallel-group study had moderate to severe asthma that was poorly controlled by current asthma therapies, prescribed according to best standard care (BSC). BSC included ICS and long-acting β_2-agonists (LABAs). The study included adults and adolescents receiving high-dose ICS (BDP or equivalent $\geq$800 µg/day adults, $\geq$400 µg/day adolescents). Poor control was defined as $\geq$1 emergency room visit or hospitalization and $\geq$1 additional course of oral corticosteroids for asthma in the year preceding the study. The primary efficacy variable was the annualized mean number of asthma-deterioration-related incidents (ADRIs) recorded in patient daily diaries and defined as at least one of the following events due to asthma: course of systemic corticosteroids or antibiotics for $\geq$2 days, $\geq$2 missed school or work days, unscheduled physician visit, hospitalization or emergency room visit. Of 312 patients enrolled, 38.8% were receiving a daily dose of 2000 µg BDP, 30.1% a daily dose of 1000 µg BDP, and 16.0% a daily dose of 4000 µg BDP at baseline. In addition, 77.9% of patients were receiving concomitant LABAs, and 21.2% were receiving systemic corticosteroids at baseline. The 206 patients randomized to receive BSC with omalizumab experienced a reduced ADRI rate compared with the 106 patients receiving BSC alone (4.92 vs. 9.76 per patient year, $p < 0.001$). The asthma exacerbation rate decreased with omalizumab (2.86 placebo vs. 1.12 omalizumab per patient year, $p < 0.001$); the significant reduction in asthma exacerbations with omalizumab therapy was not affected by concomitant medication with LABAs or anti-leukotrienes (Fig. 10). Compared with BSC alone, add-on therapy with omalizumab also increased the proportion of patients requiring less than one day per week of rescue medication (20.7% vs. 41.4%, $p < 0.001$), improved FEV_1 (2.28 vs. 2.48 L, $p = 0.02$), and reduced symptom scores (−0.7 vs. −6.5, $p < 0.001$). In addition, omalizumab decreased the mean asthma exacerbation rate irrespective of the concomitant asthma medications used (such as LABAs).

Current guidelines recommend the use of LABAs in addition to ICS therapy for the long-term preventive management of step 3 (moderate persistent) and 4 (severe persistent) asthma in adults and children over five years old (70). Given this widespread LABA use, it is important to evaluate the added benefits of omalizumab alongside concomitant LABA medication.

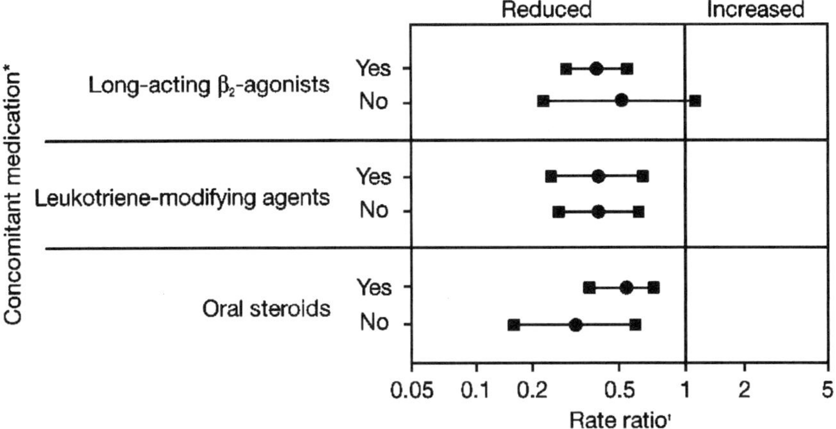

*Classification based on whether ever used during the study
'Patient-year rate analysis with protocol-specified imputation; point estimates and 95% CIs

Figure 10 The effect of concomitant asthma medications on relative asthma exacerbation rates in patients with poorly controlled moderate to severe asthma receiving omalizumab therapy. *Source*: From Ref. 75.

In the Ayres study, above (75), a similar proportion (78%) of patients in the omalizumab and BSC groups were receiving LABAs. The reduction in exacerbation rate with omalizumab was similar whether patients were also receiving LABAs or not: Rate ratios with LABAs versus without LABAs were 0.41 versus 0.35. Similarly, leukotriene-modifying agents and oral steroids did not affect the efficacy of omalizumab. These results suggest that the benefits of omalizumab are independent of concomitant medication use.

Taken together, the results from these studies indicate that patients benefiting most from omalizumab add-on therapy are those high-risk patients with more severe disease whose asthma is poorly controlled despite the best available therapies. This corresponds to a considerable burden, as the overall rate of asthma-related hospitalizations is considerable [19.5 per 10,000 population in the United States in 1995 with an average stay length of 3.7 days (76)]. In these patients, omalizumab has the potential to substantially improve disease control and symptoms.

To confirm this, a multicenter, randomized, double-blind, and placebo-controlled, parallel-group trial is currently in progress to evaluate the efficacy of add-on therapy with omalizumab in adults and adolescents with poorly controlled severe persistent allergic asthma. A total of 420 patients with serious symptoms of allergic asthma (frequent asthma exacerbations) who were inadequately controlled by GINA step 4 treatment [high-dose ICS (BDP > 1000 μg/day), long-acting β₂-agonists, and other concomitant asthma therapy, including oral corticosteroids] were randomized. Exacerbation rates, asthma symptoms, QoL, and lung function will be studied over the 28-week double-blind treatment period to provide information regarding the efficacy of omalizumab in this most severe asthma population that, despite all available therapies, continues to be poorly controlled and experience frequent asthma exacerbations.

VII. Studies in Other IgE-Mediated Allergies

Although allergic asthma is an extremely prevalent condition, globally affecting 100 to 150 million people (77), other IgE-mediated reactions are also major public health concerns. These include intermittent allergic rhinitis, which can be seasonal (SAR), persistent allergic rhinitis (PAR), latex allergy, and peanut- and tree-nut-induced anaphylaxis. These diseases often coexist (78) and have many pathophysiological features in common. Indeed, concomitant rhinitis is linked with more severe asthma, and in a retrospective study in 4944 patients with allergic asthma, patients treated for allergic rhinitis had approximately half the risk of subsequent asthma-related hospitalizations or emergency room visits ($p = 0.001$) (79). It seems likely, therefore, that appropriate treatment of one disease may confer improvements in the other.

In the United States alone, approximately 40 million people have SAR (80), while PAR affects 20 to 40 million people (81). SAR and PAR are characterized by ocular and nasal symptoms that can have a considerable detrimental effect on patients' QoL (82). Omalizumab has been shown to be effective in the treatment of both conditions. In an eight-week randomized, double-blind, and placebo-controlled trial in 251 adult patients with a history of SAR, average daily nasal symptom severity scores were unchanged throughout treatment during the pollen season in patients receiving omalizumab (0.71 at baseline vs. 0.70 overall), while they increased in placebo recipients (0.78 at baseline vs. 0.98 overall) ($p < 0.001$) (83). Average daily ocular symptom severity scores decreased from baseline (0.47 vs. 0.43), in contrast to an increase in placebo recipients (0.43 vs. 0.54) ($p = 0.031$). The average number of tablets of rescue antihistamine taken per day (0.59 vs. 1.37) and the proportion of days on which rescue medication was taken (49% vs. 28%) was lower in the omalizumab group versus placebo (both $p < 0.001$). QoL was improved in the omalizumab group versus placebo for all domains of the rhinitis quality of life questionnaire (RQLQ) (84), as well as the total score, and clinically relevant improvements [>0.05 units (85)] were observed in total score and the four domains of activities, nasal symptoms, non-nose–eye symptoms, and practical problems. Patients' assessments of treatment effectiveness favored omalizumab over placebo ($p = 0.001$).

A 12-week multicenter, randomized, double-blind, and dose-ranging, placebo-controlled trial was conducted in 536 patients aged 12 to 75 years with a history of moderate to severe ragweed-induced SAR (86). Patients received 50, 150, or 300 mg omalizumab or placebo subcutaneously every three to four weeks, depending on baseline IgE levels. Nasal symptoms were less severe in patients receiving the 300 mg dose of omalizumab than in the placebo group ($p = 0.002$). The reduction in nasal symptoms correlated with reductions in IgE [≤ 50 ng/mL, 20.8 IU/mL (59)] and rescue antihistamine use (all $p < 0.05$), and rescue antihistamine use was reduced in the 300 mg dose group compared with placebo ($p = 0.005$). In addition, RQLQ scores were consistently improved across the domains in patients receiving the 300 mg dose of omalizumab compared with placebo ($p < 0.05$ for activities, sleep, non-nasal and emotions domains, and overall).

A 16-week, randomized, double-blind, placebo-controlled trial of omalizumab in 289 adults and adolescents (aged 12 to 70 years) demonstrated its efficacy in moderate to severe symptomatic PAR (87). A dose of at least 0.016 mg/kg/IgE (IU/mL) per four weeks reduced average daily nasal severity scores throughout treatment versus placebo ($p < 0.001$). Again, average rescue-antihistamine use and proportion of days on which it was taken were both lower in the omalizumab group (both $p \leq 0.005$). Patients randomized to omalizumab experienced greater improvements in rhinoconjunctivitis-specific quality of life (RQoL) scores, and patients' global evaluation of treatment efficacy favored omalizumab versus placebo ($p < 0.001$).

Concomitant asthma and rhinitis is common and correlates with more severe asthma (79). The efficacy of omalizumab in a comorbid population of patients with asthma and rhinitis was investigated in a 28-week, multicenter, randomized, double-blind, and parallel group, placebo-controlled trial (88). A total of 405 adults and adolescents with concomitant moderate to severe allergic asthma (history of at least one year) and moderate to severe persistent PAR (history of at least two years) receiving moderate- to high-dose ICS (BDP $\geq 400\mu$g/day) were randomized. The coprimary efficacy variables were the incidence of asthma exacerbations during the 28-week treatment period and the proportion of patients who responded to treatment with a ≥ 1.0 point improvement in both asthma and rhinitis QoL scores. Omalizumab was given to 209 patients as add-on therapy to existing treatment regimens and placebo to 196. Omalizumab reduced the incidence of asthma exacerbations compared with placebo (20.6% patients vs. 30.1%, respectively, $p = 0.02$), and resulted in more responders (≥ 1.0 point improvement in both AQLQ and RQLQ scores) than placebo (57.7% vs. 40.6%, $p < 0.001$). Omalizumab treatment also improved total Wasserfallen symptom scores for asthma (treatment difference -1.8, $p = 0.023$), and rhinitis (-3.53, $p < 0.001$) compared with placebo. Exacerbation rates were similar in patients receiving and not receiving LABAs. These results show that, in patients with concomitant asthma and rhinitis, omalizumab is effective in reducing symptoms of both diseases when added to standard asthma and rhinitis therapies. These results are consistent with previous suggestions that coordinated management of asthma and rhinitis achieves optimal disease control. As both diseases share the common mechanism of IgE-mediated immune pathology, anti-IgE therapy is of particular benefit in comorbid patients.

In addition to treating rhinitis, omalizumab has demonstrated potential efficacy in the treatment of other IgE-mediated allergic diseases. Latex allergy primarily affects health care workers because they are frequently exposed to latex gloves and other latex-containing medical supplies. Their exposure to latex is ongoing and product avoidance is difficult. Symptoms may be local and/or systemic and include debilitating conjunctivitis, rhinitis, urticaria, and bronchospasm in addition to anaphylaxis. Prevalence among health care workers as high as 17% has been reported (89), but more representative figures today would be 5% to 10%. A 16-week, randomized, placebo-controlled trial evaluated the efficacy of omalizumab in 18 health care workers with latex allergy (90). The primary efficacy variable was the conjunctival challenge test score and all participants had a positive test score at baseline. Participants receiving omalizumab (150–750 mg/mo according to body weight and total serum IgE) showed improvements in conjunctival test scores at the end of the study compared with placebo ($p = 0.019$). Placebo recipients subsequently treated with open-label omalizumab also had improved scores. Anti-IgE is a promising strategy for latex allergy and further studies are required.

Peanut- and tree-nut-induced anaphylaxis is potentially life threatening. It is estimated to affect 1.5 million people in Britain (91) and about three million Americans (92). The prevalence in developed countries is estimated as 0.6% to 1.0% (93). Peanut avoidance can be impracticable in the current era of convenience foods and supermarket food shopping. As peanut-induced anaphylaxis is mediated by IgE, prophylactic treatment with an anti-IgE antibody could protect sufferers from anaphylaxis. A 20-week, randomized, double-blind, placebo-controlled, dose-ranging study of a humanized anti-IgE IgG1 monoclonal antibody (very similar to omalizumab) was conducted in 84 patients with a history of immediate hypersensitivity to peanut (94). Patients received placebo, 150, 300, or 450 mg of the antibody subcutaneously every four weeks, and underwent a final oral food challenge four weeks after the last dose and a final evaluation at week 20. In patients receiving 450 mg doses, the mean threshold of sensitivity to peanut at the final oral food challenge increased from a baseline of 178 mg (equivalent to approximately half a peanut) in a dose-responsive manner to a maximum of 2805 mg (equivalent to approximately nine peanuts) ($p < 0.001$). These results suggest that anti-IgE therapy could be a beneficial new treatment option for patients with this life-threatening condition.

VIII. Anti-inflammatory Actions of Omalizumab

Clinical studies have provided some indirect evidence of the anti-inflammatory actions of omalizumab, as patients have been able to reduce their dose of inhaled corticosteroids or withdraw completely from inhaled corticosteroid treatment. To further explore the mechanisms involved, a number of studies have been conducted with the aim of defining the markers, factors, and mediators affected by omalizumab in the immunological and cellular reactions of the inflammatory cascade. Together the data suggest that omalizumab may act on multiple components of the inflammatory cascade.

As previously discussed, a study in allergic individuals showed that omalizumab down-regulates FcεRI expression on basophils by reducing serum levels of free IgE (55), and this process attenuates the EAR. This was again demonstrated in a study of 24 subjects with ragweed-induced allergic rhinitis (56). Alongside a decline in IgE levels ($>95\%$), there was a reduction in FcεRI expression on basophils at 7, 14, 28, and 42 days after starting 72-hour omalizumab treatment as compared with baseline ($p < 0.0001$) and placebo ($p < 0.01$), and the maximum reduction occurred within 14 days (median change -73%).

Similarly to its effect on FcεRI expression on basophils, omalizumab was found to reduce dendritic cell FcεRI expression in patients with allergic rhinitis within 14 days (median change -78%, $p = 0.004$) (95). Dendritic cells are central to allergen presentation and the induction of Th2 responses in the LAR. The demonstration that an anti-IgE antibody inhibits proliferation of allergen-specific T cells, even at low allergen concentrations (96), reaffirmed this. In addition to the interaction of allergen-bound IgE with FcεRI on dendritic cells, the interaction of allergen-bound IgE with FcεRII RII on B cells is important in T-cell activation, and the effects of omalizumab may have been due, in part, to this. Further studies are needed to assess the role of omalizumab in reducing dendritic-cell-mediated antigen presentation.

Other inflammatory mediators are also reduced in patients with asthma receiving omalizumab treatment. In a multicenter, randomized, placebo-controlled study of 35 patients with moderate to severe asthma, circulating levels of IL-13 decreased after 16 weeks of omalizumab treatment compared to the placebo group (-2.4 pg/mL; $p < 0.01$), and non significant reductions were seen in IL-5 (-2.65 pg/mL) and IL-8 (-1.64 pg/mL) (97). No differences were detected for IL-6, IL-10, or s-ICAM throughout the study. As IL-13 and IL-5 are produced by Th2 cells, eosinophils, mast cells, and basophils, while IL-6 and IL-10 are produced by Th1/Th2 cells, macrophages and endothelial cells, these results reflect the proposed mechanisms of action of omalizumab. The authors also found that, after 16 and 52 weeks of omalizumab treatment, blood eosinophils were decreased compared with placebo (-25% and -50%, respectively, both $p < 0.01$).

Eosinophilia is one established feature of inflammation (29,30), and interaction between IgE and FcϵRII expressed on the surface of eosinophils may play an important role (34–36). A study in 74 asthma patients with disease severity ranging from intermittent to mild-to-moderate and severe persistent asthma, and 22 healthy non-atopic control subjects, was conducted to investigate the association between airways inflammation and disease severity (29). Using the method of induced sputum, asthma severity was monitored alongside sputum eosinophilia and eosinophil cationic protein (ECP). Sputum eosinophil counts were higher in patients from across the spectrum of asthma severity than in control subjects, and increased with asthma severity ($p \leq 0.05$). ECP concentration also increased with asthma severity ($p \leq 0.05$). Lung function parameters, symptom scores, and the inflammatory index PC_{20} in asthma patients all correlated with eosinophil count and ECP concentration. These results indicated that eosinophilic inflammation, which occurs during the LAR, can be used as a marker of asthma severity.

Similar results were obtained in a randomized, placebo-controlled trial that compared the efficacy of asthma management by normalization of induced sputum eosinophil count with that by standard British Thoracic Society guidelines (30). In 74 patients with moderate to severe asthma treated with corticosteroids, there were fewer asthma exacerbations (35 vs. 109, $p = 0.01$) and fewer asthma-related hospitalizations (1 vs. 6, $p = 0.047$) during the 12-month study period in those in the sputum management group compared with those in the BTS management group. Eosinophilia is therefore a valuable indicator of asthma control.

As eosinophilia correlates with asthma severity, it was hypothesized that reducing IgE in the airway mucosa would reduce airway inflammation. The effect of omalizumab on the eosinophil-mediated part of the inflammatory cascade was tested in a 16-week, five-center, double-blind, and placebo-controlled, parallel-group study by Djukanović et al. (98). To avoid interference from concomitant ICS, the 45 patients in this study were selected to have mild asthma that did not require ICS. Previous studies on eosinophils had included patients receiving ICS (57,97). The primary outcome measure was the effect of omalizumab on sputum eosinophilia. The mean percentage sputum eosinophil count decreased from 6.6% to 1.7% in 21 omalizumab recipients analyzed ($p < 0.001$), a reduction greater ($p = 0.05$) than in the 22 placebo recipients (8.5–7.0%) (Fig. 11A). There was a concomitant reduction in epithelial and submucosal eosinophils, as measured by immunohistochemical analysis of bronchial biopsies, from 8.0 cells/mm^2 to 1.5 cells/mm^2 ($p < 0.001$) in the 10 omalizumab recipients analyzed, compared to the nonsignificant change from 6.3 cells/mm^2 to 6.4 cells/mm^2 ($p = 0.03$) observed in the placebo group (Fig. 11B). These findings indicate that omalizumab does indeed act on the eosinophil-mediated component of airways inflammation in asthma. This considerably

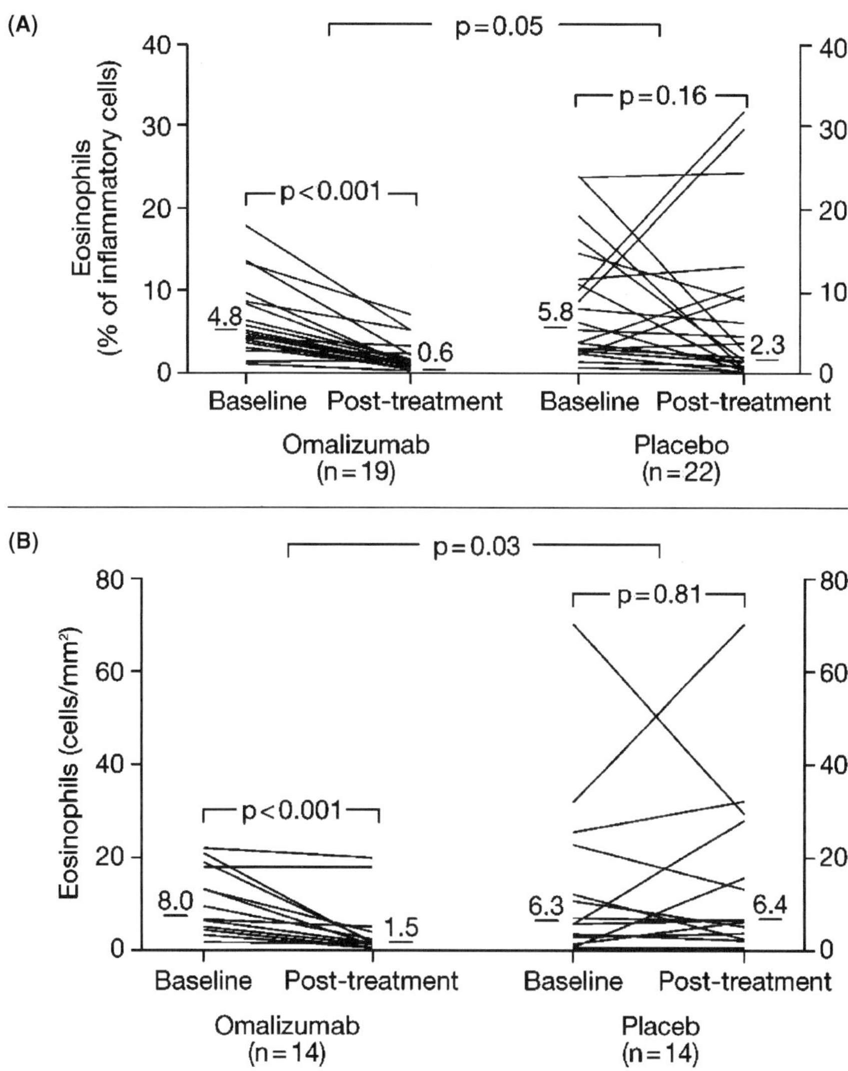

Figure 11 The effect of 16 weeks of omalizumab treatment on airway eosinophil counts. (**A**) Percentages of eosinophils in induced sputum. (**B**) Eosinophil counts in the bronchial submucosa. Horizontal bars represent medians. *Source*: From Ref. 98.

improves the understanding of the role of IgE in allergic asthma. It provides insights into the mechanisms of airways inflammation, and those by which omalizumab reduces asthma exacerbations and other asthma outcomes in more severe asthma. Anti-inflammatory effects may provide a mechanistic link between a direct reduction in IgE, reductions in eosinophil accumulation, and reductions in IL-4. In the Djukanović et al. study (98), omalizumab decreased cell surface IL-4 compared with placebo ($p < 0.001$), and expression of cell-associated IL-4 and submucosal eosinophils (Spearman's rank correlation $R_s = 0.78$, $p < 0.001$). IL-4 activates B cells for IgE production and is known to facilitate the endothelial adhesion of eosinophils (99), and is produced by Th2 cells in response to allergen challenge. This finding therefore suggests that omalizumab may mediate eosinophil reduction via IL-4. As IL-4 is also produced by mast cells, basophils, and eosinophils, the effects of omalizumab on eosinophils could result indirectly from its action on Th2 cells (via altered antigen presentation from affected dendritic cells, a process which is also enhanced by IL-4 or due to inhibition of mast cell or basophil degranulation). Taken together the results of these studies provide convincing evidence for the significant anti-inflammatory effects of omalizumab.

IX. Tolerability of Omalizumab

Since the first clinical trials in 1999, a total of 4127 patients have received omalizumab in completed studies, of whom 3224 received omalizumab in controlled studies, and 2845 received omalizumab in phase IIB/III clinical studies. The majority of adverse events with omalizumab were of short duration and mild-to-moderate intensity. In the phase IIB/III studies, adverse events with omalizumab were similar to those in control patients, regardless of asthma severity (Table 2). These 2845 patients each received at least 12 weeks of omalizumab treatment, while 2060 received more than 24 weeks, 688 more than 36 weeks, and 555 more than 52 weeks. In all controlled studies, three patients experienced anaphylactic reactions associated with subcutaneous treatment. One case was attributed to antibiotic use, and the other two resolved with therapy following discontinuation of omalizumab. No evidence of immune complex syndrome has been observed in any controlled study. Only one case of a patient developing anti-omalizumab antibodies has been reported, and this occurred during a Phase-I pilot study assessing the feasibility of administering omalizumab by aerosol inhalation. No other patient serum sample had detectable immunoreactivity to omalizumab in any study to date. As it has been postulated that IgE has a classic role in the immune defense against parasitic infestation (100), the incidence of parasitic infections was also monitored, but no increase was observed with omalizumab treatment over placebo, supporting the notion that the IgE-antibody response seen to helminthes has no or little role in an immune defense. Although expert opinion is divided as to whether IgE is involved in immune-defense mechanisms against cancer, detailed analyses into the occurrence of neoplasia have found no evidence to suggest any link with omalizumab treatment. Malignant neoplasms were observed in 20 of 4127 (0.5%) omalizumab-treated patients compared with five of 2236 (0.2%)

Table 2 Combined Safety Data from Controlled (Phases IIB and III) Studies on Omalizumab

Preferred term	All controlled studies (%)		Allergic asthma controlled studies (%)	
	Omalizumab ($n = 3224$)	Control ($n = 2019$)	Omalizumab ($n = 2076$)	Control ($n = 1383$)
Any AE	74.8	75.8	80.5	78.1
Infection viral	19.8	22.6	23.3	26.3
Headache	17.0	17.2	15.4	15.6
Pain back	5.4	5.8	6.9	7.0
Respiratory AEs				
Upper respiratory tract infection	18.2	18.7	20.0	20.5
Sinusitis	12.8	15.1	16.4	17.6
Pharyngitis	10.3	9.3	10.7	10.3
Rhinitis	7.2	9.0	9.1	10.6
Coughing	6.7	8.0	6.5	7.3
Bronchitis	6.2	7.4	8.8	10.3

The table shows adverse events (AEs) occurring in $\geq 5\%$ of patients.

control patients in clinical studies of asthma and other allergic disorders. The observed malignancies in omalizumab-treated patients were a variety of types, with breast, non-melanoma skin, prostate, melanoma, and parotid occurring more than once, and five other types occurring once each. The majority of patients were observed for less than one year.

X. Future Directions

IgE plays a central role in the initiation and propagation of the inflammatory cascade and therefore in the allergic response. The concept of attenuating allergic disease by specifically inhibiting IgE and the development of omalizumab, the first agent capable of achieving this, were major breakthroughs in the management of allergic asthma. Specific binding of IgE by omalizumab has been shown in clinical trials to diminish both early and late asthmatic responses, and reduce symptoms of IgE-mediated allergy irrespective of the allergen. Clinical studies have shown that the benefits of omalizumab therapy have been particularly highlighted in patients at high risk of exacerbations, patients with poorly controlled asthma, patients with severe asthma, and patients with IgE-mediated comorbidities.

Future studies will continue to explore the anti-inflammatory mechanisms of anti-IgE therapy. As many of these mechanisms are common to all IgE-mediated, allergic diseases, the efficacy of omalizumab in other allergic diseases needs to be further considered. Several large studies have already established efficacy in allergic rhinitis (83,86,87), and preliminary investigations have already shown efficacy in other IgE-mediated diseases such as peanut allergy (94) and latex allergy (90). Future studies are likely to evaluate omalizumab in patients with severe allergic asthma and with concomitant rhinitis and eczema. In the latter case, pretreatment, e.g., with pimecrolimus and antibiotics, could drastically reduce total IgE levels and thus lead to a situation where anti-IgE treatment had a realistic chance to eliminate IgE antibodies relevant for the allergic disease.

Another interesting application of anti-IgE therapy would be as a temporary cover during intermittent allergic diseases, e.g., seasonal asthma and rhinitis. The effect of the anti-IgE injection is already demonstrable within days to weeks, but once circulating IgE is captured in the immune complexes and the numbers of FcεR on mast cell and basophil cell surfaces are down-regulated, it takes months to restore the allergy reactive "capacity" again. Thus, one or two injections before the pollen season could keep the patient symptom-free for the entire season.

In addition to treating allergy, anti-IgE injections could be a most valuable tool to prevent IgE-mediated side effects of allergen-specific immunotherapy (ASIT). Side effects during the initial stage of uptitration of the allergen dose in ASIT are not uncommon, and even cases of severe allergic anaphylaxis have been reported. One or two injections of anti-IgE could, most likely, be an effective ASIT "umbrella," allowing a safe and faster way to reach maintenance allergen doses.

As the field of medicine continues to evolve, there is a growing trend toward the ideal of tailoring therapy to the individual. There is a need for likely responders to anti-IgE therapy to be identified on the basis of their genetic and environmental predispositions and serological profiles. Based on our present understanding of the role of IgE in allergic inflammation it is obvious that an anti-IgE therapy will only be valid if the asthma really is an IgE-mediated allergic asthma, as declared by the FDA. Thus, if no IgE antibodies can be detected in serum the potential therapeutic effect of anti-IgE therapy is questionable. In addition, it seems logical that if these IgE antibodies represent a significant percentage of all IgE molecules in circulation the anti-IgE therapy will be most efficient; there is less ballast IgE to eliminate. Although, during anti-IgE treatment, the IgE molecules in circulation are part of circulating IgE/anti-IgE immune complexes, it is possible, at least with the best immunoassays for IgE antibody on the market, to detect and quantitate individual IgE antibody specificities. Since these immune complexes are treated by the body as IgG complexes they have a half-life in the order of three weeks. Thus, the IgE antibody that is found in serum is a result of an allergen stimulation some three weeks ago.

It is also possible to evaluate any residual allergen sensitivity of the basophils of patients on anti-IgE treatment (101) using allergen threshold stimulation. In a subgroup of a previous study (72), basophils of patients on omalizumab for more than three years were found to have a very weak allergen sensitivity (approximately 1–2% of non-treated patients). However, even though almost non-sensitive, the basophils were still reactive; clinically irrelevant, high doses of the same allergens resulted in a significant up-regulation of basophil, histamine-related surface marker CD63 (SGO Johansson, unpublished observation).

We have good reasons to believe that the future will provide new opportunities for therapeutic monitoring based on IgE serology and allergen-specific inflammatory markers. Thus, it will be possible not only to identify anti-IgE drug responders but also to ensure adequate dosing over time. However, all the exciting future aspects discussed need further studies before they can be recommended for routine patient care.

References

1. Johansson SGO, O'B Hourihane J, Bousquet J, Bruijnzeel-Koomen C, Dreborg S, Haatela T, Kowalski ML, Mygind N, Ring J, van Cauwenberge P, et al. A revised nomenclature for allergy. An EAACI position statement from the EAACI nomenclature task force. Allergy 2001; 56:813–824.
2. Johansson SGO, Bieber T, Dahl R, Friedmann PS, Lanier BQ, Lockey RF, Motala C, Ortega Martell JA, Platts-Mills TA, Ring J, et al. HC. Revised nomenclature for allergy for global use: Report from the Nomenclature Review Committee of the World Allergy Organization, October 2003. J Allergy Clin Immunol 2004; 113:832–836.
3. Bennich HH, Ishizaka K, Johansson SGO, Rowe DS, Stanworth DR Terry WD. Immunoglobulin E, a new class of human immunoglobulins. Bull World Health Organ 1968; 38:151–152.
4. Johansson SGO, Nopp A, van-Hage M, Olofsson N, Lundahl J, Wehlin L, Söderström T, Stiller V, Öman H. Passive IgE-sensitization by blood transfusion. Allergy 2005 inpress.
5. Seagroatt V, Anderson SG. The second international reference preparation for human serum immunoglobulin E and the first British standard for human serum immunoglobulin E. J Biol Stand 1981; 9:431–437.
6. Barbee RA, Halonen M, Lebowitz M, Burrows B. Distribution of IgE in a community population sample: correlations with age, sex, and allergen skin test reactivity. J Allergy Clin Immunol 1981; 68:106–111.
7. Johansson SGO. Serum IgND levels in healthy children and adults. Int Arch Allergy 1968; 34:1–8.
8. Johansson SGO. Raised levels of a new immunoglobulin class (IgND) in asthma. Lancet 1967; 2:951–953.
9. Wittig HJ, Belloit J, De Fillippi I, Royal G. Age-related serum immunoglobulin E levels in healthy subjects and in patients with allergic disease. J Allergy Clin Immunol 1980; 66:305–313.

10. Öhman S, Johansson SGO, Juhlin L. Immunoglobulins in atopic dermatitis. In: Proceedings of the VIII European Congress of Allergology 1971. Excerpta Medica Int Congr Ser 251:119–126.

11. Nordbring F, Johansson SGO. IgM in cytomegalovirus mononucleosis. Scand J Infect Dis 1971; 3:87–90.

12. Gerrard JW, Heiner DC, Ko CG, Mink J, Meyers A, Dosman JA. Immunoglobulin levels in smokers and non-smokers. Ann Allergy 1980; 44:261–262.

13. Ringdén O, Persson U, Johansson SGO, Wilczek H, Gahrton G, Groth CG, Lundgren G, Lonnquist B, Moller E. Markedly elevated serum IgE levels following allogenic and syngenic bone marrow transplantation. Blood 1983; 61:1190–1195.

14. Stanworth DR, Humphrey JH, Bennich H, Johannsson SG. Inhibition of Prausnitz-Kustner reaction by proteolytic-cleavage fragments of a human myeloma protein of immunoglobulin class E. Lancet 1968; 2:17–18.

15. Dolovich J, Hargreave FE, Chalmers R, Shier KJ, Gauldie J, Bienenstock J. Late cutaneous allergic responses in isolated IgE-dependent reactions. J Allergy Clin Immunol 1973; 52:38–46.

16. Maurer D, Ebner C, Reininger B, Fiebiger E, Kraft D, Kinet JD, Stingl G. The high affinity IgE receptor (Fc epsilon RI) mediates IgE-dependent allergen presentation. J Immunol 1995; 154:6285–6290.

17. Maurer D, Fiebiger E, Reininger B, Wolff-Winiski B, Jouvin MH, Kilgus O, Kinet JP, Stingl G. Expression of functional high affinity immunoglobulin E receptors (FcepsilonRI) on monocytes of atopic individuals. J Exp Med 1994; 179:745–750.

18. Wang B, Rieger A, Kilgus O, Ochiai K, Maurer D, Fodinger D, Kinet JP, Stingl G. Epidermal langerhans cells from normal human skin bind monomeric IgE via Fc epsilon RI. J Exp Med 1992; 175:1353–1365.

19. Maurer D, Fiebiger S, Ebner C, Reininger B, Fischer GF, Wichlas S, Jouvin MH, Schmitt-Egenolf M, Kraft D, Kinet JP, et al. Peripheral blood dendritic cells express Fc epsilon RI as a complex composed of Fc epsilon RI alpha- and Fc epsilon RI gamma-chains and can use this receptor for IgE-mediated allergen presentation. J Immunol 1996; 157:607–616.

20. Campbell AM, Vachier I, Chanez P, Vignola AM, Lebel B, Kochan J, Godard P, Bousquet J. Expression of the high-affinity receptor for IgE on bronchial epithelial cells of asthmatics. Am J Respir Cell Mol Biol 1998; 19:92–97.

21. Hasegawa S, Pawankar R, Suzuki K, Nakahata T, Furukawa S, Okumura K, Ra C. Functional expression of the high affinity receptor for IgE (Fcepsilon RI) in human platelets and its intracellular expression in human magalokaryocytes. Blood 1999; 93:2543–2551.

22. Gounni AS, Lamkhioued B, Ochiai K, Tanaka Y, Delaporte E, Capron A, Kinet JP, Capron M. High-affinity IgE receptor on eosinophils is involved in defence against parasites. Nature 1994; 367:183–186.

23. Zheng Y, Shopes B, Holowka D, Baird B. Conformations of IgE bound to its receptor Fc epsilon RI and in solution. Biochemistry 1991; 30:9125–9132.

24. Bonnefoy JY, Lecoanet-Henchoz S, Gauchat JF, Graber P, Aubry JP Jeannin P, Plater-Zyberk C. Structure and functions of CD23. Int Rev Immunol 1997; 16:113–128.

25. Yokota A, Yukawa K, Yamamoto A, Sugiyama K, Suemura M, Tashiro Y, Kishimoto C, Kikutani H. Two forms of the low-affinity Fc receptor for IgE differentially mediate endocytosis and phagocytosis: identification of the critical cytoplasmic domains. Proc Natl Acad Sci USA 1992; 89:5030–5034.

26. Abdelaziz MM, Devalia LJ, Khair OA, Calderon M, Sapsford RJ, Davis RJ. The effect of conditioned medium from cultures of human bronchial epithelial cells on eosinophil and neutrophil chemotaxis and adherence in vitro. Am J Respir Cell Mol Biol 1995; 13:728–737.

27. Bradding P. The role of the mast cell in asthma: a reassessment. Curr Opin Clin Immunol 2003; 3:45–50.

28. Holgate ST. The role of mast cells and basophils in inflammation. Clin Exp Allergy 2000; 30(Suppl 1):28–32.

29. Louis R, Lau RC, Bron AO, Roldaan AC, Radermecker M, Djukanovic R. The relationship between airways inflammation and asthma severity. Am J Respir Crit Care Med 2000; 161:9–16.

30. Green RH, Brightling CE, McKenna S, Hargadon B, Parker D, Bradding P, Wardlaw AJ, Pavord ID. Asthma exacerbations and sputum eosinophil counts: a randomised controlled trial. Lancet 2002; 360:1715–1721.

31. Leckie MJ, ten Brinke A, Khan J, Diamant Z, O'Connor BJ, Walls CM, Mathur AK, Cowley HC, Chung KF, Djukanovic R, et al. Effects of an interleukin-5 blocking monoclonal antibody on eosinophils, airway hyper-responsiveness, and the late asthmatic response. Lancet 2000; 356:2144–2148.

32. Prussin C, Metcalfe DD. IgE, mast cells, basophils and eosinophils. J Allergy Clin Immunol 2003; 111:S486–494.

33. Kay AB. T lymphocytes and their products in atopic allergy and asthma. Int Arch Allergy Appl Immunol 1991; 94:189–193.

34. Alevy YG, Compas MB, Shaffer A, Rup B, Kahn LE. Regulation of human IgE synthesis by soluble factors. Papain treatment of a FcE receptor-positive B-cell line (RPMI-1788) releases regulatory factors for IgE synthesis. Int Arch Allergy Appl Immunol 1988; 86:125–130.

35. Yu P, Kosco-Vilbois M, Richards M, Kohler G, Lamers MC. Negative feedback regulation of IgE synthesis by murine CD23. Nature 1994; 369:753–756.

36. Yang P-C, Berin MC, Yu LCH, Conrad DH, Perdue MH. Enhanced intestinal transepithelial antigen transport in allergic rats is mediated by IgE and CD23 (FcεRII). J Clin Invest 2000; 106:879–886.

37. Hakonarson H, Carter C, Kim C, Grunstein MM. Altered expression and action of the low-affinity IgE receptor FcεRII (CD23) in asthmatic airway smooth muscle. J Allergy Clin Immunol 1999; 104(3pt1):575–584.

38. Stingl G, Maurer D. IgE-mediated allergen presentation via Fc epsilon RI on antigen-presenting cells. Int Arch Allergy Immunol 1997; 113:24–29.

39. Bonnefoy J-Y, Aubry J-P, Gauchat J-R, Gaber P, Life P, Flores-Romo L, Mazzei G. Receptors for IgE. Curr Opin Immunol 1993; 5:944–949.

40. Shibaki A. FcepsilonRI on dendritic cells: a receptor, which links IgE mediated allergic reaction and T-cell mediated cellular response. J Dermatol Sci 1998; 20:29–38.

41. Humbert M, Grant JA, Taborda-Barata L, Durham SR, Pfister P, Menz G, Barkans J, Ming S, Kay AB. High-affinity IgE receptor (FcepsilonRI)-bearing

cells in bronchial biopsies from atopic and nonatopic asthma. Am J Respir Crit Care Med 1996; 153:1931–1937.

42. Mudde GC, Van Reijsen FC, Boland GJ, de Gast GC, Bruijnzeel PL, Bruijnzeel-Koomen CA. Allergen presentation by epidermal Langerhans cells from patients with atopic dermatitis is mediated by IgE. Immunology 1990; 69:335–341.

43. Jahnsen FL, Moloney ED, Hogan T, Upham JW, Burke CM, Holt PG. Rapid dendritic cell recruitment to the bronchial mucosa of patients with atopic asthma in response to local allergen challenge. Thorax 2001; 56:823–826.

44. Upham JW, Denburg JA, O'Byrne PM. Rapid response of circulating myeloid dendritic cells to inhaled allergen in asthmatic subjects. Clin Exp Allergy 2002; 32:818–823.

45. Tunon-de-Lara JM, Redington AE, Bradding P, Church MK, Hartley JA, Semper AE, Holgate ST. Dendritic cells in normal and asthmatic airways: expression of the alpha subunit of the high affinity immunoglobulin E receptor (FcεRI-α). Clin Exp Allergy 1996; 26:648–655.

46. Jurgens M, Wollenberg A, Hanau D, de la Salle H, Bieber T. Activation of human epidermal Langerhans cells by engagement of the high-affinity receptor for IgE, Fc epsilon RI. J Immunol 1995; 155:5184–5189.

47. Geiger E, Magerstaedt R, Wessendorf JHM, Kraft S, Hanau D, Bieber T. IL-4 induces the intracellular expression of the alpha chain of the high-affinity receptor for IgE in in vitro-generated dendritic cells. J Allergy Clin Immunol 2000; 105:150–156.

48. Upham JW. The role of dendritic cells in immune regulation and allergic airway inflammation. Respirology 2003; 8:140–148.

49. Holt PG, Macaubras C, Stumbles PA, Sly PD. The role of allergy in the development of asthma. Nature 1999; 402(suppl):B12–B17.

50. MacGlashan DW. Releasability of human basophils: cellular sensitivity and maximal histamine release are independent variables. J Allergy Clin Immunol 1993; 91:605–615.

51. Presta LG, Lahr SJ, Shields RL, Porter JP, Gorman CM, Fendly BM Jardieu PM. Humanization of an antibody directed against IgE. J Immunol 1993; 151:2623–2632.

52. Shields RL, Whether WR, Zioncheck K, O'Connell L, Fendly B, Presta LG, Thomas D, Saban R, Jardieu P. Inhibition of allergic reactions with antibodies to IgE. Int Arch Allergy Immunol 1995; 107:308–312.

53. Liu J, Lester P, Builder S, Shire SJ. Characterization of complex formation by humanized anti-IgE monoclonal antibody and monoclonal human IgE. Biochemistry 1995; 34:10474–10482.

54. Casale TB, Bernstein IL, Busse WW, LaForce CF, Tinkelman DG, Stoltz RR, Dockhorn RJ, Reimann J, Su JQ, Fick RB Jr, et al. Use of an anti-IgE humanized monoclonal antibody in ragweed-induced allergic rhinitis. J Allergy Clin Immunol 1997; 100:110–121.

55. MacGlashan DW, Bochner BS, Adelman DC, Jardieu PM, Togias A, McKenzie-White J, Sterbinsky SA, Hamilton RG, Lichtenstein LM. Down-regulation of FcεRI expression on human basophils during in vivo treatment of atopic patients with anti-IgE antibody. J Immunol 1997; 158: 1438–1445.

56. Lin H, Boesel KM, Griffith DT, Prussin C, Foster B, Romero FA, Townley R, Casale TB. Omalizumab rapidly decreases nasal allergic response and FcepsilonRI on basophils. J Allergy Clin Immunol 2004; 113:297–302.

57. Fahy JV, Fleming HE, Wong HH, Liu JT, Su JQ, Reimann J, Fick RB Jr, Boushey HA. The effect of an anti-IgE monoclonal antibody on the early-phase and late-phase responses to allergen inhalation in asthmatic subjects. Am J Respir Crit Care Med 1997; 155:1828–1834.

58. Boulet LP, Chapman KR, Côté J, Kalra S, Bhagat R, Swystun VA, Laviolette M, Cleland LD, Deschesnes F, Su JQ, et al. Inhibitory effects of an anti-IgE antibody E25 on allergen-induced early asthmatic response. Am J Respir Crit Care Med 1997; 155:1835–1840.

59. Hochhaus G, Brookman L, Fox H, Johnson C, Matthews J, Ren S, Deniz Y. Pharmacodynamics of omalizumab: implications for optimized dosing strategies and clinical efficacy in the treatment of allergic asthma. Curr Med Res Op 2003; 19:491–498.

60. Busse W, Corren J, Lanier BQ, McAlary M, Fowler-Taylor A, Della Cioppa G, vanAs A, Gupta N. Omalizumab, anti-IgE recombinant humanized monoclonal antibody, for the treatment of severe allergic asthma. J Allergy Clin Immunol 2001; 108:184–190.

61. Solèr M, Matz J, Townley R, Buhl R, O'Brien J, Fox H, Thirlwell J, Gupta N, Della Cioppa G. The anti-IgE antibody omalizumab reduces exacerbations and steroid requirement in allergic asthmatics. Eur Respir J 2001; 18: 254–261.

62. Milgrom H, Berger W, Nayak A, Gupta N, Pollard S, McAlary M, Fowler-Taylor A, Rohane P. Treatment of childhood asthma with anti-immunoglobulin E antibody (omalizumab). Pediatrics 2001; 108:E36.

63. Lanier WB, Corren J, Lumry W, Liu J, Fowler-Taylor A, Gupta N. Omalizumab is effective in the long-term control of severe allergic asthma. Ann Allergy Asthma Immunol 2003; 91:154–159.

64. Buhl R, Soler M, Matz J, Townley R, O'Brien J, Noga O, Champain K, Fox H, Thirlwell J, Della Cioppa G. Omalizumab provides long-term control in patients with moderate-to-severe allergic asthma. Eur Respir J 2002; 20:73–78.

65. Finn A, Gross G, van Bavel J, Lee T, Windon H, Everhard F, Fowler-Taylor A, Liu J, Gupta N. Omalizumab improves asthma-related quality of life in patients with severe allergic asthma. J Allergy Clin Immunol 2003; 111:278–284.

66. Buhl R, Hanf G, Soler M, Bensch G, Wolfe J, Everhard F, Champain K, Fox H, Thirlwell J. The anti-IgE antibody omalizumab improves asthma-related quality of life in patients with allergic asthma. Eur Respir J 2002; 20:1088–1094.

67. Lemanske RF, Nayak A, McAlary M, Everhard F, Fowler-Taylor A, Gupta N. Omalizumab improves asthma-related quality of life in children with allergic asthma. Pediatrics 2002; 110:e55.

68. Juniper EF, Guyatt GH, Epstein RS, Ferrie PJ, Jaeschke R, Hiller TK. Evaluation of impairment of health-related quality of life in asthma: development of a questionnaire for use in clinical trials. Thorax 1992; 47:76–83.

69. Juniper EF, Guyatt GH, Willan A, Griffith LE. Determining a minimal important change in a disease-specific Quality of Life Questionnaire. Thorax 1994; 47:81–87.

70. Global Initiative for Asthma (GINA). Global strategy for asthma management and prevention. NHLBI/WHO workshop report. NIH publication number 02-3659. Issued January 1995 (updated 2002, 2003). The 2002 and 2003 reports are available on www.ginasthma.com.

71. Corren J, Casale T, Deniz Y, Ashby M. Omalizumab, a recombinant humanized anti-IgE antibody, reduces asthma-related emergency room visits and hospitalizations in patients with allergic asthma. J Allergy Clin Immunol 2003; 111:87–90.

72. Holgate ST, Chuchalin AG, Hebert J, Lotvall J, Persson GB, Chung KF, Bousquet J, Kerstjens HA, Fox H, Thirlwell J, et al. Efficacy and safety of a recombinant anti-IgE antibody (omalizumab) in severe allergic asthma. Clin Exp Allergy 2004; 34:632–638.

73. Holgate S, Bousquet J, Wenzel S, Fox H, Liu J, Castellsague J. Efficacy of omalizumab, an anti-immunoglobulin E antibody, in patients with allergic asthma at high risk of serious asthma-related morbidity and mortality. Curr Med Res Opin 2001; 17:233–240.

74. Bousquet J, Wenzel S, Holgate S, Lumry W, Freeman P, Fox H. Predicting response to omalizumab, an anti-immunoglobulin E antibody, in patients with allergic asthma. Chest 2004; 125:1378–1386.

75. Ayres JG, Higgins B, Chilvers ER, Ayre G, Blogg M, Fox H. Efficacy and tolerability of anti-immunoglobulin E therapy with omalizumab in patients with poorly controlled (moderate-to-severe) allergic asthma. Allergy 2004; 59:701–708.

76. National Institutes of Health, National Heart, Lung and Blood Institute. Data Fact Sheet January 1999.

77. World Health Organization. Bronchial asthma. Fact Sheet no 206. Geneva: WHO 2000.

78. Kapsali T, Horowitz E, Diemer F, et al. Rhinitis is ubiquitous in allergic asthmatics (abstract). J Allergy Clin Immunol 1997; 99:S138.

79. Crystal-Peters J, Neslusan C, Crown WH, Torres A. Treating allergic rhinitis in patients with comorbid asthma: the risk of asthma-related hospitalizations and emergency department visits. J Allergy Clin Immunol 2002; 109:57–62.

80. Meltzer EO. The prevalence and medical and economic impact of allergic rhinitis in the United States. J Allergy Clin Immunol 1997; 99(6 pt 2): S805–S828.

81. Weiss KB, Sullivan SD. The health economics of asthma and rhinitis. I. Assessing the economic impact. J Allergy Clin Immunol 2001; 107:3–8.

82. Meltzer EO, Nathan RA, Selner JC, Storms W. Quality of life and rhinitic symptoms: results of a nationwide survey with the SF-36 and RQLQ questionnaires. J Allergy Clin Immunol 1997; 99:S815–S819.

83. Ädelroth E, Rak S, Haahtela T, Aasand G, Rosenhall L, Zetterstom O, Byrne A, Champain K, Thirlwell J, Della Cioppa G, et al. Recombinant humanized mAb-E25, an anti-IgE mAb, in birch pollen-induced seasonal allergic rhinitis. J Allergy Clin Immunol 2000; 106:253–259.

84. Juniper EF, Guyatt GH. Development and testing of a new measure of health status for clinical trials in rhinoconjuncitivits. Clin Exp Allergy 1991; 21: 77–83.

85. Juniper EF, Guyatt GH, Griffith LE, Ferrie PJ. Interpretation of rhinoconjunctivitis quality of life questionnaire data. J Allergy Clin Immunol 1996; 98:843–845.

86. Casale TB, Condemi J, LaForce C, Nayak A, Rowe M, Watrous M, McAlary M, Fowler-Taylor A, Racine A, Gupta N, Fick R, et al. Effect of omalizuumab on symptoms of seasonal allergic rhinitis. A randomised controlled trial. JAMA 2001; 286:2956–2967.

87. Chervinsky P, Casale T, Townley R, Tripathy I, Hedgecock S, Fowler-Taylor A, Shen H, Fox H. Omalizumab, an anti-IgE antibody, in the treatment of adults and adolescents with perennial allergic rhinitis. Ann Allergy Asthma Immunol 2003; 91:160–167.

88. Vignola AM, Humbert M, Bousquet J, Boulet LP, Hedgecock S, Blogg S, Fox H, Surrey K. Efficacy and tolerability of anti-immunoglobulin E therapy with omalizumab in patients with concominant allergic asthma and persistent allergic rhinitis: SOLAR. Allergy 2004; 59:709–717.

89. Agarwal S, Gawkrodger DJ. Latex allergy: a health care problem of epidemic proportions. Eur J Dermatol 2002; 12:311–315.

90. Leynadier F, Doudou O, Gaouar H, Le Gros V, Bourdeix I, Guyomarch-Cocco L, Trunet P. Effect of omalizumab in health care workers with occupational latex allergy. J Allergy Clin Immunol 2004; 113:360–361.

91. Tariq SM, Stevens M, Matthews S, Ridout S, Twiselton R, Hide DW. Cohort study of peanut and tree nut sensitisation by age of 4 years. Br Med J 1996; 313:514–517.

92. Sicherer SH, Munoz-Furlong A, Sampson HA. Prevalence of peanut and tree nut allergy in the United States determined by means of a random digit dial telephone survey: a 5-year follow-up study. J Allergy Clin Immunol 2003; 112:1203–1207.

93. Al-Muhsen S, Clarke AE, Kagan RS. Peanut allergy: an overview. CMAJ 2003; 168:1279–1285.

94. Leung DY, Sampson HA, Yunginger JW, Burks AW Jr, Schneider LC, Wortel CH, Davis FM, Hyun JD, Shanahan WR Jr. Effect of anti-IgE therapy in patients with peanut allergy. N Engl J Med 2003; 348:986–993.

95. Prussin C, Griffith DT, Boesel KM, Lin H, Foster B, Casale TB. Omalizumab treatment downregulates dendritic cell FcεRI expression. J Allergy Clin Immunol 2003; 112:1147–1154.

96. van Neerven RJJ, van Roomen CPAA, Thomas WR, de Boer M, Knol EF, Davis FM. Humanized anti-IgE mAb Hu-901 prevents the activation of allergen-specific T cells. Int Arch Allergy Immunol 2001; 124:400–402.

97. Noga O, Hanf G, Kunkel G. Immunological changes in allergic asthmatics following treatment with omalizumab. Int Arch Allergy Immunol 2003; 131:46–52.

98. Djukanović R, Wilson S, Kraft M, Jarjour N, Steel M, Chung KF, Bao W, Fowler-Taylor A, Matthews J, Busse W, Holgate S, Fahy JV. Effects of treatment with anti-immunoglobulinE antibody (omalizumab) treatment in airways inflammation in allergic asthma. Am J Respir Crit Care Med 2004; 170:583–593.

99. Rajakulasingam K, Till S, Ying S, Humbert M, Barkans J, Sullivan M, Meng Q, Corrigan CJ, Bungre J, Grant JA, et al. Increased expression of high affinity IgE (FcεRI) receptor-α chain mRNA and protein-bearing eosinophils in human allergen-induced atopic asthma. Am J Respir Crit Care Med 1998; 158: 233–240.
100. Rihet P, Demeure CE, Bourgois A, Prata A, Dessein AJ. Evidence for an association between human resistance to *Schistosoma mansoni* and high anti-larval IgE levels. Eur J Immunol 1991; 21:2679–2686.
101. Nopp A, Johansson SGO, Lundberg M, Ankerst J, Bylin G, Cardell L-O, Grönneberg R, Irander K, Palmqvist M, Öman H. Basophil allergen threshold sensitivity. A useful approach to anti-IgE treatment efficacy evaluation. Submitted.

10

Immunosuppressive and Other Alternate Treatments for Asthma

MARK S. DYKEWICZ

Division of Allergy and Immunology, Department of Internal Medicine, Saint Louis
    University School of Medicine
St. Louis, Missouri, U.S.A.

I. Introduction

Most patients with persistent asthma can be well controlled with minimal
toxicity employing strategies that include avoidance of clinically relevant
allergens, pharmacotherapy, allergen immunotherapy in selected patients,
and control of comorbid conditions such as rhinosinusitis and gastroesophageal reflux that can otherwise negatively impact asthma. Nonetheless,
even with the broadening repertoire of agents now approved as asthma
treatments (inhaled and systemic corticosteroids, leukotriene modifiers,
cromolyn, nedocromil, β-agonists, methylxanthines, and omalizumab),
and increasing use of regimens that combine several agents that have com-
plementary mechanisms, there remains a subset of patients who either do
not respond adequately to available agents or develop significant toxicities
to them. Consequently, there is still an important need for additional pharmacologic agents for asthma. In addition to the development of new therapies, there are alternate agents that are currently available for human use, that
have undergone at least some clinical trials for asthma, but are approved for
indications or uses other than for asthma, such as rheumatologic disease

"

or suppression of transplant rejection. Generally, these available alternate agents have known immunosuppressive or other immune-modulating effects that, at least in concept, might benefit the inflammatory basis of asthma. Specifically, these agents include gold, methotrexate, azathioprine, hydroxychloroquine, dapsone, nebulized lidocaine, inhaled furosemide, cyclosporine, intravenous immunoglobulin, and troleandomycin (1–4).

II. Patient Candidates for Alternate Asthma Treatments

Because of the potential toxicity of some proposed alternate treatments for asthma, asthma patients who might be considered candidates for therapy with alternate agents are often the most problematic of asthma patients. These patients may fall into several subsets. First, there are patients who do respond to systemic corticosteroids, but are termed steroid dependent because they require chronic administration of systemic corticosteroids, often at doses that have the potential to cause significant side effects such as osteoporosis, cushionoid features, or glucose intolerance. Second, there are patients who are termed steroid resistant who, by definition, fail to respond to a 7- to 14-day course of daily prednisone as measured by less than a 15% improvement in morning prebronchodilator FEV_1 following the glucocorticoid course (5). Furthermore, two types of steroid-resistant asthma have been defined. Type-I steroid resistant asthma is acquired and is associated with abnormally reduced glucocorticoid receptor (GCR) ligand and DNA-binding affinity (6). Type-II steroid-resistant asthma appears to be due to a constitutive defect and is associated with low numbers of GCRs. An important distinction between these two types of steroid-resistant asthma is that the GCR defect in Type I, but not Type II, steroid-resistant asthma is reversible in culture (and to some degree clinically) and is sustained by incubation with combination IL-2 and IL-4. This latter finding is consistent with the possibility that different patterns of cytokine expression and immune activation alter the response to corticosteroid therapy.

Other studies have identified differences in asthma patients in terms of cell populations that contribute to airway inflammation. While some data show that in subjects with moderate to severe asthma, lymphocytes and eosinophils constitute most of the inflammatory cells infiltrating the bronchial mucosa, neutrophils may become more prevalent in severe, corticosteroid-dependent asthma patients with nocturnal symptoms (7,8). Consequently, different patient subsets with asthma may have different profiles of inflammatory cells that would be targets for anti-inflammatory therapy.

In the context of considering alternate treatments for more problematic, severe asthma patients, recognition that there are different phenotypic subsets of severe asthma patients is important for several reasons. First, elucidation of the pathologic mechanisms that underlie different asthma phenotypes may lead to development of new therapeutic interventions that specifically target the pathologic mechanisms that distinguish one subset of asthma patients from another. Second, it should be expected conceptually that if patients with similar severe asthma severity can differ in their response to corticosteroids, patients might also differ in their responses to other agents. Consequently, trials of a new agent for asthma must include sufficient numbers of patients to ensure sufficient statistical power to detect clinical efficacy that may be present in only a subset of patients (2). If this is not done, one may incorrectly conclude that an agent has no value in asthma treatment, even though it may be of value to a patient subset.

III. Caveats in Interpreting Asthma Trial Data

In reviewing trials that attempt to assess the clinical efficacy of new, alternate, or experimental therapies for asthma, study results must be viewed with an awareness that the natural history of asthma is highly variable. Dykewicz et al. retrospectively reviewed the natural history of 40 patients who had been treated with inhaled steroids but still required systemic steroids (mean dose 11.7 mg/day prednisone) for at least one year (mean duration 6.2 years) (9). During 12 to 32 months of follow up, 25% tolerated discontinuation of oral steroids, and 7.5% tolerated significant reductions of oral steroids. Although 60% had no change in long-term steroid-dose requirements, one-third of these patients were able to discontinue prednisone for extended periods (mean 3.2 years) during follow up, only to again require steroid doses similar to the original requirements. Consequently, studies without placebo-control groups that report a reduction in oral-steroid requirements in association with use of investigational therapies for asthma may be merely demonstrating the natural history of asthma in such patients, and not that the studied therapy truly has clinical effectiveness. During a clinical trial in which physician investigator judgment is required to assess whether there can be reduction in the dose of oral corticosteroids, single-blind studies can be open to bias if the treatment allocation is known to the investigator.

These considerations underscore the importance of using double-blinded, controlled, long-term studies to definitively assess efficacy of putative treatments for asthma. Unfortunately, for some agents proposed as possible alternate treatments for asthma, efficacy has been studied only in uncontrolled, open trials. Moreover, many of the studies investigating alternate therapies for asthma have been conducted in relatively small numbers of subjects, or for relatively short periods of time.

IV. Gold

A. Background

Gold preparations have long been used for their anti-inflammatory effect in rheumatoid arthritis. Although the clinically relevant mechanisms of action are incompletely understood, gold agents have been shown to have multiple immunomodulatory effects, including inhibition of IL-5 enhancement of eosinophil survival, inactivation of C1 (complement), and reduction in neutrophil and macrophage phagocytosis, lymphocyte reactivity to antigenic stimulation, IgE-mediated release of histamine from isolated basophils and lung mast cells, prostaglandin, and leukotriene production in vitro, antibody production, and lysosomal enzyme release from phagocytic leukocytes (14,82–86). A parenteral preparation of aurothioglucose and an oral preparation of auranofin are available. Pharmacokinetically, a steady state is reached after 8 to 12 weeks of continued administration, which might suggest that several months of therapy may be required before efficacy can be assessed. It has been stated that the minimum duration of a valid trial of therapy is probably six months (3).

B. Clinical Studies

Several double-blind studies in asthma have reported benefit, with some patients being able to discontinue oral steroids (10–12). The largest study, the Auranofin Multicenter Drug Trial (12), studied 275 patients with daily oral prednisone requirements of ≥ 10 mg. Patients were randomized to auranofin, 3 mg twice daily, or placebo for six months. The study had limitations including a high dropout rate of $\geq 40\%$ in both groups, but did conclude that patients treated with gold were able to reduce their daily oral-corticosteroid dose by $\geq 50\%$ compared to those receiving placebo (60% vs. 32%, respectively; $p < 0.001$). However, there were no significant differences in objective measurements of pulmonary function or symptoms. Auranofin treatment was also associated with statistically significant reductions in serum IgE levels. Data from this trial were included with two others in a Cochrane review looking at the addition of gold compared to placebo in adult steroid-dependent asthmatics (13). The review confirmed that there was a small but significant treatment effect for gold in terms of steroid-dose reduction [Peto odds ratio (POR) 0.51, 95% confidence intervals (CI) 0.31, 0.83]. No meta-analysis could be done for measures of lung function, although overall there were few changes suggesting a positive benefit for gold. There were trends suggestive of adverse effects but no significant changes for gold-treated patients with respect to proteinuria (POR 1.4, 95% CI 0.6, 3.3) and dermatitis/eczema (POR 2.1, 95% CI 0.9, 4.7). The review concluded that because the changes seen in these trials are small and probably of limited clinical significance, and gold is associated with toxicity and requires monitoring, the use of gold as a steroid-sparing agent in asthma cannot be recommended. In contrast, it has been argued that the relative lack of severe side effects with gold therapy, compared to methotrexate therapy, make it a preferable agent for the treatment of severe, glucocorticoid-dependent asthma (14).

C. Adverse Events

In widespread usage for rheumatoid arthritis, more common side effects of gold agents include rash (26% auranofin and 39% aurothioglucose), diarrhea (43% auranofin and 13% aurothioglucose), stomatitis (13% auranofin and 18% aurothioglucose), other GI side effects, proteinuria (3–9%), and bone marrow suppression (leukopenia, thrombocytopenia 1%). Accordingly, periodic monitoring of laboratory tests to detect hematologic or renal toxicities is recommended.

V. Methotrexate

A. Background

Methotrexate is a folic acid antagonist that is cytotoxic to rapidly dividing cells in S phase (15). Although the exact mechanism of action is uncertain, it is used for treatment of rheumatoid arthritis, psoriasis, and some malignancies, including lymphoma.

B. Clinical Studies

The methotrexate doses used in asthma studies (5–25 mg weekly), are similar to those used in rheumatoid arthritis. While some double-blind, placebo-controlled studies have reported benefit in asthma, whereas other studies report no benefit versus placebo (15–17), meta-analyses conclude some benefit with longer term (≥ 3 months) use (18,19). One meta-analysis reported a 6% pooled improvement in FEV_1 and a 8.2% reduction in oral-steroid dose (19). In another meta-analysis, methotrexate was associated with a 23.7% decrease in oral-steroid doses with the greatest benefit noted in trials of at least six months of therapy (18).

A Cochrane review of 10 trials of at least 12 weeks duration found that there was a reduction in oral-corticosteroid dose favoring methotrexate in parallel trials (weighted mean difference -4.1 mg/day, 95% CI -6.8–1.3) and also in cross-over trials (weighted mean difference -2.9 mg/day, 95% CI -5.9–0.2) (20). However, there was no difference between methotrexate and placebo for forced expiratory volume in one minute (weighted mean difference 0.12 L, 95% CI -0.21–0.45). Hepatotoxicity was a common adverse effect with methotrexate compared to placebo [odds ratio (OR) 6.9, 95% CI 3.1–15.5]. The reviewers concluded that while methotrexate may have a small steroid-sparing effect in adults with asthma who are dependent on oral corticosteroids, the overall reduction in daily steroid use is probably not large enough to reduce steroid-induced adverse effects.

C. Adverse Events

The more serious side effects of methotrexate are leukopenia, hepatic fibrosis, pulmonary toxicity, and immunosuppression with infection (pneumocystis, cytomegalovirus, and varicella). The most frequent reasons for cessation of methotrexate therapy for asthma have been abnormal liver function tests and symptomatic GI side effects (e.g., nausea, heartburn, and diarrhea) (21). There must be periodic monitoring of blood counts and liver function.

VI. Azathioprine

A. Background

Azathioprine is reduced in the presence of glutathione to 6-mercaptopurine and then metabolized into active metabolites that interfere with purine metabolism. It has immunosuppressive effects that have been used for transplant rejection and severe rheumatoid arthritis.

B. Clinical Studies

Although azathioprine has been proposed as a treatment for asthma for decades (87) and has been studied in a number of trials, only two small randomized, placebo-controlled studies that recruited a total of 23 subjects have been published (22). These studies were limited by several factors, including the possible presence of comorbid lung disease, inadequate washout (in one study), and no data reporting about oral-steroid consumption (23). No significant differences were observed in the studies for FEV_1, FVC, PaO_2, and symptoms. One study reported a statistically significant difference in sGaw (specific airway conductance).

C. Adverse Events

Based upon experience in disease states other than asthma, azathioprine can induce leukopenia, thrombocytopenia and gastroinstestinal toxicity, including cholestatic hepatotoxicity. In addition to an increased risk of infection, evidence for mutagenicity has been reported.

VII. Hydroxychloroquine

A. Background

Hydroxychloroquine is widely used for treatment of rheumatoid arthritis, collagen vascular diseases, and malaria. Although its mechanisms are uncertain, there is evidence that it inhibits phospholipase A_2 and phagocytosis, and decreases stimulation of CD4+ lymphocytes.

B. Clinical Studies

In an open study of 11 asthma patients, hydroxychloroquine treatment was associated with an increase in pulmonary function, a decrease in symptom scores, and a decrease in oral-steroid dose by about 50% in seven patients (24). Mean IgE levels were reported to decrease in 10 patients to about half their pretreatment level. However, in a double-blind, placebo-controlled trial of nine asthmatic subjects over eight weeks, hydroxychloroquine had no more corticosteroid-sparing properties than placebo (25).

C. Toxicity

Because hydroxychloroquine can cause irreversible retinal damage, patients should be monitored for ocular changes at baseline and every 6 to 12 months thereafter.

VIII. Dapsone

A. Background

Dapsone is a sulfone used in pemphigoid, pemphigus, bullous SLE, and leprosy. It has been shown to block integrin-mediated neutrophil migration and inhibit antibody adherence to neutrophils (26,27).

B. Clinical Studies

In one open study by Berlow et al. for up to 20 months at a dose of 100 mg twice daily, 7 of 10 patients were able to decrease or discontinue oral corticosteroids after 6 to 13 months (28). Symptoms and pulmonary functions were unchanged. To date, there are no published controlled studies of dapsone in asthma (29).

C. Adverse Events

In the Berlow trial, dose-dependent hemolytic anemia occurred in nine patients and theophylline toxicity in four. Other toxic reactions including malaise, rash, and thrombocytopenia were observed. Based upon experience in other disorders, side effects of dapsone include dose-related hemolysis with nearly all patients experiencing a loss of 1–2 g of hemoglobin (with a greater risk in G6PD deficiency). Less common or rare side effects include agranulocytosis and aplastic anemia, peripheral neuropathy that is usually reversible, rash, a fatal mononucleosis-like syndrome, lymphadenopathy, and hepatic necrosis. Monitoring for hematologic and liver function abnormalities should be performed.

IX. Nebulized Lidocaine

A. Background

Interest in using nebulized lidocaine for asthma developed when it was found that lidocaine inhibits eosinophil survival in bronchoalveolar lavage fluid (30). Studies have also shown that lidocaine can have an inhibitory effect on T cells from patients with allergic asthma (31). Local anesthetic agents can also acutely inhibit bronchial reactivity and reflex bronchoconstriction (32,33).

B. Clinical Studies

One placebo-controlled trial of nebulized lidocaine in mild–moderate asthma has been published, although no placebo-controlled trials in severe asthma have been published. In the controlled study of mild–moderate asthma by Hunt et al. all patients were treated with daily inhaled glucocorticoids (but not systemic glucocorticoids) and bronchodilators for at least two months (34). At initiation, subjects inhaled either nebulized placebo (saline) or lidocaine (4%, 100 mg) four times daily. Subjects were instructed to reduce their inhaled glucocorticoid dosage by one half each week for three weeks, then discontinue glucocorticoid treatment at week 4, and continue the nebulized lidocaine or placebo for a total of eight weeks. The lidocaine-treated group showed statistically significant benefits in FEV_1, nighttime awakenings, symptoms, bronchodilator use, and blood eosinophil counts. Conversely, the nebulized placebo group showed decreases in FEV_1, increased symptom scores and bronchodilator use, and blood eosinophil counts. Subjects in both groups reduced use of inhaled glucocorticoids comparably. In an uncontrolled trial of nebulized lidocaine [2–3 mL lidocaine 2% (40–60 mg) up to 2.5–4 mL lidocaine (100–160 mg) qid] in 20 adult asthmatics who were corticosteroid dependent (mean prednisone dose of 24 mg for 6.5 years), three patients were able to discontinue prednisone, and four were able to tolerate significant prednisone dose reductions (35). In an small, exploratory open study of severe asthma in children treated with nebulized lidocaine (0.8–2.5 mg/kg/dose tid to qid), five of six patients completely discontinued oral steroids within an average of 3.4 months (range 1–7 months) (36).

C. Adverse Events

Lidocaine toxicity occurs when serum levels exceed 5–6 µg/mL and includes muscle twitching, seizures, arrhythmias, paresthesias, and respiratory arrest (37). In the placebo-controlled trial by Hunt, no signs of lidocaine toxicity were observed in the treated subjects by using a 4% concentration and a total dosage of 100 mg per use (34). Serum levels of greater than 1 µg/mL are not reached until greater than 300–400 mg is administered to the airway, either by direct instillation or nebulization (34). Occasionally, subjects have dropped out of studies because of lidocaine intolerance (oral and pharyngeal hypoethesia). Reduced airflow not related to histamine responsiveness has been observed in a minority of patients, but albuterol has been demonstrated to prevent this (34–38).

X. Inhaled Furosemide

A. Background

Long used as a loop diuretic, interest in furosemide developed for asthma treatment after studies in exercise-induced bronchospasm examined the role of changes in surface osmolarity and water concentration of the airway epithelium (39). Studies have identified multiple mechanisms in which furosemide might affect asthma, including reduction in apical chloride channel activity with consequent decrease in the potential difference and short-circuit current in airway epithelial cells (40,41), inhibition of the release of eosinophil mediators through inhibition of chloride transport (42), inhibition of release of histamine and leukotrienes from passively sensitized human lung (43), modulatory effects in animal models studying presynaptic neuropeptide release from non-cholinergic, non-adrenergic sensory nerves and cholinergic neural responses (44), and effects on prostaglandin production (45,46,88).

B. Clinical Studies

Furosemide is not effective against asthma when administered orally at the usual diuretic doses but rather must be inhaled (20–40 mg doses) for significant antiasthma effects (39). Although a number of clinical trials have examined the positive effects of furosemide on abrogating responses to various bronchoconstrictor agents in asthma patients, and several studies have investigated inhaled furosemide in acute asthma exacerbations, there have been only two clinical trials using furosemide therapy for the treatment of chronic asthma. One studied a combination of lysine acetylsalicylate (LASA) and furosemide on a small group of patients with severe steroid-dependent asthma for 10 to 28 weeks, and found a significant steroid-sparing effect (47). In a follow-up, double-blind, randomized, cross-over trial, nine patients with mild to moderate asthma receiving standard therapy were treated with sequential inhaled doses of LASA, furosemide, or placebo twice daily (48). After approximately two months with scheduled reductions in inhaled corticosteroid therapy as tolerated, treatment with furosemide/LASA was associated with a mean dose reduction of $71 \pm 7\%$ in the amount of inhaled beclomethasone required for asthma control, and two patients were able to discontinue inhaled steroid therapy.

C. Adverse Events

In clinical trials using inhaled furosemide for asthma, no diuresis has been noted (presumably because of lack of absorption of significant amounts of furosemide into the general circulation), and no significant adverse effects have been reported.

XI. Cyclosporine

A. Background

Cyclosporine has been widely used as an immunosuppressive agent in transplantation. Its principal action is to bind cyclophilin, thereby inhibiting cytokine messenger RNA transcription and CD4+ T-cell activation (49). Cyclosporine has been demonstrated to decrease production of granulocyte macrophage colony–stimulating factor and IL-5 from stimulated monocytes with consequent inhibition of eosinophil proliferation and survival activity (50,51). It has also been found to reduce production and release of proinflammatory mediators from mast cells and basophils; decrease B-cell IgE synthesis and release; decrease macrophage synthesis of IL-1, tumor necrosis factor, superoxide, and hydrogen peroxide; and decrease neutrophil chemotaxis, IL-2 levels, and serum soluble IL-2 receptor concentrations (14,52–56).

B. Clinical Studies

Cyclosporine has been reported to result in improvement in airway hyperresponsiveness (57). Several prospective, randomized trials have studied the effect of cyclosporine in asthma patients. In a 12-week cross-over trial of 33 steroid-dependent asthma patients, cyclosporine (initial dose, 5 mg/kg/day) compared to placebo was associated with statistically significant greater benefit with a 12% increase in morning peak expiratory flow rates (PEFRs), a 17.6% increase in FEV_1, and a 48% reduction in exacerbations requiring increased steroid dosing ($p < 0.02$) compared to those receiving placebo (55). Of special note is that several steroid-resistant patients had improvement of clinical symptoms on cyclosporine. A similar but smaller study of 16 patients with severe asthma for 36 weeks found that cyclosporine (initial dose, 5 mg/kg/day) was associated with a statistically significant reduction in median daily prednisolone dosage (62% vs. 25% with placebo) and improvements in PEFR (58). However, a study of 34 severe asthma patients and longer follow-up period failed to find that cyclosporine had significant effects on pulmonary function and steroid-sparing effects (59). A Cochrane review of available cyclosporine trials analyzed data from 98 patients, and found a small but significant treatment effect for cyclosporine in steroid-dose reduction (SMD -0.5, 95% CI -1.0, -0.04) (60). No meta-analyses could be performed for measures of lung function. The review assessed that the clinical changes in asthma with cyclosporine are small and of questionable clinical significance.

C. Adverse Events

Side effects from cyclosporine include irreversible renal toxicity (focal interstitial fibrosis with tubular dysfunction), reversible increases in BUN and alkaline phosphatase, hypertension, hyperkalemia, transient peripheral neuropathy, and hirsutism. Based upon experience with cyclosporine use in transplantation, less renal toxicity occurs with low doses (2–5 mg/kg/day) than with high doses (15 mg/kg/day). Regular monitoring of renal function, blood pressure, and blood concentrations of cyclosporine is required.

XII. Intravenous Immunoglobulin (IVIG)

A. Background

Intravenous immunoglobulin (IVIG) is thought to have immunomodulatory activity through a variety of mechanisms, including Fc receptor blockade on monocytes and macrophages, inhibition of IL-2 and IL-4 cytokine production and cytokine-dependent lymphocyte proliferation in vitro, and induction of suppressor T cells (61–64). Additionally, there is evidence that IVIG can enhance glucocorticoid receptor binding affinity, as well as synergize corticosteroid-induced suppression of lymphocytes, even in patients with prior steroid resistance (64,65).

B. Clinical Studies

In an open label, six-month trial of monthly administration of high-dose IVIG in eight children with severe steroid-dependent asthma, IVIG was associated with a threefold decrease in oral-corticosteroid requirement, a reduction in symptom scores, and decreases in serum total IgE levels and skin test reactivity to allergens (65). In small case series of adult and pediatric asthma patients, IVIG was reported to have steroid-sparing effects (66,67). In a controlled study of 38 patients with severe steroid-dependent asthma, subjects were randomized to receive either a 2 g/kg loading dose of IVIG followed by a regimen of 400 mg/kg IVIG every three weeks or IV albumin, with subsequent efforts to reduce oral-corticosteroid doses. Of 28 patients who completed the study (seven patients withdrew from the protocol), there was no overall difference in the amount of steroid reduction (68). However, a post hoc subgroup analysis found that patients who had required high-dose, long-term corticosteroid therapy (i.e., >2000 mg in the year prior to study entry) had a statistically greater reduction in oral glucocorticoid requirements with IVIG treatment compared to placebo subjects (median reduction, 16.4 vs. 3 mg/day; $p = 0.0078$). In another trial of 40 adult and pediatric patients with severe asthma, subjects were randomized to IVIG doses of 2 g/kg/mo, 1 g/kg/mo, or 2 g IV albumin/mo (69). The study was ended early after three patients in the high-dose IVIG group were hospitalized with aseptic meningitis. Interim analysis concluded that there was no significant difference between groups in steroid dose reductions, pulmonary function results, or the number of clinical exacerbations.

C. Adverse Events

Although high-dose IVIG is costly, it is generally well tolerated except for infusion-related events such as fever, chills, nausea, back pain, and, infrequently, anaphylaxis. Rarely IVIG is associated with aseptic meningitis and interstitial nephritis. Although current commercial preparations should have no risk of transmission of viral hepatitis, there remains the remote possibility with IVIG.

XIII. Troleandomycin

A. Background

For several decades, the macrolide antibiotic troleandomycin (TAO) had been used for concomitant administration with methylprednisone as a "steroid sparing" agent for corticosteroid-dependent asthma (70). TAO prolongs the half-life and bioavailability of methylprednisolone by decreasing hepatic metabolism and excretion (but not some other commonly used corticosteroids such as prednisone), an effect that is thought to account for much of the reported benefit of the drug (71–73). Patient improvement has not been associated with reduced infection assessed by sputum culture, and it is not thought that TAO has a direct antimicrobial effect that is relevant to its effect on asthma (73).

B. Clinical Studies

In an open trial of steroid-dependent asthma patients using 14 mg/kg/day TAO (maximum dose, 1 g) and methylprednisolone, 62 of 74 patients had improvement in clinical symptoms and/or a reduction in corticosteroid dosage (70). Several case series found similar effects (74,75). A subsequent study reduced the starting TAO dose to 250 mg once or twice daily with a rapid methylprednisolone taper to alternate-day dosing for > 4 to 8 days, and found that steroid-related and GI side effects could be reduced (76).

In one large prospective, double-blind, randomized, placebo-controlled trial of TAO, 75 steroid-dependent asthma patients were randomized to TAO, 250 mg daily, or placebo, with attempted tapering of methylprednisolone as tolerated (77). The study was hampered by a high patient dropout rate (TAO group: seven patients at one year, 20 patients at two years; placebo group: 11 patients at one year, 30 patients at two years.) Those TAO patients continuing on the study did tolerate lower steroid doses at one year ($p < 0.03$), but they did not have a significant reduction in the number of hospitalizations and emergency department visits, and had more cases of bone loss ($p < 0.01$) and higher cholesterol levels ($p < 0.05$) than did placebo subjects. The study concluded that TAO offered no advantage for asthma outcome, and was associated with greater steroid-related side effects. In a Cochrane review of aggregate data from three randomized trials in which 112 patients were recruited, data from 90 patients were analyzed (78). Addition of TAO was not associated with benefits in lung function.

C. Adverse Events

Even with reduced doses of TAO, progression of osteoporosis, cushionoid features, hyperglycemia, and other typical corticosteroid side effects are common. GI complaints and liver toxicity may also occur, particularly at higher doses (79–81). Decreased IgG levels were identified in the TAO group ($p < 0.05$) by Nelson et al. (77) and one case of varicella zoster has been reported (75).

XIV. Conclusions

In reviewing available data about the efficacy and safety of immunosuppressive and other alternate therapies for asthma treatment, it is clear that many agents that have shown promise in exploratory uncontrolled series have failed to demonstrate effectiveness when subjected to more extensive, controlled trials. This experience provides several lessons. First, it can be difficult to predict whether an agent will have clinical efficacy in asthma based upon its known or assumed mechanisms of drug activity. Second, the natural history of the asthma syndrome and differences between asthma phenotypes require that large, well-controlled trials of significant duration are absolutely necessary to properly assess whether an agent has efficacy in asthma. Third, experience with use of agents in other disease states generally accurately predicts the toxicity profile of these drugs when used for asthma. Finally, the majority of available immunosuppressive agents that have been studied in asthma do not have a favorable therapeutic index for asthma treatment. Those few alternate agents that currently appear to have a more favorable therapeutic index for asthma (e.g., nebulized lidocaine) deserve further investigation in larger, well-controlled studies.

References

1. Szefler SJ, Nelson HS. Alternative agents for anti-inflammatory treatment of asthma. J Allergy Clin Immunol 1998; 102:S23–S35.
2. Dykewicz MS. Newer and alternative non-steroidal treatments for asthmatic inflammation. Allergy Asthma Proc 2001; 22:11–15.
3. Corrigan CJ. Asthma refractory to glucocorticoids: the role of newer immuno-suppressants. Am J Respir Med 2002; 1:47–54.
4. Niven AS, Argyros G. Alternate treatments in asthma. Chest 2003; 123:1254–1265.
5. Nimmagadda SR, Spahn JD, Leung DY, Szefler SJ. Steroid-resistant asthma: evaluation and management. Ann Allergy Asthma Immunol 1996; 77:345–355.
6. Leung DY, Szefler SJ. New insights into steroid resistant asthma. Pediatr Allergy Immunol 1998; 9:3–12.
7. Chakir J, Hamid Q, Bosse M, Boulet LP, Laviolette M. Bronchial inflammation in corticosteroid-sensitive and corticosteroid-resistant asthma at baseline and on oral corticosteroid treatment. Clin Exp Allergy 2002; 32:578–582.
8. Wenzel SE, Szefler SJ, Leung DY, Sloan SI, Rex MD, Martin RJ. Broncho-scopic evaluation of severe asthma. Persistent inflammation associated with high dose glucocorticoids. Am J Respir Crit Care Med 1997; 156:737–743.
9. Dykewicz MS, Greenberger PA, Patterson R, Halwig JM. Natural history of asthma in patients requiring long-term systemic corticosteroids. Arch Int Med 1986; 146:2369–2372.
10. Muranaka MM, Miyamoto T, Shida T, Kabe J, Makino S, Okumura H, Takeda K, Suzuki S, Horiuchi Y. Gold salt in the treatment of bronchial asthma: a dou-ble blind study. Ann Allergy 1978; 40:132–137.
11. Nierop G, Gijzel WP, Bel EH, Zwinderman AH, Dijkman JH. Auranofin in the treatment of steroid dependent asthma: a double blind study. Thorax 1992; 47:349–354.
12. Bernstein IL, Bernstein DI, Dubb JW, Faiferman I, Wallin B. A placebo-controlled multicenter study of auranofin in the treatment of patients with corticosteroid-dependent asthma: auranofin multicenter drug trial. J Allergy Clin Immunol 1996; 98:317–324.
13. Evans DJ, Cullinan P, Geddes DM. Gold as an oral corticosteroid sparing agent in stable asthma. Cochrane Database Syst Rev 2001; 2:CD002985.
14. Ledford DK. Treatment of steroid-resistant asthma. Immunol Allergy Clin North Am 1996; 16:777–796.
15. Mullarkey MF, Blumenstein BA, Andrade WP, Bailey GA, Olason I, Wetzel CE. Methotrexate in the treatment of corticosteroid-dependent asthma. N Engl J Med 1988; 318:603–607.
16. Stewart GE, Diaz JD, Lockey RF, Seleznick MJ, Trudeau WL, Ledford DK. Comparison of oral pulse methotrexate with placebo in the treatment of severe glucocorticosteroid-dependent asthma. J Allergy Clin Immunol 1994; 94:482–489.
17. Erzurum SC, Leff JA, Cochran JE, Ackerson LM, Szefler SJ, Martin RJ, Cott GR. Lack of benefit of methotrexate in severe, steroid-dependent asthma. Ann Intern Med 1991; 114:353–360.

18. Marin MG. Low-dose methotrexate spares steroid usage in steroid-dependent asthmatic patients: a meta-analysis. Chest 1997; 112:29–33.

19. Aaron SD, Dales RE, Pham B. Management of steroid-dependent asthma with methotrexate: a meta-analysis of randomized clinical trials. Respir Med 1998; 92:1059–1065.

20. Davies H, Olson L, Gibson P. Methotrexate as a steroid sparing agent for asthma in adults. Cochrane Database Syst Rev 2000; 2:CD000391.

21. Shulimzon TR, Shiner RJ. A risk-benefit assessment of methotrexate in corticosteroid dependent asthma. Drug Safety 1996; 15:283–290.

22. Hodges NG, Brewis RA, Howell JB. An evaluation of azathioprine in severe chronic asthma. Thorax 1971; 26:734–739.

23. Dean T, Dewey A, Bara A, Lasserson TJ, Walters EH. Azathioprine as an oral corticosteroid sparing agent for asthma. Cochrane Database Syst Rev 2004; 1:CD003270.

24. Charous JH. Open study of hydroxychloroquine in the treatment of severe symptomatic or corticosteroid-dependent asthma. Ann Allergy 1990; 65: 53–58.

25. Roberts JA, Gunneberg A, Elliott JA, Thomson NC. Hydroxychloroquine in steroid dependent asthma. Pulm Pharmacol 1988; 1:59–61.

26. Booth SA, Moody CE, Dahl MV, Herron MJ, Nelson RD. Dapsone suppresses integrin-mediated neutrophil adherence function. J Invest Dermatol 1992; 98:135–140.

27. Thuong-Nguyen V, Kadunce DP, Hendrix JD, Gammon WR, Zone JJ. Inhibition of neutrophil adherence to antibody by dapsone: a possible therapeutic mechanism of dapsone in the treatment of IgA dermatoses. J Invest Dermatol 1993; 100:349–355.

28. Berlow BA, Liebhaber MI, Dyer Z, Spiegel TM. The effect of dapsone in steroid-dependent asthma. J Allergy Clin Immunol 1991; 87:710–715.

29. Dewey A, Bara A, Dean T, Walters H. Dapsone as an oral corticosteroid sparing agent for asthma. Cochrane Database Syst Rev 2002; 4:CD003268.

30. Ohnishi T, Kite H, Mayeno AN, Okada S, Sur S, Broide DH, Gleich GJ. Lidocaine in bronchoalveolar lavage fluid (BALF) is an inhibitor of eosinophil-active cytokines. Clin Exp Immunol 1996; 104:325–331.

31. Tanaka A, Minoguchi K, Oda N, Yokoe T, Matsuo H, Okada S, Tasaki T, Adachi M. Inhibitory effect of lidocaine on T cells from patients with allergic asthma. J Allergy Clin Immunol 2002; 109:485–490.

32. Ohnishi T, Kita H, Mayeno AN, Okada S, Sur S, Broide DH, Gleich GJ. Lidocaine in bronchoalveolar lavage fluid (BALF) is an inhibitor of eosinophil-active cytokines. Clin Exp Immunol 1996; 104:325–331.

33. Harrison TW, Tattersfield AE. Effect of single doses of inhaled lignocaine on FEV_1 and bronchial reactivity in asthma. Respir Med 1998; 92:1359–1363.

34. Hunt LW, Frigas E, Butterfield JH, Kita H, Blomgren J, Dunnette SL, Offord KP, Gleich GJ. Treatment of asthma with nebulized lidocame: a randomized, placebo-controlled study. J Allergy Clin Immunol 2004; 113: 853–859.

35. Hunt LW, Swedlund HA, Gleich GJ. Effect of nebulized lidocaine on severe corticosteroid-dependent asthma. Mayo Clinic Proc 1996; 71:361–368.

36. Decco ML, Neeno TA, Hunt LW, O'Connell EJ, Yunginger JW, Sachs MI. Nebulized lidocaine in the treatment of severe asthma in children: a pilot study. Ann Allergy Asthma Immunol 1999; 82:29–32.

37. Boye NP, Bredesen JE. Plasma concentrations of lidocaine during inhalation anaesthesia for fiberoptic bronchoscopy. Scand J Respir Dis 1979; 60:105–108.

38. Groeben H, Silvanus M-T, Beste M, Peters J. Combined lidocaine and salbutamol inhalation for airway anesthesia markedly protects against reflex bronchoconstriction. Chest 2000; 118:509–515.

39. Bianco S, Vaghi A, Robuschi M, Pasargiklian M. Prevention of exercise-induced bronchoconstriction by inhaled furosemide. Lancet 1988; 2:252–255.

40. Welsh MJ. Inhibition of chloride secretion by furosemide in canine tracheal epithelium. J Membr Biol 1993; 71:218–226.

41. Alton EW, Kingsleigh-Smith DJ, Munkonge FM, Smith SN, Lindsay AR, Gruenert DC, Jeffery PK, Norris A, Geddes DM, Williams AJ. Asthma prophylaxis agents alter the function of an airway epithelial chloride channel. Am J Respir Cell Mol Biol 1996; 14:380–387.

42. Perkins R, Dent G, Chung KF, Barnes PJ. Effect of anion transport inhibitors and extracellular Cl-concentrations on eosinophil respiratory burst activity. Biochem Pharmacol 1992; 107:481–488.

43. Anderson SD, Wei HE, Temple DM. Inhibition by furosemide of inflammatory mediators from lung fragments [letter]. N Engl J Med 1991; 324:131.

44. Elwood W, Lotvall JO, Barnes PJ, Chung KF. Loop diuretics inhibit cholinergic and non-cholinergic nerves in guinea pig airways. Am Rev Respir Dis 1991; 143:1340–1344.

45. Barnes PJ. Diuretics and asthma. Thorax 1993; 48:195–196.

46. Levasseur-Acker GM, Molimard M, Regnard J, Naline E, Freche C, Lockhart A. Effect of furosemide on prostaglandin synthesis by human nasal and bronchial epithelial cells in culture. Am J Respir Cell Mol Biol 1994; 10: 378–383.

47. Bianco S, Robuschi M, Vaghi A, Pasargiklian M. Steroid sparing effect of inhaled lysine-aspirin and furosemide in steroid-dependent asthma. In: Melillo G, O'Byrne PH, Marone G, eds. Respiratory Allergy. Amsterdam, The Netherlands: Elsevier, 1993:261–269.

48. Bianco S, Vaghi A, Robuschi M, Refini RM, Pieroni MG, Sestini P. Steroid-sparing effect of inhaled lysine acetylsalicylate and furosemide in high-dose beclomethasone-dependent asthma. J Allergy Clin Immunol 1995; 95:937–943.

49. Sihra BS, Kon OM, Durham SR, Walker S, Barnes NC, Kay AB. Effect of cyclosporin A on the allergen-induced late asthmatic reaction. Thorax 1997; 52:447–452.

50. Sano T, Nakamura Y, Matsunaga Y, Takahashi T, Azuma M, Okano Y, Shimizu E, Ogushi F, Sone S, Ogura T. FK506, and cyclosporin A inhibit granulocyte/macrophage colony-stimulating factor production by mononuclear cells in asthma. Eur Respir J 1995; 8:1473–1479.

51. Mori A, Suko M, Nishizaki Y, Kaminuma O, Kobayashi S, Matsuzaki G, Yamamoto K, Ito K, Tsuruoka N, Okudaira H. IL-5 production by CD4+ T cells of asthmatic patients is suppressed by glucocorticoids and the immunosuppressants FK506 and cyclosporine A. Int Immunol 1995; 7:449–457.

52. Calderon E, Lookey RF, Bukants SC, Coffey RG, Ledford DK. Is there a role for cyclosporine in asthma? J Allergy Clin Immunol 1992; 89:629–636.

53. Bourgeres PF, Carel JC, Castano L, Boitard C, Gardin IP, Landais P, Hors J, Mihatsch MJ, Paillard M, Chaussain JL. Factors associated with early remission of type I diabetes in children treated with cyclosporine. N Engl J Med 1988; 318:663–670.

54. Frew AJ, Plummeridge MJ. Alternative agents in asthma. J Allergy Clin Immunol 2001; 108:3–10.

55. Alexander AG, Barnes NC, Kay AB. Trial of cyclosporin in corticosteroid-dependent chronic severe asthma. Lancet 1992; 339:324–328.

56. Alexander AG, Barnes NC, Kay AB, Corrigan CJ. Clinical response to cyclosporin in chronic severe asthma is associated with reduction in serum soluble interleukin-2 receptor concentrations. Eur Respir J 1995; 8:574–578.

57. Fukuda T, Asakawa J, Motojima S, Makino S. Cyclosporine A reduces T lymphocyte activity and improves airway hyperresponsiveness in corticosteroid-dependent chronic severe asthma. Ann Allergy Asthma Immunol 1995; 75:65–72.

58. Lock SH, Kay AB, Barnes NC. Double-blind, placebo-controlled study of cyclosporin A as a corticosteroid-sparing agent in corticosteroid-dependent asthma. Am J Respir Crit Care Med 1996; 153:509–514.

59. Nizankowska E, Soja J, Pinnis G, Bochenek G, Sladek K, Domagala B, Pajak A, Szczeklik A. Treatment of steroid-dependent bronchial asthma with cyclosporin. Eur Respir J 1995; 8:1091–1099.

60. Evans DJ, Cullinan P, Geddes DM. Cyclosporin as an oral corticosteroid sparing agent in stable asthma. Cochrane Database Syst Rev 2001; 2:CD002993.

61. Mazer BD, Gielas PC, Gelfand EW. Immunomodulatory effects of intravenous immunoglobulin in severe steroid-dependent asthma. Clin Immunol Immunopathol 1989; 53:S156–S163.

62. Amran D, Renz H, Lack G, Bradley K, Gelfand EW. Suppression of cytokine-dependent human T-cell proliferation by intravenous immunoglobulin. Clin Immunol Immunopathol 1994; 73:180–186.

63. Leung DY, Burns J, Newburger J, Geha RS. Reversal of immunoregulatory abnormalities in Kawasaki syndrome by intravenous gammaglobulin. J Clin Invest 1987; 79:468–472.

64. Spahn JD, Leung DY, Chan MT, Szefler SJ, Gelfand EW. Mechanisms of glucocorticoid reductions in asthmatic patients treated with intravenous immunoglobulin. J Allergy Clin Immunol 1999; 103:421–426.

65. Mazer BD, Gelfand EW. An open label study of high dose intravenous immunoglobulin in severe childhood asthma. J Allergy Clin Immunol 1991; 87:976–983.

66. Jakobsson T, Croner S, Kjellman N, Pettersson A, Vassella C, Bjorksten B. Slight steroid-sparing effects of intravenous immunoglobulin in children and adolescents with moderately severe bronchial asthma. Allergy 1994; 49:413–420.

67. Landwehr LP, Jeppson ID, Katlan MG, Esterl B, McCormick D, Hamilos DL, Gelfand EW. Benefits of high-dose IV immunoglobulin in patients with severe steroid-dependent asthma. Chest 1998; 114:1349–1356.

68. Salmun LM, Barlan I, Wolf HM, Eibl M, Twarog FJ, Geha RS, Schneider LC. Effect of intravenous immunoglobulin on steroid consumption in patients with severe asthma: a double-blind, placebo-controlled, randomized trial. J Allergy Clin Immunol 1999; 103:810–815.

69. Kishiyama JL, Valacer D, Curmingham-Rundles C, Sperber K, Richmond GW, Abramson S, Glovsky M, Stiehm R, Stocks J, Rosenberg L, Shames RS, Com B, Shearer WT, Bacot B, DiMaio M, Tonetta S, Adelman DC. A multi-center, randomized, double-blind, placebo-controlled trial of high-dose intravenous immunoglobulin for oral corticosteroid-dependent asthma. Clin Immunol 1999; 91:126–133.

70. Spector SL, Katz FH, Fair RS. Troleandomycin: effectiveness in steroid dependent asthma and bronchitis. J Allergy Clin Immunol 1974; 54: 367–379.

71. Szefler SJ, Rose JQ, Ellis EF, Spector SL, Green AW, Jusko WJ. The effect of troleandomycin on methylprednisolone elimination. J Allergy Clin Immunol 1980; 66:447–451.

72. Townley RG, Selenke WM. Metabolic effects of macrolide antibiotics on bronchial asthma, experimental anaphylaxis and corticosteroid metabolism. In: Ninth International Congress of Allergy. Vol. 144. Excerpta Medica, Hillsborough, NJ: 1967:90.

73. Itkin IH, Menzel ML. The use of macrolide antibiotic substances in the treatment of asthma. J Allergy 1970; 45:146–162.

74. Siracusa A, Brugnami G, Fiordi, T, Areni S, Severini C, Marabini A. Troleandomycin in the treatment of difficult asthma. J Allergy Clin Immunol 1993; 92:677–682.

75. Zeiger RS, Schatz M, Sperling W, Simon RA, Stevenson DD. Efficacy of troleandomycin in outpatients with severe, corticosteroid-dependent asthma. J Allergy Clin Immunol 1980; 66:438–446.

76. Wald JA, Friedman BF, Farr RS. An improved protocol for the use of troleandomycin (TAO) in the treatment of steroid-requiring asthma. J Allergy Clin Immunol 1986; 78:36–43.

77. Nelson HS, Hamilos DL, Corsello PR, Levesque NV, Buchmeier AD, Bucher BL. A double-blind study of troleandomycin and methylprednisolone in asthmatic subjects who require daily corticosteroids. Am Rev Respir Dis 1993; 147:398–404.

78. Evans DJ, Cullinan P, Geddes DM. Troleandomycin as an oral corticosteroid steroid sparing agent in stable asthma. Cochrane Database Syst Rev 2001; 2:CD002987.

79. Dasgupta A, Marcoux JP. Hepatic abnormalities associated with long-term use of troleandomycin in asthma: a case report. Ann Allergy 1978; 41: 297–298.

80. Larrey D, Amouyal G, Danan G, Degott C, Pessayre D, Benhamou JP. Prolonged cholestasis after troleandomycin-induced acute hepatitis. J Hepatol 1987; 4:327–329.

81. Uzzan B, Vassy R, Nicholas P, Chapman A, Perret G. Troleandomycin hepatotoxicity: a case report of overt jaundice and a placebo-controlled trial. Therapie 1993; 48:61–62.

82. Suzuki S, Okubo M, Kaise S, Ohara M, Kasukawa R. Gold sodium thiomalate selectively inhibits interleukin-5-mediated eosinophil survival. J Allergy Clin Immunol 1995; 96:251–256.

83. Walz DT, DiMartino MJ, Griswold DE, Intoccia AP, Flanagan TL. Biologic actions and pharmacodynamic studies of auranofin. Am J Med 1983; 75: 90–108.

84. Columbo M, Galeone D, Guidi G, Kagey-Sobotka A, Lichtenstein LM, Pettit GR, Marone G. Modulation of mediator release from human basophils and pulmonary mast cells and macrophages by auranofin. Biochem Pharmacol 1990; 39:285–291.

85. Parente J, Wong K, David P, Burka JF, Percy JS. Effects of gold compounds on leukotriene B4, leukotriene C4 and prostaglandin E2 production by polymorphonuclear leukocytes. J Rheumatol 1986; 3:47–51.

86. Bernstein DI, Bernstein IL, Bodenheimer SS, Pietrusko RG. An open study of auranofin in the treatment of steroid-dependent asthma. J Allergy Clin Immunol 1988; 81:6–16.

87. Kaiser HB, Beall GN. Azathioprine (imuran) in chronic asthma. Ann Allergy 1966; 24:369–370.

88. Miyanoshita A, Terada M, Endou H. Furosemide directly stimulates prostaglandin E2 production in the thick ascending limb of Henle's loop. J Pharmacol Exp Ther 1989; 251:1155–1159.

11

Specific Immunotherapy for Asthma

ANTHONY J. FREW

University of Southampton School of Medicine, Southampton General Hospital
Southampton, U.K.

I. Introduction

Asthma and allergic disorders are both becoming increasingly common, and unlike most of the other disorders that have also increased in recent years, asthma predominantly affects children and young adults. Two key themes emerge from epidemiological work on allergies and asthma: first, the importance of early-life environmental conditions in the development of allergic sensitization, and second, the role of allergic sensitization as a risk factor for asthma. Once asthma has developed, some patients clearly have episodes triggered by allergic exposure, while in other asthmatics allergy appears to be less important. Targeting allergic sensitization should therefore be a sensible tactic both for preventing the development of asthma and for managing some, but perhaps not all, patients with established asthma. Since current forms of allergen avoidance have not proved very successful in managing established asthma, there is considerable interest in using specific allergen immunotherapy to treat asthma. But a decision to use immunotherapy to treat asthma must take into account both the potential benefits and the known risks of treatment, and has to be made on a case by case basis.

A. The Importance of Allergy in Asthma

There is a strong familial component to asthma, eczema, and rhino-conjunctivitis, the so-called atopic cluster. While this argues for a genetic component to asthma, the rapid increase in the prevalence of asthma means that something in the environment must be responsible. The current consensus is that environmental factors act on genetically susceptible individuals, stimulating the production of specific IgE antibodies against otherwise harmless environmental antigens, such as pollen, house dust mite, and animal dander proteins. Not everyone who develops IgE antibodies will go on to experience clinical symptoms. Indeed, only half of the people with detectable levels of antibody against grass pollen will have any sort of hay fever. Nevertheless, the more IgE antibody someone has, the more likely they are to have associated clinical symptoms. Usually, there is a progression of allergic disease, sometimes termed the allergic march, in which children first suffer with atopic eczema, then they get allergic rhinitis, and afterwards they may progress to develop asthma. But this pattern is certainly not universal, and many children who develop asthma have not had significant eczema or rhinitis. Intriguingly, genetic analysis of asthma and eczema have implicated different chromosomal loci, suggesting that whether an atopic individual develops asthma may depend on the susceptibility of the target organ rather than simply be a consequence of allergic sensitization.

Following extensive research into risk factors for the development of asthma and atopy, it has now been established conclusively that allergic sensitization to common environmental allergens (house dust mites, cockroach, domestic animals, etc.) is a major risk factor for the development of childhood asthma (1–3). The tendency to produce IgE antibodies is regulated by T lymphocytes. Naïve B lymphocytes capable of recognizing allergenic proteins start life with a full complement of immunoglobulin heavy-chain genes. When they first encounter the antigenic determinant that they recognize, they differentiate into two cell types: antibody-producing cells that produce IgM antibodies and antigen-specific memory cells. Upon subsequent exposure, the memory cells are triggered to produce a secondary response that consists of higher affinity antibodies than the initial (primary) response. Depending on the context of this secondary stimulation, the memory cells switch over from producing IgM antibodies towards IgG, IgA, or IgE antibodies (4,5). In order to make an IgE response, T cells must recognize the antigen and interact with the B cell to provide "T-cell help," which comprises two signals: a direct contact with ligands on the memory B-cell surface and a signal delivered by soluble mediators (cytokines) (4). The contact signal for IgE switching is an interaction between

CD40 and its ligand, while the soluble signal is delivered by either IL-4 or IL-13 (5). This process is partly controlled by the context in which the allergenic antigen is encountered, and partly by genetic predisposition, with some individuals being more likely to develop allergic antibody responses than others, despite similar levels of allergen exposure (5,6). In individuals predisposed to making IgE responses, their T cells may be skewed towards production of the cytokines IL-4 and IL-5 (the so-called Th2 phenotype), which, respectively, facilitate memory B cells to switch over to make IgE (5) and promote eosinophilic inflammation (7). Th2-type cytokines have also been implicated directly in the pathogenesis of asthma: IL-4 activates vascular endothelial cells and stimulates mucus production, while IL-13 has multiple actions on epithelium, smooth muscle, and fibroblasts, which may alter airways structure and responsiveness (8,9). Thus, the association between Th2 cytokines and asthma is complex, and may not simply be attributable to the effect of IL-4 on IgE switching (10).

When sensitized individuals are exposed to relevant allergens they may develop clinical symptoms, including rhinitis and asthma. However, by no means all sensitized individuals will have clinical symptoms. Many population studies have shown that for every patient with allergic symptoms there is at least one individual who remains asymptomatic despite being sensitized (as judged by allergy skin tests). Moreover, the relationship between sensitization and symptoms is not simple. Data from Australia has shown a doubling in the proportion of patients reporting asthma and hay fever between 1971 and 1981, without any change in the proportion of patients with positive skin tests to grass pollen or house dust mite (11). The implication is that the likelihood of the sensitization being translated into symptoms has increased, although this increase could also reflect increased willingness to label symptoms as being due to asthma or hay fever.

Conversely, although patients with seasonal allergic rhinitis will almost always be sensitized to seasonal airborne allergens, up to half of adult patients with clinical asthma have no evidence of specific allergic sensitization. These observations call for some caution in postulating a link between allergic sensitization and disease: if patients can have asthma without any evidence of allergy, then presumably the mechanisms operating in these patients might also apply in some patients who happen to be sensitized. In other words, allergy is not necessarily responsible for asthma in all asthmatic patients who show skin-test sensitization.

In summary, the link between allergy and asthma is well established and the majority of patients with asthma have evidence of IgE-mediated hypersensitivity to airborne allergens (12). This is especially true of children with asthma, among whom over 85% will show positive skin tests to one or more airborne allergens (13). While IgE-mediated allergy is clearly an important risk factor for the development of asthma, it is less clear how important allergic triggers are in exacerbations of the disease or in the maintenance of ongoing asthma. In children, most exacerbations of asthma correspond with episodes of viral upper respiratory tract infection (14), while in adults about 50% of exacerbations are associated with rhinovirus infection (15). Anecdotally, exposure to cats or horses can trigger severe acute episodes of asthma, but the role of pollens in triggering acute episodes seems less certain. Asthma admissions to U.K. hospitals are actually lower during the grass pollen hay fever season than in the three months preceding or following the hay fever season (16), although epidemics of acute asthma associated with thunderstorms are probably triggered by inhalation of fragmented pollen grains (17).

Before embarking on allergen-specific therapies for asthma, we therefore need to be confident that allergy is important in the individual patient. We do not know for sure whether IgE-mediated allergy, viral infection, and occupational sensitization are alternative triggers for some final common pathway that presents clinically as asthma. We know that there are similar histological pictures in allergic, non-allergic, and occupational asthma (18–22), and also in children (23), suggesting that at least part of the inflammatory process in asthma is independent of allergy. Understanding these points will be critical in determining whether we should pursue better forms of immunotherapy for asthma, or look elsewhere for a solution.

B. Strategies for Allergen Avoidance

At face value, allergen avoidance should be an attractive strategy for managing asthma in patients for whom allergic triggers predominate. This approach is predicated on the relevance of particular allergens to the continuing symptoms of asthma, and requires that there should be a simple method to eliminate the relevant allergens or to reduce them to a level at which symptoms will improve. In other words, if there is a threshold level of allergen exposure that you need to get below to achieve benefit, this must be achievable by affordable and practical means. While it is true that extreme forms of avoidance have achieved significant clinical benefits (24), the approaches used in conventional clinical practice have led to only modest reductions in nonspecific bronchial responsiveness (25) and the overall degree of clinical improvement has been disappointing (26). In the context of occupational asthma, where complete allergen avoidance is definitely achievable, it is clear that some patients improve markedly on ceasing exposure, but others continue to have asthmatic symptoms for many years, even though they are no longer exposed to the allergen that induced their asthma (27). Factors that have been associated with the persistence of occupational asthma include the duration of exposure before developing symptoms, the duration of continuing exposure after the onset of asthma, and the persistence of airways eosinophilia (28). So, while it remains an article of faith that reducing allergen load will reduce the inflammatory process in allergic asthma, it is clear that other factors also contribute to the maintenance of established allergic inflammation and clinical symptoms of asthma.

II. Specific Allergen Immunotherapy for Asthma

Specific allergen immunotherapy (SIT) has been used for over a century to treat allergic disorders. Treatment regimes vary, but the general principle is to give a prolonged course of extracts of allergens that are thought to be relevant to the particular patient's illness. Allergen is usually given by subcutaneous injection, starting with a very low dose and escalating in a logarithmic sequence until the top dose is reached. At this stage, the interval between doses is extended, and maintenance therapy is given for about three years. A number of alternative routes have been tried, among which the sublingual route is the most popular.

There are two distinct ways in which SIT could be used to treat asthma. These are first to use SIT to prevent the development of asthma in patients who are sensitized to allergens but do not have asthma, and second to use SIT to treat established asthma.

III. SIT to Prevent Asthma

Specific immunotherapy may modify the natural history of asthma in children, who are known to be atopic but have not yet developed asthma. Studies from the 1960s and 1970s indicate that between 5% and 10% of atopic children and young adults with allergic rhinitis will develop asthma symptoms each year, although the epidemiological context is changing and these data will need updating (29). In children with allergic rhinitis and a limited range of sensitivities, SIT with house dust mite extract has been shown to reduce the probability of developing new sensitivities (i.e., new positive skin tests to allergens other than the one used for therapy) (30). An ongoing major multicenter study is assessing whether SIT is able to prevent allergic children aged 7 to 13 years from going on to develop asthma. After three years of therapy 28% fewer children had asthma symptoms compared to the control group, and this difference has been maintained up to five years, suggesting that SIT does indeed affect the clinical outcome of allergic sensitization (31). As the subjects in this study are followed up, we will eventually learn whether SIT prevents asthma completely, or just postpones its onset.

IV. SIT to Manage Established Asthma

Immunotherapy has been widely used to treat allergic asthma, but with the introduction of more effective inhaled therapies and increased concerns about the side effects of SIT, questions have been raised about the place of SIT in managing asthma.

The efficacy of SIT in adult asthma has been assessed in many trials over the last 50 years. Some of the earlier studies are difficult to interpret, because poor quality allergen extracts were used or the studies were poorly designed. A Cochrane review of allergen immunotherapy for asthma considered 75 trials published up to June 2001, including all available randomized, controlled trials that had used SIT to treat asthma and had reported at least one clinical outcome (32). These trials included nearly 3200 patients with asthma. Thirty-six of the trials were of SIT for house mite allergy, 20 for pollen allergy, 10 for animal dander allergy, two for mold allergy, one for latex allergy, and six for mixed allergens. Unfortunately, concealment of treatment allocation was judged adequate in only 15 of these 75 trials and there was significant heterogeneity in the number of comparisons. The review found a significant reduction in asthma symptoms and medication usage, as well as an improvement in bronchial hyper-reactivity following SIT. The review calculated that it was necessary to treat four patients to prevent one from having a deterioration in asthma symptoms and to treat five patients to prevent one from requiring increased antiasthma medication. Airways responses to inhaled allergen improved more than nonspecific bronchial reactivity and there was no change in formal measures of lung function. The meta-analysis concluded that SIT is effective in asthma, but should only be used in carefully selected patients (32).

Clinical trials have confirmed the efficacy of SIT in patients with grass pollen asthma, and in those with asthma caused by cat allergy (33). Greater benefits are observed for specific responses to allergen inhalation than for nonspecific airways reactivity. An important recent study of SIT for ragweed allergy found that patients who received active injections had an improvement in peak flow rates during the pollen season as well as reduced hay fever symptoms and reduced sensitivity to laboratory challenge with ragweed-pollen extracts (34). In addition, the active group required much less antiasthma medication. However, the parallel economic analysis indicated that the saving on costs of asthma drugs was less than the additional costs of giving SIT.

V. Comparison of SIT with Other Types of Treatment for Asthma

Most clinical trials of SIT for asthma have compared SIT either with historical controls or with a matched group treated with placebo. Very few studies have compared specific SIT with conventional management of asthma using allergen avoidance measures and conventional inhaled or oral drugs. A recent study of SIT in asthmatic children receiving conventional drug therapy found no additional benefit in patients whose drug therapy was already optimized (35). This study had significant design flaws and further work in this area is needed before one could draw any final conclusions about the pharmaco-economics of SIT. Such trials should also include analysis of cost-benefit and cost-effectiveness since purchasers of health care are increasingly demanding this evidence before agreeing to fund therapies or agree to changes in clinical practice.

Work from the 1950s and 1960s using mixed allergen extracts suggested that SIT may increase the rate of remission for children with asthma, and may also reduce the severity of symptoms in those who remain symptomatic (36). In contrast, a study that investigated withdrawal of therapy found rapid recurrence of asthma symptoms after stopping SIT, although there was more sustained relief for rhinitis symptoms (37).

VI. Risks of Allergen Immunotherapy in Asthma

The main issue that prevents the widespread adoption of SIT for asthma is the risk of serious adverse reactions. In the United Kingdom, between 1957 and 1986, 26 fatal reactions due to SIT were reported to the Committee on Safety of Medicines (38). In 17 of the fatal cases, the indication for SIT was documented, and 16 of these 17 patients were receiving SIT to treat their asthma. Similarly, in the American Academy of Allergy Asthma and Immunology confidential inquiry into SIT-associated deaths, asthma appeared to be the mode of death in virtually all the fatal cases (39). In those where asthma was not cited as a contributory factor, bronchospasm was a cardinal feature of the clinical course of the anaphylactic reactions that led to death. The incidence of systemic reactions in patients receiving SIT for asthma varies between series and has been reported to range from 5% to 35%. The central issue in using safety as an endpoint is to recognize that all treatments carry risks. Where differential risks exist between therapies, a more risky therapy can only be justified if that therapy offers substantial additional benefit over the safer therapy.

VII. Future Directions

There is definitely scope to improve conventional SIT. Possible approaches include using recombinant allergens, using modified allergens, or using new or better adjuvants. Recombinant technology might allow us to achieve better standardization of allergen vaccines, and could lead to tailoring of vaccines for individual patients. Work is needed to assess whether the non-allergen components of current allergen extracts offer any useful adjuvant effect for SIT. Most natural allergen extracts contain a variety of polysaccharide and lipid components that may act in the immune system, and it will be interesting to see whether recombinant vaccines will be as effective as natural extracts, or whether perhaps the extraneous elements in natural extracts contribute to the clinical efficacy of current extracts.

Recombinant molecular technology also makes it possible to develop novel forms of allergenic molecules that may have reduced allergenic activity, but retain the T-cell epitopes required for the beneficial effects of SIT (40,41). Other possible approaches include the use of aldehyde-inactivated allergoids or peptide vaccines to induce T-cell tolerance (42,43).

Linking immunostimulatory DNA sequences to allergenic proteins could also prove to be a useful option. If oligonucleotide sequences containing the motif CpG are coupled to allergenic proteins, this enhances their immunogenicity and leads to a Thl-type response against the allergen, while at the same time reducing the protein's allergenicity (44). Initial clinical trials have confirmed that the hybrid vaccine elicits a Thl-pattern response (45) and attenuates nasal inflammatory responses (46). Allergen-specific naked DNA sequences could also be used as vaccines. Although this technology is in its infancy, preliminary data suggests that administration of naked DNA encoding allergenic proteins leads to production of allergens within airways epithelial cells (47,48). As endogenous and exogenous allergens are handled differently, the endogenously produced allergens elicit a Thl-type response. If this process can be reproduced in allergic humans, it might prove effective in allergic disease, without carrying any significant risk of side effects. Initial animal studies support the concept (49) but need to be progressed into man before further conclusions can be drawn. Another area of interest is to use monoclonal antibodies directed against IgE in combination with SIT. Anti-IgE could reduce the risk of side effects, but might also redirect the injected allergenic material so that it is handled through different pathways. Since anti-IgE has beneficial effects in its own right on moderate to severe asthma (50,51), any trial of SIT and anti-IgE in asthma would need to be large and very carefully designed.

VIII. Conclusions

In summary, SIT has some efficacy in selected patients with asthma. Before using SIT to treat patients with established asthma, the physician needs to carefully consider whether the patient's symptoms are genuinely exacerbated and maintained by specific allergens. Allergic sensitization is clearly a risk factor for developing asthma, but finding skin-test evidence of allergic sensitization in an asthmatic does not guarantee that their asthma will be improved by SIT. A careful risk–benefit estimate is needed, based on an understanding of the likelihood of improvement, which in turn largely depends on the degree of allergic sensitization and the number of allergens to which the patient is sensitized. Broadly speaking, the larger the number of positive skin tests, the lower the probability that any individual allergen is critically responsible for the patient's asthma. Careful consideration is also needed to safety issues since the risks of SIT are clearly increased in patients with asthma. Current evidence suggests that conventional pharmacotherapy is the best option for patients with mild-allergic asthma, and yet these are the patients in whom one might have the greatest chance of influencing the natural history of the disease. There is an urgent need for proper comparative studies of best current SIT versus best current drug therapy, with robust endpoints including symptoms, objective measures of lung function, evaluation of cost, benefit ratios, safety, and quality of life. Further clinical trials are also indicated in mild to moderate childhood asthma and in patients with atopic rhinitis who have not yet developed asthma but are at high risk of progression to asthma.

Finally, advances in our understanding of the biology of allergy and asthma are leading to the development of novel forms of SIT, which may offer increased efficacy and reduced risks compared to conventional SIT.

References

1. Sporik R, Holgate ST, Platts-Mills TAE, Cogswell JJ. Exposure to house dust mite allergen (Derp1) and the development of asthma in childhood: a prospective study. N Engl J Med 1990; 323:502–507.
2. Platts-Mills TAE, Sporik RB, Chapman MD, Heymann PW. The role of indoor allergens in asthma. Allergy 1995; 50(S22):5–12.
3. Wahn U, Lau S, Bergmann R, Kulig M, Forster J, Bergmann K, Bauer CP, Guggenmoos-Holzmann I. Indoor allergen exposure is a risk factor for sensitization during the first three years of life. J Allergy Clin Immunol 1997; 99:763–769.
4. Li Z, Woo CJ, Iglesias-Ussel MD, Ronai D, Scharff MD. The generation of antibody diversity through somatic hypermutation and class switch recombination. Genes Dev 2004; 18:1–11.
5. Hajoui O, Janani R, Tulic M, Joubert P, Ronis T, Hamid Q, Zheng H, Mazer BD. Synthesis of IL-13 by human B lymphocytes: regulation and role in IgE production. J Allergy Clin Immunol 2004; 114:657–663.
6. Illi S, von Mutius E, Lau S, Nickel R, Niggemann B, Sommerfeld C, Wahn U. The pattern of atopic sensitization is associated with the development of asthma in childhood. J Allergy Clin Immunol 2001; 108:709–714.
7. Gleich GJ, Adolphson CR, Leiferman KM. The biology of the eosinophilic leukocyte. Annu Rev Immunol 1993; 44:85–101.
8. Zhu Z, Homer RJ, Wang Z, Chen Q, Geba GP, Wang J, Zhang Y, Elias JA. Pulmonary expression of IL-13 causes inflammation, mucus hypersecretion, subepithelial fibrosis, physiolgic abnormalities and eotaxin production. J Clin Invest 1999; 103:779–788.
9. Laporte JC, Moore PE, Baraldo S, Jouvin MH, Church TL, Schwartzman IN, Panettieri RA Jr, Kinet JP, Shore SA. Direct effects of IL-13 on signalling pathways for physiological responses in cultured human airway smooth muscle cells. Am J Respir Crit Care Med 2001; 164:141–148.

10. Corrigan CJ. Elevated IL-4 secretion by T-lymphocytes: a feature of atopy or asthma? Clin Exp Allergy 1995; 25:485–487.

11. Peat JK, Haby M, Spijker J, Berry G, Woolcock AJ. Prevalence of asthma in adults in Busselton, Western Australia. Br Med J 1992; 305:1326–1329.

12. Burrows B, Martinez FD, Halonen M, Barbee RA, Cline MG. Association of asthma with serum IgE levels and skin test reactivity to allergens. N Engl J Med 1989; 320:271–277.

13. Martinez FD, Wright AL, Taussig LM, Holberg CJ, Halonen M, Morgan WJ. Asthma and wheezing during the first 6 years of life. N Engl J Med 1995; 332:133–138.

14. Johnston SL, Pattemore PK, Sanderson G, Smith S, Lampe F, Josephs L, Symington P, O'Toole S, Myint SH, Tyrrell DAJ, et al. Community study of the role of virus infections in exacerbations of asthma in school children in the community. Br Med J 1995; 310:1225–1229.

15. Corne JM, Marshall C, Smith S, Schreiber J, Sanderson G, Holgate ST, Johnston SL. Frequency, severity, and duration of rhinovirus infections in asthmatic and non-asthmatic individuals: a longitudinal cohort study. Lancet 2002; 359:831–834.

16. Adams RJ, Smith BJ, Ruffin RE. Factors associated with hospital admissions and repeat emergency department visits for adults with asthma. Thorax 2000; 55:566–573.

17. Davidson AC, Emberlin J, Cook AD, Venables KM. A major outbreak of asthma associated with a thunderstorm. Br Med J 1996; 312:601–604.

18. Bentley AM, Menz G, Storz C, Robinson DS, Bradley B, Jeffery PK, Durham SR, Kay AB. Identification of T lymphocytes, macrophages and activated eosinophils in the bronchial mucosa in intrinsic asthma. Relationship to symptoms and bronchial responsiveness. Am Rev Respir Dis 1992; 146:500–506.

19. Walker C, Bode E, Boer L, Hansel TT, Blaser K, Virchow JC. Allergic and nonallergic asthmatics have distinct patterns of T-cell activation and cytokine production in peripheral blood and bronchoalveolar lavage. Am Rev Respir Dis 1992; 146:109–115.

20. Humbert M, Grant JA, Taborda-Barata L, Durham SR, Pfister R, Menz G, Barkans J, Ying S, Kay AB. High affinity IgE receptor-bearing cells in bronchial biopsies from atopic and nonatopic asthma. Am J Respir Crit Care Med 1996; 153:1931–1937.

21. Bentley AM, Maestrelli P, Fabbri LM, Menz G, Storz C, Bradley B, Jeffery PK, Durham SR, Kay AB. Activated T lymphocytes and eosinophils in the bronchial mucosa in isocyanate-induced asthma. J Allergy Clin Immunol 1992; 89:821–829.

22. Frew AJ, Chan H, Lam S, Chan-Yeung M. Bronchial inflammation in occupational asthma due to western red cedar. Am J Respir Crit Care Med 1995; 151:340–344.

23. Stevenson EC, Turner G, Heaney LG, Schock BC, Taylor R, Gallagher T, Ennis M, Shields MD. Bronchoalveolar lavage findings suggest two different forms of childhood asthma. Clin Exp Allergy 1997; 27:1027–1035.

24. Platts-Mills TAE, Tovey ER, Mitchell EB, Moszoro H, Nock P, Wilkins SR. Reduction of bronchial hyperreactivity during prolonged allergen avoidance. Lancet 1982; 2:675–678.

25. Ehnert B, Lau-Schadendorf S, Weber A, Buettner P, Schou C, Wahn U. Reducing domestic exposure to dust mite allergen reduces bronchial hyperreactivity in sensitive children with asthma. J Allergy Clin Immunol 1992; 90:135–138.
26. Woodcock A, Forster L, Matthews E, Martin J, Letley L, Vickers M, Britton J, Strachan D, Howarth P, Altmann D, et al. Control of exposure to mite allergen and allergen-impermeable bed covers for adults with asthma. N Engl J Med 2003; 349:225–236.
27. Chan-Yeung M, Lam S, Koener S. Clinical features and natural history of occupational asthma due to western red cedar (thuja plicata). Am J Med 1982; 72:411–415.
28. Frew AJ. What can we learn about asthma from studying occupational asthma? Ann Allergy Asthma Immunol 2003; 90(Suppl):7–10.
29. Horak F. Manifestation of allergic rhinitis in latent sensitized patients. A prospective study. Arch. Otorhinolaryngol 1985; 242:242–249.
30. Des Roches A, Paradis L, Menardo JL, Bouges S, Daures JP, Bousquet J. Immunotherapy with a standardized Dermatophagoides pteronyssinus extract. VI. Specific immunotherapy prevents the onset of new sensitizations in children. J Allergy Clin Immunol 1997; 99:450–453.
31. Moller C, Dreborg S, Ferdousi HA, Halken S, Host A, Jacobsen L, Koivikko A, Koller DY, Niggemann B, Norberg LA, Wahn U, et al. Pollen immunotherapy reduces the development of asthma in children with seasonal rhinoconjunctivitis (the PAT-study). J Allergy Clin Immunol 2002; 109:251–256.
32. Abramson MJ, Puy RM, Weiner JM. Allergen immunotherapy for asthma (Cochrane Review). In: The Cochrane Library, Issue 2. Chichester, UK: Wiley, 2004.
33. Lilja G, Sundin B, Graff-Lonnevig V, Hedlin G, Heilborn H, Norrlind K, Pegelow KO, Lowenstein H. Immunotherapy with partially purified and standardized animal dander extracts. IV. Effects of 2 years of treatment. J Allergy Clin Immunol 1989; 83:37–44.
34. Creticos PS, Reed CE, Norman PS, Khoury J, Adkinson NF, Buncher CR, Busse WW, Bush RK, Gadde J, Li JT, et al. Ragweed immunotherapy in adult asthma. N Engl J Med 1996; 334:501–506.
35. Adkinson NF, Eggleston PA, Eney D, Goldstein EO, Schuberth KC, Bacon JR, Hamilton RG, Weiss ME, Arshad H, Meinert CL, et al. A controlled trial of immunotherapy for asthma in allergic children. N Engl J Med 1997; 336: 324–331.
36. Johnstone DE, Dutton A. The value of hyposensitization therapy for bronchial asthma in children. A 14 year study. Pediatrics 1968; 42:793–802.
37. Shaikh WA. Immunotherapy vs inhaled budesonide in bronchial asthma: an open parallel comparative trial. Clin Exp Allergy 1997; 27:1279–1284.
38. Committee on the Safety of Medicines. CSM update: immunotherapy. Br Med J 1986; 293:948.
39. Stewart GE, Lockey RF. Systemic reactions from allergen immunotherapy. J Allergy Clin Immunol 1992; 90:567–578.
40. Vrtala S, Hirtenlehner K, Susani M, Akdis M, Kussebi F, Akdis CA, Blaser K, Hufnagl P, Binder BR, Politou A, et al. Genetic engineering of a hypoallergenic trimer of the major birch pollen allergen Betv 1. FASEB J 2001; 15:2045–2047.

41. Vrtala S, Akdis CA, Budak F, Akdis M, Blaser K, Kraft D, Valenta R. T-cell epitope-containing hypoallergenic recombinant fragments of the major birch pollen allergen, Bet v 1, induce blocking antibodies. J Immunol 2000; 165: 6653–6659.

42. Klimek L, Dormann D, Jarman ER, Cromwell O, Riechelmann H, Reske-Kunz AB. Short-term preseasonal birch pollen allergoid immunotherapy influences symptoms, specific nasal provocation and cytokine levels in nasal secretions, but not peripheral T-cell responses in patients with allergic rhinitis. Clin Exp Allergy 1999; 29:1326–1335.

43. Fasler S, Aversa G, de Vries JE, Yssel H. Antagonistic peptides specifically inhibit proliferation, cytokine production, CD40L expression and help for IgE synthesis by Der pl-specific human T-cell clones. J Allergy Clin Immunol 1998; 101:521–530.

44. Tighe H, Takabayashi K, Schwartz D, van Nest G, Tuck S, Eiden JJ, Kagey-Sobotka A, Creticos PS, Lichtenstein LM, Spiegelberg HL, et al. Conjugation of immunostimulatory DNA to the short ragweed allergen Amb al enhances its immunogenicity and reduces its allergenicity. J Allergy Clin Immunol 2000; 106:124–134.

45. Creticos PS, Eiden JJ, Broide D, Balcer-Whaley SL, Schroeder JT, Khattignavong A, Li H, Norman PP, Hamilton RG. Immunotherapy with immunostimulatory oligonucleotides linked to purified ragweed Amb a 1 allergen: effects on antibody production, nasal allergen provocation and ragweed seasonal rhinitis. J Allergy Clin Immunol 2002; 109:743–744.

46. Tulic MK, Fiset PO, Christodoulopoulos P, Vaillancourt P, Desrosiers M, Lavigne F, Eiden J, Hamid Q. Amb al-immunostimulatory oligodeoxynucleotide conjugate immunotherapy decreases the nasal inflammatory response. JACI 2004; 113:235–241.

47. Hsu CH, Chua KY, Tao MH, Lai YL, Wu HD, Huang SK, et al. Immunoprophylaxis of allergen-induced IgE synthesis and airway hyperresponsiveness in vivo by genetic immunisation. Nature Med 1996; 2:540–544.

48. Hartl A, Kiesslich J, Weiss R, Bernhaupt A, Mostbock S, Scheiblhofer S, Ebner C, Ferreira F, Thalhamer J. Immune responses after immunisation with plasmid DNA encoding Bet v 1, the major allergen of birch pollen. J Allergy Clin Immunol 1999; 103:107–113.

49. Hartl A, Hochreiter R, Stepanoska T, Ferreira F, Thalhamer J. Characterisation of the protective and therapeutic efficiency of a DNA vaccine encoding the major birch pollen allergen Bet vla. Allergy 2004; 590:65–73.

50. Buhl R, Hanf G, Soler M, Bensch G, Wolfe J, Everhard F, Champain K, Fox H, Thirlwell J. Omalizumab provides long-term control in patients with moderate to severe asthma. Eur Respir J 2002; 20:73–78.

51. Finn A, Gross G, van Bavel J, Lee T, Windom H, Everhard F, Fowler-Taylor A, Liu J, Gupta N. Omalizumab improves asthma-related quality of life in patients with severe allergic asthma. J Allergy Clin Immunol 2003; 111:278–284.

12

Outpatient Pharmacotherapy

GUY G. BRUSSELLE and ROMAIN A. PAUWELS

Department of Respiratory Diseases, Ghent University Hospital
Ghent, Belgium

I. Introduction

Asthma is defined by the Global Initiative for Asthma (GINA) as a chronic inflammatory disorder of the airways, causing an increase in airway hyper-responsiveness that leads to recurrent episodes of wheezing, breathlessness, chest tightness, and coughing. These episodes are usually associated with widespread but variable airflow obstruction that is often reversible (1,2). This revised definition emphasizes two crucial characteristics of asthma: first, the central role of chronic airway inflammation in the pathophysiology of asthma, and second, the variable nature of the disease. Appreciation of the key role of the underlying inflammation in asthma implies that anti-inflammatory agents are the cornerstone of asthma therapy. Recognition of the variable nature of asthma implies that a flexible approach is needed in the management of this disease.

The goals of successful asthma management include achieving and maintaining asthma control. A patient's asthma is under control if the patient has minimal (ideally no) chronic symptoms, has no limitations on activities, experiences neither exacerbations nor emergency visits, and attains and maintains lung function close to normal, while avoiding adverse events from asthma medications. Good control of asthma can be achieved in a majority of patients if exposure to risk factors (e.g., smoking) is avoided and if the currently available antiasthma drugs are used properly. However, the Asthma Insights and Reality surveys demonstrated that a significant proportion of patients worldwide continue to have symptoms and lifestyle restrictions and to require emergency care (3–6). Moreover, the use of anti-inflammatory preventative medication was low, even in patients with severe persistent asthma. These surveys thus point out that in many patients worldwide, asthma control is still suboptimal, despite the availability of effective therapies.

In this chapter we still divide the pharmacotherapy of asthma in reliever therapy using rescue medications on the one hand, and maintenance therapy using controller medications on the other hand. As will be discussed later, the use of the rapid- and long-acting inhaled β_2-agonist formoterol as both a reliever and controller medication already underlined that this distinction has become rather artificial. The advent of the combination formoterol/budesonide in a single inhaler further closes the gap between reliever and controller therapy, since this combination is currently under investigation as single-inhaler therapy in patients with persistent asthma of different levels of severity. However, for reasons of clarity, we still find it useful to discuss the pharmacotherapy of reliever and controller medications separately. It is also imperative to educate the asthmatic patient about the different treatments as part of an asthma (self-) management plan, and the words "reliever" and "controller" remain useful in educational terms.

II. Reliever Therapy

Reliever medications are medications that act quickly to relieve bronchoconstriction and the accompanying acute symptoms such as shortness of breath, chest tightness, wheezing, and cough. These quick-relief or rescue medicines include rapid-acting inhaled β_2-agonists, inhaled anticholinergics, systemic glucocorticosteroids, short-acting theophylline, and short-acting oral β_2-agonists (Table 1).

Rapid-acting inhaled β_2-agonists are the cornerstone for treatment of episodic bronchoconstriction and acute exacerbations of asthma, and should be available to every asthmatic patient suffering from mild to severe persistent asthma to provide rapid relief of symptoms. These rapid-acting inhaled β_2-agonists, such as albuterol (salbutamol) and terbutaline, should be used as required for symptom control ("as needed") instead of as regularly scheduled therapy four times daily (7). They are also indicated for the pretreatment of exercise-induced asthma (8). It is important to keep in mind, both for asthmatic patients and their treating physicians, that the

Table 1 Reliever Medications

Rapid-acting inhaled β_2-agonists
   Short-acting: salbutamol (albuterol), fenoterol, pirbuterol, and terbutaline
   Long-acting: formoterol
Combination formoterol/budesonide in a single inhaler
Inhaled anticholinergics: ipratropium bromide, and oxitropium bromide
Systemic glucocorticosteroids: predniso(lo)ne and methylprednisolone
Short-acting theophylline
Short-acting oral β_2-agonists

---

increased use of rapid-acting inhaled β_2-agonists, especially during the night, is a warning of worsening of asthma, indicating the need to start or to augment a maintenance anti-inflammatory therapy.

Since formoterol has both a rapid onset and a long duration of action, this inhaled β_2-agonist can also be used "as needed" (9). In patients with moderate persistent asthma who are taking regular inhaled corticosteroids (ICS), the use of formoterol as rescue medication improved asthma control compared to as-needed use of terbutaline (10). In a large international real-life asthma study (the RELIEF study), use of formoterol as needed had a similar safety profile to salbutamol, and its use as a reliever therapy was associated with fewer asthma symptoms and exacerbations (11). Interestingly, reductions of exacerbations with as-needed formoterol versus salbutamol increased with increasing age and asthma severity. However, the open label design of the study might introduce a significant potential for bias (12), implying that further studies are needed to identify the role of formoterol as a reliever therapy.

The combination of formoterol and the inhaled corticosteroid budesonide has been made available as a convenient fixed combination of these agents, marketed under the product name Symbicort®. Although this formoterol/budesonide combination in a single inhaler was first launched for the maintenance treatment of moderate and severe persistent asthma, the rapid action of both compounds also offers the opportunity to use Symbicort as a rescue therapy. Indeed, budesonide is an ICS with significant acute effects in improving lung function (13,14). As stated above, the long-acting β_2-agonist formoterol has also a fast onset of action, comparable to the short-acting salbutamol. Consequently, the combination of formoterol/budesonide has a faster onset of action than salmeterol/fluticasone, improving shortness of breath and lung function already three minutes after administration (15).

Triggers are factors that cause asthma symptoms by provoking acute bronchoconstriction or precipitate asthma exacerbations by inducing airway inflammation. Interestingly, most triggers, including allergens, respiratory infections (e.g., rhinovirus), air pollutants (e.g., passive smoking), and weather changes, can provoke both acute symptoms due to bronchoconstriction and acute exacerbations of asthma due to enhanced inflammation of the airways (16,17). From a pathophysiological point of view, it is thus logical to use both the rapid-acting inhaled β_2-agonist formoterol and the ICS budesonide in case of asthma symptoms triggered by one of these risk factors. Indeed by using the formoterol/budesonide combination as rescue therapy it is expected that not only the acute symptoms due to the bronchoconstriction will be rapidly relieved (by the formoterol component), but that also the possibly ensuing exacerbation will be prevented (by the budesonide component, preventing an escalation of the inflammatory changes in the airways). Thus, by promptly increasing the number of inhalations of the combination formoterol/budesonide when experiencing an onset of worsening symptoms, asthmatic patients could prevent the development of an exacerbation. It is, however, not known if increasing the number of inhalations of the combination formoterol/budesonide from a single inhaler is more efficacious than increasing both drugs separately in the treatment of an acute exacerbation. Convenience comes at a price, but higher efficacy of the single-inhaler therapy in this clinical situation needs further documentation.

Short-acting theophylline may be considered for relief of symptoms, but as a bronchodilator theophylline is less effective than an inhaled β_2-agonist, and its onset of action is significantly slower than that of a rapid-acting β_2-agonist (18). Moreover, since theophylline has the potential for severe adverse effects, short-acting theophylline should not be administered to patients who are already on long-term treatment with slow-release theophylline, unless the serum concentration of theophylline is known.

Short-acting oral β_2-agonists could be used as rescue therapy in the few patients who are unable to use aerosolized medications appropriately. However, adverse side effects such as cardiac arrhythmia, tachycardia, tremor, and hypokalemia occur more frequently with this oral therapy compared to treatment with inhaled rapid-acting β_2-agonists. Administering the rapid-acting β_2-agonists by inhalation is thus preferred, since this route of administration has the advantage of delivering effectively high concentrations of medications directly to the airways, while the systemic side effects are minimized.

Last, systemic glucocorticosteroids are the "final" rescue therapy, since they are crucial in the treatment of severe acute exacerbations (19,20). Systemic corticosteroids such as prednisolone or methylprednisolone prevent the progression of an asthma exacerbation, decreasing the need for hospitalization or emergency department visit. Even after emergency treatment of an acute asthma attack, systemic corticosteroids prevent early relapse. The pharmacotherapy of asthma attacks, including the use of systemic glucocorticosteroids, is discussed in greater detail in chapter 8.

III. Maintenance Pharmacotherapy

The choice of therapy depends upon the severity of a patient's asthma, but is also influenced by the availability and cost of antiasthma medications, and by the characteristics of the individual patient.

A. Intermittent Asthma

If over a period of at least three months a patient experiences less than once a week symptoms of cough, dyspnea, or wheezing, the patient has intermittent asthma. Nocturnal asthma symptoms are rare and occur less than twice a month. The patient is asymptomatic in between exacerbations and has a normal lung function (peakflow as well as FEV_1). No maintenance treatment with a controller medication is recommended for intermittent asthma. Patients with intermittent asthma who experience rare but severe exacerbations, however, should be treated as having moderate persistent asthma (see section Combination Therapy as Maintenance Treatment of Moderate to Severe Persistent Asthma).

B. Persistent Asthma

If a patient experiences symptoms more than once a week over a three-month period, or has nocturnal asthma symptoms more than twice a month, the patient has persistent asthma. Patients with persistent asthma require controller medication every day (Table 2).

Monotherapy as Maintenance Treatment of Mild Persistent Asthma

Inhaled Corticosteroids

ICS are the cornerstone therapy for patients with persistent asthma at all levels of severity, and are considered the most effective anti-inflammatory therapy. Numerous studies have demonstrated that treatment with ICS decreases the pathological signs of airway inflammation in asthmatics (21–23), reduces the airway hyper-responsiveness (24), and improves lung function. More importantly, both symptoms and the frequency and severity of exacerbations are reduced in patients with persistent asthma treated with ICS (25,26). Even in patients with mild persistent asthma of recent onset, once-daily treatment with low-dose budesonide significantly decreased the risk of severe exacerbations and improved asthma control (27). In this inhaled steroid treatment as regular therapy in early asthma (START) study, ICS treatment also resulted in more symptom-free days and better lung function measurements compared to placebo (27).

The ideal inhaled glucocorticoid should display maximal antiasthmatic effects, without systemic bioactivity. The main determinants of

Table 2 Controller Medications

Inhaled glucocorticosteroids (ICS)
  Beclomethasone dipropionate
  Budesonide
  Ciclesonide
  Flunisolide
  Fluticasone propionate
  Mometasone furoate
  Triamcinolone acetonide
Systemic glucocorticosteroids
Cromones: sodium cromoglycate and nedocromil sodium
Theophylline (sustained-release)
Long-acting inhaled β_2-agonists: formoterol and salmeterol
Combination formoterol/budesonide or salmeterol/fluticasone in a single inhaler
Long-acting oral β_2-agonists
Leukotriene modifiers
  5-lipoxygenase inhibitors: zileuton
  cysteinyl leukotriene receptor antagonists: montelukast, pranlukast, and
  zafirlukast

efficacy are dose and potency of the compound, and the percentage of lung deposition from the delivery device. Both the receptor affinity and intrinsic activity determine the potency of a glucocorticoid (28). On the other hand, adverse effects of ICS result from systemic exposure, implicating that the main determinants of safety are the oral and pulmonary bioavailability of the drug (29). The therapeutic ratio is the ratio of safety (risk) to efficacy (benefit), and is shifted into the favorable range if the receptor affinity and lung tissue affinity of an ICS are high and the oral bioavailability— due to a rapid metabolic inactivation—is low. The glucocorticoids flunisolide and triamcinolone have a less favorable therapeutic ratio, since both ICS have a low receptor and lung tissue affinity and a high oral bioavailability ($\pm 20\%$) (30). The newer ICS fluticasone propionate, mometasone furoate, and ciclesonide have a high receptor and lung tissue affinity and a very low oral bioavailability (less than 1%), so that a favorable therapeutic ratio can be expected (31–33). Moreover, the systemic availability of fluticasone propionate is substantially less in patients with moderate to severe asthma than in healthy controls, indicating that ICS with minimum oral bioavailability that are absorbed through the lungs need to be assessed in patients who are receiving doses appropriate for disease severity, and not (only) in normal volunteers (34,35). On the other hand, in mild or moderate asthma, maximal clinical benefit is already attained with lower doses of highly potent corticosteroids. Further increase of dose does not add to efficacy, but compromises safety in the milder spectrum of the disease (36).

Alternative Maintenance Treatments of Mild Persistent Asthma

Several other medications, including theophylline, leukotriene modifiers, and cromones, can be used instead of ICS in the treatment of patients with mild asthma (Table 3). Sustained-release theophylline can be used as a second-line controller medication in asthma. In patients with mild persistent asthma, monotherapy with sustained-release theophylline is effective in controlling asthma symptoms and improving lung function. Although theophylline is usually less effective than low doses of ICS (37,38), it is less expensive. While dose–response studies showed an increasing bronchodilator response of theophylline above plasma concentrations of 10 mg/L, the anti-inflammatory effects of theophylline are seen at concentrations that are usually less than 10 mg/L (39). At these low doses (plasma concentration 5–10 mg/L) theophylline is easier to use, side effects are uncommon, and the problems of drug interaction are less of an issue. Moreover, the side effects of theophylline may be reduced by gradually increasing the dose until therapeutic—anti-inflammatory—concentrations are achieved.

Leukotriene modifiers, including the 5-lipoxygenase inhibitor zileuton and the cysteinyl leukotriene receptor antagonists (montelukast, pranlukast, and zafirlukast), could serve as an alternative to ICS in patients with mild chronic asthma. Leukotriene modifiers have, indeed, a small and variable bronchodilator effect, improving lung function and reducing asthma symptoms (40,41). However, the effect of leukotriene modifiers as monotherapy in mild persistent asthma is less than that of low doses of ICS (42). Moreover, the effect of leukotriene receptor antagonists as single-agent asthma treatment on asthma exacerbations is small (43), and less than that obtained by ICS at doses equivalent to 400 µg/day beclomethasone (44). Since leukotriene modifiers are administered as a tablet, this route of administration is an advantage in asthma patients who are unable to use aerosolized medications (metered-dose inhalers, dry powder inhalers, and nebulized aerosols) correctly. A second indication for leukotriene modifiers are patients with aspirin-sensitive asthma who may respond well to this new class of antiasthma drugs, but these patients often have more

Table 3 Maintenance Treatment for Mild Persistent Asthma

Daily controller medication: inhaled corticosteroid
 ≤ 500 µg beclomethasone dipropionate or equivalent
Alternative treatment regimens
 Theophylline (sustained-release), or
 Cromone, or
 Leukotriene modifier

---

severe persistent asthma, needing a combination of several drug classes to control their asthma (45).

The cromones sodium cromoglycate or nedocromil may be used as controller therapy in mild persistent asthma. Since cromones produce only minimal side effects and do not influence growth velocity, they are of special interest in children with mild allergic asthma. However, both nedocromil and sodium cromoglycate are less effective than ICS (46). Since cromones prevent the acute airflow limitation induced by exercise, they can be administered prophylactically before sporting. A major drawback to using cromones as a maintenance treatment, however, is the fact that they need to be administered three to four times a day, which is inconvenient for both asthmatic children and their parents, thereby decreasing therapy compliance and thus endangering clinical effectiveness.

Several patient groups, including children, pregnant women, and the older adult asthmatics, need special consideration when the management of asthma is discussed. We will focus here on the management of asthma in pregnant women and in women who want to become pregnant. The greatest risk to pregnant patients with asthma and to their babies is poorly controlled asthma, since this can result in low birth weight, increased prematurity, and increased perinatal mortality (47,48). The inhaled corticosteroids beclomethasone dipropionate and budesonide, inhaled short-acting β_2 agonists, theophylline (at therapeutic levels), and sodium cromoglycate are not associated with an increased incidence of fetal abnormalities (49–51). It is important to reassure pregnant patients with asthma that these treatments are both safe and necessary (52). ICS remain the cornerstone of pharmacotherapy of persistent asthma in pregnant women, and have been demonstrated to prevent exacerbations of asthma specifically in pregnancy. Since the majority of the safety data and experience concerns beclomethasone dipropionate and budesonide, we recommend to use these ICS in pregnant women with chronic persistent asthma.

Combination Therapy as Maintenance Treatment of Moderate to Severe Persistent Asthma

Combination of an ICS and a Long-Acting β_2-Agonist

When low to medium doses of ICS fail to achieve control of asthma, long-acting inhaled β_2-agonists (formoterol or salmeterol) should be added before increasing the dose of ICS (Table 4). Numerous clinical studies have demonstrated that—in patients with moderate to severe asthma—the addition of long-acting inhaled β_2-agonists to a daily therapy with ICS improves symptoms, increases lung function, decreases the rate of asthma exacerbations, and is more effective than increasing the dose of ICS twofold or more (53–57). Indeed, most of the therapeutic benefit of ICS is achieved with a total daily dose of $\leq$500 μg/day beclomethasone dipropionate ($\leq$400 μg/

Table 4 Maintenance Treatment for Moderate to Severe Persistent Asthma

Daily controller medication: combination of a long-acting inhaled β_2-agonist and an inhaled corticosteroid (200–1.000 µg BDP or equivalent in moderate asthma; > 1.000 µg BDP or equivalent in severe asthma)

Alternative treatment regimens for *moderate asthma*:

*Combination of inhaled corticosteroid (500–1000 µg BDP or equivalent) and sustained-release theophylline, *or*

long-acting oral β_2-agonist, *or*

leukotriene modifier

*Monotherapy with inhaled corticosteroid at higher doses (>1.000 µg BDP or equivalent)

In *severe asthma* one or more of the following medications can be added to the combination of a long-acting inhaled β_2-agonist and high dose inhaled corticosteroid, if needed:

    sustained-release theophylline, *and/or*

    long-acting oral β_2-agonist, *and/or*

    leukotriene modifier, *and/or*

    oral glucocorticosteroid, *and/or*

    omalizumab (anti-IgE monoclonal antibody)

Abbreviation: BDP, beclomethasone dipropionate.

day budesonide or ≤ 250 µg/day fluticasone propionate), indicating a relatively flat dose–response curve of ICS in adults with asthma (58). However, since there is considerable individual variability in the response to ICS in asthma, some patients—especially the more severe asthmatics with frequent exacerbations—may obtain a greater benefit at higher doses. The greater efficacy of adding a long-acting inhaled β_2-agonist to an ICS than increasing the dose of ICS has led to the development of fixed combination inhalers (formoterol plus budesonide; salmeterol plus fluticasone).

Recently, the Gaining Optimal Asthma Control (GOAL) study demonstrated that in patients whose asthma is not controlled as defined by GINA/ NIH guidelines, asthma control was achieved more rapidly and in more patients with salmeterol/fluticasone combination therapy than with fluticasone monotherapy (59). In this one-year, randomized, double-blind, parallel-group study of more than 3400 patients with uncontrolled asthma, treatment with either fluticasone or salmeterol/fluticasone combination was stepped up until total control was achieved. Importantly, asthma control was achieved at a lower corticosteroid dose with salmeterol/fluticasone combination versus fluticasone, and patients that achieved control recorded very low rates of exacerbations (0.07–0.27/patient/yr) and near-maximal health status scores (as assessed by the Asthma Quality of Life Questionnaire) (59). Even in patients entering the GOAL study as corticosteroid-naïve, combination therapy showed greater efficacy than fluticasone monotherapy. This contrasts with the OPTIMA-A trial, in which little additional benefit was obtained with the addition of formoterol to the ICS budesonide in corticosteroid-naïve patients with mild asthma (60). However, this difference may be explained by differences in patient selection (patients with very mild asthma) in the OPTIMA-A trial versus uncontrolled moderate to severe asthmatics in the GOAL study and in primary outcome selection (single endpoint of time to first severe asthma exacerbation in the OPTIMA-A trial versus composite measure of total control in the GOAL study).

Since both short-term and long-term treatment with long-acting inhaled β_2-agonists do not influence the chronic airway inflammation in patients with asthma (61,62), it is imperative that this therapy should always be combined with ICS. Indeed, two clinical trials performed by the National Heart, Lung, and Blood Institute's Asthma Clinical Research Network clearly demonstrated the risks of monotherapy with the long-acting inhaled β_2-agonist salmeterol in adult patients with persistent asthma (63,64). In the SOCS (Salmeterol or Corticosteroids) trial, patients with moderate asthma who were treated with salmeterol alone experienced more asthma exacerbations and more treatment failures than patients treated with the ICS triamcinolone in monotherapy (63). Moreover, a similar worsening of asthma control, including an increase in asthma exacerbations and a decrease in pulmonary function, was observed in the SLIC (Salmeterol $\pm$ Corticosteroids) trial. This study examined if the addition of salmeterol on a scheduled basis in patients with moderate asthma permitted a reduction in dose (or even elimination) of ICS over time (64). Discontinuation of ICS in this SLIC trial was clearly not safe, indicating that long-acting inhaled β_2-agonists cannot be used as monotherapy in patients with persistent asthma. To ensure that the long-acting inhaled β_2-agonist is always accompanied by an ICS, the use of fixed combination inhalers, delivering corticosteroids and long-acting β_2-agonist together, is strongly recommended. Moreover, these fixed combination inhalers appear at least as effective as giving each drug separately (65–69), and are more convenient for patients, thereby increasing compliance (70).

Other Medications as Add-On Therapy to ICS in Patients with Moderate to Severe Asthma

In patients with moderate to severe asthma theophylline may be used as an add-on therapy to low or high doses of ICS when further asthma control is needed (Table 4) (71–73). Compared to long-acting inhaled β_2-agonists however, theophylline is less effective as add-on therapy and is associated with more frequent adverse effects, but it is less expensive (74–76).

Leukotriene modifiers (cysteinyl leukotriene receptor antagonists and the 5-lipoxygenase inhibitor zileuton) can be used as add-on therapy to ICS in patients whose asthma is not controlled with low or even high doses of

ICS (45,77). In these patients with moderate (to severe) asthma, adding the leukotriene receptor antagonist montelukast to the ICS budesonide was superior to adding placebo (78) and appeared as effective as doubling the dose of inhaled budesonide (79). When studying the effects of the leukotriene receptor antagonist zafirlukast on the rate of asthma exacerbations, it is important to consider the dose of zafirlukast used in the clinical studies. At the licensed dose (20 mg twice per day) adding zafirlukast to ICS was inferior to doubling the dose of ICS, whereas at higher than licensed doses (80 mg twice per day) zafirlukast as add-on therapy to ICS appeared as effective as doubling the dose of ICS (80,81). Leukotriene modifiers are less effective than long-acting inhaled β_2-agonists as add-on therapy (82), although one study suggests a similar preventative effect on asthma exacerbations when montelukast was added to low-dose fluticasone, compared to add-on therapy with salmeterol (83).

Some patients with severe persistent asthma remain inadequately controlled despite combined available therapy. These patients represent a significant unmet medical need, since they are at high risk of serious exacerbations and asthma-related mortality. Omalizumab is an anti-IgE humanized recombinant monoclonal antibody, which suppresses IgE-mediated allergic reactions by binding to free IgE (84). Results from several clinical trials have shown that omalizumab decreases the number of exacerbations and the need for emergency medical interventions in patients with severe allergic asthma on high-dose ICS or on ICS/long-acting β_2-agonist combination therapy (85–90). Moreover, significantly greater improvements were achieved with omalizumab compared with placebo in asthma symptom scores and asthma-related quality of life. Omalizumab is thus indicated for the prevention of asthma exacerbations and control of asthma symptoms when given as add-on therapy for adult and adolescent patients with severe persistent allergic asthma who remain inadequately controlled, despite daily high-dose ICS plus a long-acting inhaled β_2-agonist.

IV. Future Prospects of Asthma Pharmacotherapy

Although drug therapy is crucial in the management of patients with asthma, there is a huge variation in drug responses between individual patients. In asthmatics, this variation may be due to differences in disease severity, drug adherence, environmental exposures, or age, but genetic factors may account for 60% to 80% of the heterogeneity in treatment responsiveness. Pharmacogenetics is the study of the contribution of these genetic differences among individuals to the variability in the responses to pharmacotherapy. Until now, physicians are unable to predict in which patients a drug will work well and in whom not. Identifying the genetic variants responsible for this interindividual variability may lead to improved effectiveness in the use of existing treatments, instead of the current practice of "trial and error."

Genetic polymorphisms can produce variations in individual responses to a given pharmacotherapy by at least two different mechanisms. First, genetic variants may be associated with altered uptake, distribution, metabolism, or elimination of a given medication, leading to impaired or enhanced drug clearance. Genetic polymorphisms altering the availability of the drug at the site of action by influencing its metabolism (e.g., cytochrome P450 pathways) will determine the individual response to treatment. The second major pharmacogenetic mechanism is due to genetic variation in the drug target (e.g., the drug receptor), leading to altered drug efficacy or differences in the expression of a disease phenotype.

Recently, genetic polymorphisms in the 5-lipoxygenase (5-LO) gene and leukotriene C4 (LTC4) synthase gene have been described (91–93). Moreover, it was found that asthma in carriers of these genetic variants of the 5-LO pathway had a diminished response to treatment with antileukotriene drugs, indicating a pharmacogenetic effect of these genetic polymorphisms on responses to treatment.

Polymorphisms of the β_2-adrenergic receptor gene may similarly dictate the relative responsiveness to β_2-agonists among asthma patients. Several studies have demonstrated that β_2-adrenergic receptor single-nucleotide polymorphisms (SNPs) determine the response of asthmatics to treatment with bronchodilators (94,95). Indeed, patients with asthma who are homozygous for Gly at amino acid position 16 (Gly-16) of the β_2-adrenoreceptor are more prone to develop bronchodilator desensitization. However, when the influence of the β_2-adrenoreceptor genotype on the response of asthmatic patients to regular versus as-needed short-acting salbutamol was examined, those patients who were Arg-16 homozygous and were receiving regular salbutamol had significantly lower lung function than Arg-16 homozygous patients who took salbutamol only as needed (96,97). Moreover, homozygous Arg-16 patients also appeared susceptible to clinically important increases in asthma exacerbations during chronic dosing with the short-acting β_2-agonist salbutamol (98).

These pharmacogenetic studies are only beginning to unravel the drug response variability among asthmatic patients. In the future, by studying combinations of SNPs (i.e., haplotypes) of several drug target genes (e.g., β_2-adrenergic receptor, glucocorticosteroid receptor, and the leukotriene pathway) it might be possible to distinguish responders from nonresponders to a pharmacological agent at the start. Extensive pharmacogenetic studies, best built into drug trials, will teach us whether in the future we will be able to predict a patient's response to antiasthmatic drugs of different classes. If this proves to be true, it might be possible to tailor drug treatments to a specific patient's need (99).

V. Conclusion

Since asthma is a variable disease, all patients with asthma should be prescribed rapid-acting inhaled β_2-agonists PRN (as needed) to use as rescue therapy in case of symptoms. However, one of the goals of the management of asthma is minimal (ideally no) need for as-needed β_2-agonist, together with minimal or no chronic symptoms, no exacerbations, and no emergency visits. Therefore, as soon as patients experience symptoms at least once a week, controller medication(s) should be started on a daily basis to achieve and maintain control of their asthma. In patients with mild persistent asthma, treatment with inhaled corticosteroids at a dose of 200–500 µg beclomethasone dipropionate (200–400 µg budesonide, 100–250 µg fluticasone, or equivalent) is preferred. Alternative controller medications in patients with mild disease include sustained-release theophylline, cromones, and leukotriene modifiers. If the patient is still symptomatic despite regular use of inhaled corticosteroids, or if the patient experiences daily symptoms, the patient has moderate to severe asthma, and a long-acting inhaled β_2-agonist should be added to the inhaled corticosteroid. Fixed combinations of formoterol/budesonide or salmeterol/fluticasone in a single inhaler are not only convenient for these moderate and severe asthmatics, they also enhance drug adherence and thereby clinical effectiveness. Alternative add-on therapies to inhaled corticosteroids in patients with moderate to severe asthma include theophylline, long-acting oral β_2-agonists and leukotriene modifiers. The overall goal of asthma pharmacotherapy is to offer the patients a (near) normal life, implicating that they have no daytime nor nocturnal symptoms of asthma, and that they feel no limitations in physical or social activities.

Abbreviations

BDP	Beclomethasone dipropionate
FEV_1	Forced expiratory value in one second
ICS	Inhaled (gluco) corticosteroids
SNP	Single nucleotide polymorphism

References

1. Global Initiative for Asthma (GINA). Global strategy for asthma management and prevention. NHLBI/WHO workshop report. National Institutes of Health, National Heart, Lung and Blood Institute, National Institutes of Health publication No. 95–3659, 1995.
2. Global Initiative for Asthma. Global Strategy for asthma management and prevention. National Institutes of Health, NTH publication No. 02–3659, 2002.

3. Rabe KF, Adachi M, Lai CK, et al. Worldwide severity and control of asthma in children and adults: the global asthma insights and reality surveys. J Allergy Clin Immunol 2004; 114:40–47.

4. Rabe KF, Vermeire PA, Soriano JB, Maier WC. Clinical management of asthma in 1999: the asthma insights and reality in europe (AIRE) study. Eur Respir J 2000; 16:802–807.

5. Lai CK, De Guia TS, Kim YY, et al. Asthma control in the Asia-Pacific region: the asthma insights and reality in Asia-Pacific study. J Allergy Clin Immunol 2003; 111:263–268.

6. Adams RJ, Fuhlbrigge A, Guilbert T, Lozano P, Martinez F. Inadequate use of asthma medication in the United States: results of the asthma in America national population survey. J Allergy Clin Immunol 2002; 110:58–64.

7. Sears MR, Taylor DR, Print CG, et al. Regular inhaled beta-agonist treatment in bronchial asthma. Lancet 1990; 336:1391–1396.

8. McFadden ER Jr, Gilbert IA. Exercise-induced asthma. N Engl J Med 1994; 330:1362–1367.

9. Ringdal N, Derom E, Wahlin-Boll E, Pauwels R. Onset and duration of action of single doses of formoterol inhaled via Turbuhaler. Respir Med 1998; 92: 1017–1021.

10. Tattersfield AE, Lofdahl CG, Postma DS, et al. Comparison of formoterol and terbutaline for as-needed treatment of asthma: a randomised trial. Lancet 2001; 357:257–261.

11. Pauwels RA, Sears MR, Campbell M, et al. Formoterol as relief medication in asthma: a worldwide safety and effectiveness trial. Eur Respir J 2003; 22:787–794.

12. Jenkins C. Formoterol as relief medication in asthma: the jury is still out. Eur Respir J 2003; 22:723–724.

13. Engel T, Dirksen A, Heinig JH, Nielsen NH, Weeke B, Johansson SA. Single-dose inhaled budesonide in subjects with chronic asthma. Allergy 1991; 46: 547–553.

14. Ellul-Micallef R, Johansson SA. Acute dose-response studies in bronchial asthma with a new corticosteroid, budesonide. Br J Clin Pharmacol 1983; 15:419–422.

15. Palmqvist M, Arvidsson P, Beckman O, Peterson S, Lotvall J. Onset of bronchodilation of budesonide/formoterol vs. salmeterol/fluticasone in single inhalers. Pulm Pharmacol Ther 2001; 14:29–34.

16. Djukanovic R, Feather I, Gratziou C, et al. Effect of natural allergen exposure during the grass pollen season on airways inflammatory cells and asthma symptoms. Thorax 1996; 51:575–581.

17. Norris G, Larson T, Koenig J, Claiborn C, Sheppard L, Finn D. Asthma aggravation, combustion, and stagnant air. Thorax 2000; 55:466–470.

18. Weinberger M, Hendeles L. Theophylline in asthma. N Engl J Med 1996; 334:1380–1388.

19. Harrison BD, Stokes TC, Hart GJ, Vaughan DA, Ali NT, Robinson AA. Need for intravenous hydrocortisone in addition to oral prednisolone in patients admitted to hospital with severe asthma without ventilatory failure. Lancet 1986; 1:181–184.

20. O'Driscoll BR, Kalra S, Wilson M, Pickering CA, Carroll KB, Woodcock AA. Double-blind trial of steroid tapering in acute asthma. Lancet 1993; 341:324–327.

21. Djukanovic R, Wilson JW, Britten KM, et al. Effect of an inhaled corticosteroid on airway inflammation and symptoms in asthma. Am Rev Respir Dis 1992; 145:669–674.

22. Laitinen LA, Laitinen A, Haahtela T. A comparative study of the effects of an Inhaled corticosteroid, budesonide, and a beta 2-agonist, terbutaline, on airway inflammation in newly diagnosed asthma: a randomized, double-blind, parallel-group controlled trial. J Allergy Clin Immunol 1992; 90:32–42.

23. Wilson JW, Djukanovic R, Howarth PH, Holgate ST. Inhaled beclomethasone dipropionate downregulates airway lymphocyte activation in atopic asthma. Am J Respir Crit Care Med 1994; 149:86–90.

24. Long-term effects of budesonide or nedocromil in children with asthma. The Childhood Asthma Management Program Research Group. N Engl J Med 2000; 343:1054–1063.

25. Barnes PJ, Pedersen S, Busse WW. Efficacy and safety of inhaled corticosteroids. New developments. Am J Respir Crit Care Med 1998; 157:Sl–S53.

26. Suissa S, Ernst P, Benayoun S, Baltzan M, Cai B. Low-Dose Inhaled Corticosteroids and the Prevention of Death from Asthma. N Engl J Med 2000; 343:332–336.

27. Pauwels RA, Pedersen S, Busse WW, et al. Early intervention with budesonide in mild persistent asthma: a randomised, double-blind trial. The Lancet 2003; 361:1071–1076.

28. Williams DM. Clinical considerations in the use of inhaled corticosteroids for asthma. Pharmacotherapy 2001; 21:38S–48S.

29. Hogger P. Dose response and therapeutic index of inhaled corticosteroids in asthma. Curr Opin Pulm Med 2003; 9:1–8.

30. Derendorf H, Hochhaus G, Rohatagi S, et al. Pharmacokinetics of triamcinolone acetonide after intravenous, oral, and inhaled administration. J Clin Pharmacol 1995; 35:302–305.

31. Affrime MB, Cuss F, Padhi D, et al. Bioavailability and metabolism of mometasone furoate following administration by metered-dose and dry-powder inhalers in healthy human volunteers. J Clin Pharmacol 2000; 40:1227–1236.

32. Nave R, Bethke TD, van Marie SP, Zech K. Pharmacokinetics of [14C]ciclesonide after oral and intravenous administration to healthy subjects. Clin Pharmacokinet 2004; 43:479–486.

33. O'Connor B, Bonnaud G, Haahtela T, et al. Dose-ranging study of mometasone furoate dry powder inhaler in the treatment of moderate persistent asthma using fiuticasone propionate as an active comparator. Ann Allergy Asthma Immunol 2001; 86:397–404.

34. Brutsche MH, Brutsche IC, Munawar M, et al. Comparison of pharmacokinetics and systemic effects of inhaled fluticasone propionate in patients with asthma and healthy volunteers: a randomised crossover study. Lancet 2000; 356:556–561.

35. Harrison TW, Wisniewski A, Honour J, Tattersfield AE. Comparison of the systemic effects of fluticasone propionate and budesonide given by dry powder inhaler in healthy and asthmatic subjects. Thorax 2001; 56:186–191.

36. Busse WW, Brazinsky S, Jacobson K, et al. Efficacy response of inhaled beclomethasone dipropionate in asthma is proportional to dose and is improved

by formulation with a new propellant. J Allergy Clin Immunol 1999; 104: 1215–1222.

37. Reed CE, Offord KP, Nelson HS, Li JT, Tinkelman DG. Aerosol beclomethasone dipropionate spray compared with theophylline as primary treatment for chronic mild-to-moderate asthma. The American Academy of Allergy, Asthma and Immunology Beclomethasone Dipropionate-Theophylline Study Group. J Allergy Clin Immunol 1998; 101:14–23.

38. Dahl R, Larsen BB, Venge P. Effect of long-term treatment with inhaled budesonide or theophylline on lung function, airway reactivity and asthma symptoms. Respir Med 2002; 96:432–438.

39. Barnes PJ. Theophylline: new perspectives for an old drug. Am J Respir Crit Care Med 2003; 167:813–818.

40. Drazen JM, Israel E, O'Byrne PM. Treatment of asthma with drugs modifying the leukotriene pathway. N Engl J Med 1999; 340:197–206.

41. Lipworth BJ. Leukotriene-receptor antagonists. Lancet 1999; 353:57–62.

42. Bleecker ER, Welch MJ, Weinstein SF, et al. Low-dose inhaled fluticasone propionate versus oral zafirlukast in the treatment of persistent asthma. J Allergy Clin Immunol 2000; 105:1123–1129.

43. Barnes NC, Miller CJ. Effect of leukotriene receptor antagonist therapy on the risk of asthma exacerbations in patients with mild to moderate asthma: an integrated analysis of zafirlukast trials. Thorax 2000; 55:478–483.

44. Ducharme FM. Inhaled glucocorticoids versus leukotriene receptor antagonists as single agent asthma treatment: systematic review of current evidence. BMJ 2003; 326:621–625.

45. Dahlen B, Nizankowska E, Szczeklik A, et al. Benefits from adding the 5- lipoxygenase inhibitor zileuton to conventional therapy in aspirin-intolerant asthmatics. Am J Respir Crit Care Med 1998; 157:1187–1194.

46. Szefler SJ, Nelson HS. Alternative agents for anti-inflammatory treatment of asthma. J Allergy Clin Immunol 1998; 102:S23–S35.

47. Schatz M. Interrelationships between asthma and pregnancy: a literature review. J Allergy Clin Immunol 1999; 103:S330–S336.

48. Demissie K, Breckenridge MB, Rhoads GG. Infant and maternal outcomes in the pregnancies of asthmatic women. Am J Respir Crit Care Med 1998; 158:1091–1095.

49. Wendel PJ, Ramin SM, Barnett-Hamm C, Rowe TF, Cunningham FG. Asthma treatment in pregnancy: a randomized controlled study. Am J Obstet Gynecol 1996; 175:150–154.

50. Schatz M, Zeiger RS, Harden KM, et al. The safety of inhaled beta-agonist bronchodilators during pregnancy. J Allergy Clin Immunol 1988; 82:686–695.

51. Norjavaara E, de Verdier MG. Nonnal pregnancy outcomes in a population-based study including 2,968 pregnant women exposed to budesonide. J Allergy Clin Immunol 2003; 111:736–742.

52. Schatz M, Dombrowski MP, Wise R, et al. The relationship of asthma medication use to perinatal outcomes. J Allergy Clin Immunol 2004; 113:1040–1045.

53. Shrewsbury S, Pyke S, Britton M. Meta-analysis of increased dose of inhaled steroid or addition of salmeterol in symptomatic asthma (MIASMA). BMJ 2000; 320:1368–1373.

54. Greening AP, Ind PW, Northfield M, Shaw G. Added salmeterol versus higher-dose corticosteroid in asthma patients with symptoms on existing inhaled corticosteroid. Lancet 1994; 344:219–224.

55. Woolcock A, Lundback B, Ringdal N, Jacques L. Comparison of addition of salmeterol to inhaled steroids with doubling of the dose of inhaled steroids. Am J Respir Crit Care Med 1996; 153:1481–1488.

56. Pauwels RA, Lofdahl CG, Postma DS, et al. Effect of inhaled formoterol and budesonide on exacerbations of asthma. Formoterol and Corticosteroids Establishing Therapy (FACET) International Study Group. N Engl J Med 1997; 337:1405–1411.

57. Tattersfield AE, Postma DS, Barnes PJ, et al. Exacerbations of asthma: a descriptive study of 425 severe exacerbations. The FACET International Study Group. Am J Respir Crit Care Med 1999; 160:594–599.

58. Masoli M, Weatherall M, Holt S, Beasley R. Clinical dose-response relationship of fluticasone propionate in adults with asthma. Thorax 2004; 59:16–20.

59. Bateman ED, Boushey HA, Bousquet J, et al. Can Guideline-defined Asthma Control be Achieved? The Gaining Optimal Asthma Control Study. Am J Respir Crit Care Med 2004; 170:836–844.

60. O'Byrne PM, Barnes PJ, Rodriguez-Roisin R, et al. Low dose inhaled budesonide and formoterol in mild persistent asthma: the OPTIMA randomized trial. Am J Respir Crit Care Med 2001; 164:1392–1397.

61. Calhoun WJ, Hinton KL, Kratzenberg JJ. The effect of salmeterol on markers of airway inflammation following segmental allergen challenge. Am J Respir Crit Care Med 2001; 163:881–886.

62. Wallin A, Sue-Chu M, Bjermer L, et al. Effect of inhaled fluticasone with and without salmeterol on airway inflammation in asthma. J Allergy Clin Immunol 2003; 112:72–78.

63. Lazarus SC, Boushey HA, Fahy JV, et al. Long-acting beta2-agonist monotherapy vs continued therapy with inhaled corticosteroids in patients with persistent asthma: a randomized controlled trial. JAMA 2001; 285:2583–2593.

64. Lemanske RF Jr, Sorkness CA, Mauger EA, et al. Inhaled corticosteroid reduction and elimination in patients with persistent asthma receiving salmeterol: a randomized controlled trial. JAMA 2001; 285:2594–2603.

65. Zetterstrom O, Buhl R, Mellem H, et al. Improved asthma control with budesonide/formoterol in a single inhaler, compared with budesonide alone. Eur Respir J 2001; 18:262–268.

66. Nelson HS, Chapman KR, Pyke SD, Johnson M, Pritchard JN. Enhanced synergy between fluticasone propionate and salmeterol inhaled from a single inhaler versus separate inhalers. J Allergy Clin Immunol 2003; 112:29–36.

67. Kavuru M, Melamed J, Gross G, et al. Salmeterol and fluticasone propionate combined in a new powder inhalation device for the treatment of asthma: a randomized, double-blind, placebo-controlled trial. J Allergy Clin Immunol 2000; 105:1108–1116.

68. Aubier M, Pieters WR, Schlosser NJ, Steinmetz KO. Salmeterol/fluticasone propionate (50/500 microg) in combination in a Diskus inhaler (Seretide) is effective and safe in the treatment of steroid-dependent asthma. Respir Med 1999; 93:876–884.

69. Shapiro G, Lumry W, Wolfe J, et al. Combined salmeterol 50 microg and fluticasone propionate 250 microg in the diskus device for the treatment of asthma. Am J Respir Crit Care Med 2000; 161:527–534.

70. Stoloff SW, Stempel DA, Meyer J, Stanford RH, Carranza Rosenzweig JR. Improved refill persistence with fluticasone propionate and salmeterol in a single inhaler compared with other controller therapies. J Allergy Clin Immunol 2004; 113:245–251.

71. Evans DJ, Taylor DA, Zetterstrom O, Chung KF, O'Connor BJ, Barnes PJ. A comparison of low-dose inhaled budesonide plus theophylline and high-dose inhaled budesonide for moderate asthma. N Engl J Med 1997; 337: 1412–1418.

72. Ukena D, Harnest U, Sakalauskas R, et al. Comparison of addition of theophylline to inhaled steroid with doubling of the dose of inhaled steroid in asthma. Eur Respir J 1997; 10:2754–2760.

73. Lim S, Jatakanon A, Gordon D, Macdonald C, Chung KF, Barnes PJ. Comparison of high dose inhaled steroids, low dose inhaled steroids plus low dose theophylline, and low dose inhaled steroids alone in chronic asthma in general practice. Thorax 2000; 55:837–841.

74. Davies B, Brooks G, Devoy M. The efficacy and safety of salmeterol compared to theophylline: meta-analysis of nine controlled studies. Respir Med 1998; 92:256–263.

75. Wilson AJ, Gibson PG, Coughlan J. Long acting beta-agonists versus theophylline for maintenance treatment of asthma. Cochrane Database Syst Rev 2000; CD001281.

76. Shah L, Wilson AJ, Gibson PG, Coughlan J. Long acting beta-agonists versus theophylline for maintenance treatment of asthma. Cochrane Database Syst Rev 2003; CD001281.

77. Laviolette M, Mahmstrom K, Lu S, et al. Montelukast added to inhaled beclomethasone in treatment of asthma. Montelukast/Beclomethasone Additivity Group. Am J Respir Crit Care Med 1999; 160:1862–1868.

78. Vaquerizo MJ, Casan P, Castillo J, et al. Effect of montelukast added to inhaled budesonide on control of mild to moderate asthma. Thorax 2003; 58: 204–210.

79. Price DB, Hernandez D, Magyar P, et al. Randomised controlled trial of montelukast plus inhaled budesonide versus double dose inhaled budesonide in adult patients with asthma. Thorax 2003; 58:211–216.

80. Nathan RA, Bernstein JA, Bielory L, et al. Zafirlukast improves asthma symptoms and quality of life in patients with moderate reversible airflow obstruction. J Allergy Clin Immunol 1998; 102:935–942.

81. Ducharme FM. Anti-leukotrienes as add-on therapy to inhaled glucocorticoids in patients with asthma: systematic review of current evidence. BMJ 2002; 324:1545–1551.

82. Busse W, Nelson H, Wolfe J, Kalberg C, Yancey SW, Rickard KA. Comparison of inhaled salmeterol and oral zafirlukast in patients with asthma. J Allergy Clin Immunol 1999; 103:1075–1080.

83. Bjermer L, Bisgaard H, Bousquet J, et al. Montelukast and fluticasone compared with salmeterol and fluticasone in protecting against asthma exacerbation

in adults: one year, double blind, randomised, comparative trial. BMJ 2003; 327:891–900.

84. Fick R Jr JP. IgE and anti-IgE therapy in asthma and allergic disease. Lung Biol Health Dis 2002; 164.

85. Soler M, Matz J, Townley R, et al. The anti-IgE antibody omalizumab reduces exacerbations and steroid requirement in allergic asthmatics. Eur Respir J 2001; 18:254–261.

86. Lanier BQ, Corren J, Lumry W, Liu J, Fowler-Taylor A, Gupta N. Omalizumab is effective in the long-term control of severe allergic asthma. Ann Allergy Asthma Immunol 2003; 91:154–159.

87. Busse W, Corren J, Lanier BQ, et al. Omalizumab, anti-IgE recombinant humanized monoclonal antibody, for the treatment of severe allergic asthma. J Allergy Clin Immunol 2001; 108:184–190.

88. Vignola AM, Humbert M, Bousquet J, et al. Efficacy and tolerability of anti-immunoglobulin E therapy with omalizumab in patients with concomitant allergic asthma and persistent allergic rhinitis: SOLAR. Allergy 2004; 59:709–717.

89. Holgate ST, Chuchalin AG, Hebert J, et al. Efficacy and safety of a recombinant anti-immunoglobulin E antibody (omalizumab) in severe allergic asthma. Clin Exp Allergy 2004; 34:632–638.

90. Ayres JG, Higgins B, Chilvers ER, Ayre G, Blogg M, Fox H. Efficacy and tolerability of anti-immunoglobulin E therapy with omalizumab in patients with poorly controlled (moderate-to-severe) allergic asthma. Allergy 2004; 59:701–708.

91. Wechsler ME, Israel E. Pharmacogenetics of treatment with leukotriene modifiers. Curr Opin Allergy Clin Immunol 2002; 2:395–401.

92. Sampson AP, Siddiqui S, Buchanan D, et al. Variant LTC(4) synthase allele modifies cysteinyl leukotriene synthesis in eosinophils and predicts clinical response to zafirlukast. Thorax 2000; 55(suppl 2):S28–S31.

93. Drazen JM, Yandava CN, Dube L, et al. Pharmacogenetic association between ALOX5 promoter genotype and the response to anti-asthma treatment. Nat Genet 1999; 22:168–170.

94. Raby BA, Weiss ST. Beta2-adrenergic receptor genetics. Curr Opin Mol Ther 2001; 3:554–566.

95. Drysdale CM, McGraw DW, Stack CB, et al. Complex promoter and coding region beta 2-adrenergic receptor haplotypes alter receptor expression and predict in vivo responsiveness. Proc Natl Acad Sci U S A 2000; 97: 10483–10488.

96. Drazen JM, Israel E, Boushey HA, et al. Comparison of regularly scheduled with as-needed use of albuterol in mild asthma. Asthma Clin Res Network. N Engl J Med 1996; 335:841–847.

97. Israel E, Drazen JM, Liggett SB, et al. The effect of polymorphisms of the beta(2)-adrenergic receptor on the response to regular use of albuterol in asthma. Am J Respir Crit Care Med 2000; 162:75–80.

98. Taylor DR, Drazen JM, Herbison GP, Yandava CN, Hancox RJ, Town GI. Asthma exacerbations during long term beta agonist use: influence of beta(2) adrenoceptor polymorphism. Thorax 2000; 55:762–767.

99. Holgate ST. Pharmacogenetics: the new science of personalizing treatment. Curr Opin Allergy Clin Immunol 2004; 4:37–38.

13

Pharmacotherapy in the Emergency Department, Hospital Floor, and Intensive Care Unit

AJEET G. VINAYAK, J. P. KRESS, and JESSE HALL

Section of Pulmonary and Critical Care Medicine, University of Chicago Hospitals
Chicago, Illinois, U.S.A.

I. Introduction

Asthma is a chronic inflammatory disorder of the airways. In the chronic disease state, asthma severity can be classified based on symptom frequency, spirometric evaluation, or rescue medication usage (1). Worsening disease occurs as a result of increased bronchial smooth muscle contraction, increased airway edema, and/or a higher burden of intraluminal mucus (1). The hallmark features of an acute asthma (AA) attack are wheezing, coughing, chest tightness, and dyspnea. These attacks are associated with variable obstruction to airflow with an inconsistent degree of reversibility.

All patients with asthma are at risk for severe exacerbation that requires urgent medical attention and places them at risk for respiratory failure. Significant asthma morbidity and mortality occur during these intense episodes. Proper assessment of severity and aggressive initiation of therapy may improve outcomes (2,3). These hyperacute, acute, or even subacute events are referred to as severe asthma, status asthmaticus, or AA. The purpose of this chapter is to review the epidemiology, assessment, and treatment of AA in the emergency department (ED), hospital, and intensive care unit (ICU).

II. Epidemiology

Recent estimates place the cost of asthma in the United States at roughly $6 billion a year (4,5). Direct treatment costs account for up to 88% of this total. Nearly half of all costs related to asthma are due to hospitalization (4,5). Given that the minority of asthmatics require ED and hospital care, cost analysis suggests that 20% of all asthmatics utilize 80% of all resources. This $6 billion amount is roughly 1% of the direct medical costs for all diseases nationally and 13% of direct costs for respiratory diseases (4). Therefore, the economic burden of asthma is sizable, but if prevention measures, outcomes research, and awareness advocacy can direct a larger proportion of treatment to the ambulatory setting, these costs may be reducible.

The overall prevalence of asthma and associated hospitalizations in the United States has steadily increased over the last four decades (6–8). The prevalence trends appeared to plateau over the last few years of the last century and the first several years of the current century (Fig. 1) (9,10). It is estimated that approximately 5% or 15 million Americans meet criteria for a diagnosis of asthma (11). Adults over the age of 18 years make up two-thirds of this group (11). The most recently reported data suggest that ED visits continued to increase during the 1990s. By 1999 there were two million visits to the ED with women comprising the slight majority. African American patients, while still accounting for the overall minority of these visits, were largely overrepresented. Comparative rates of ED entry among white and African American patients were 59 per 10,000 versus 174 per 10,000 persons (9).

Hospitalization and mortality rates at the end of the last decade have not increased in the way apparent from 1970 to 1990 (8,12,13) (Fig. 1) The number of hospitalizations in 1999 was approximately one-half million, and the overall mortality rate was 17.2 per 1,000,000 people in the general population. This last value represents a decrease from the prior years in part due to changes associated with the use of the new coding system (ICD-10) (9). Regardless of this change in recording systems, the interpretation of these trends is that hospitalization and mortality may have reached a plateau, halting alarming increases seen over the previous decade and a half. African American asthmatics were disproportionately represented in those hospitalized for or succumbing to asthma (8,12,13).

III. Emergency Department Assessment

Paramount in the evaluation of AA is determination of attack severity and the risk of respiratory failure. Patients with AA at presentation to the ED or clinic are often in considerable visible distress. Dyspnea and wheezing are common elements in an asthma exacerbation. Among the myriad of other

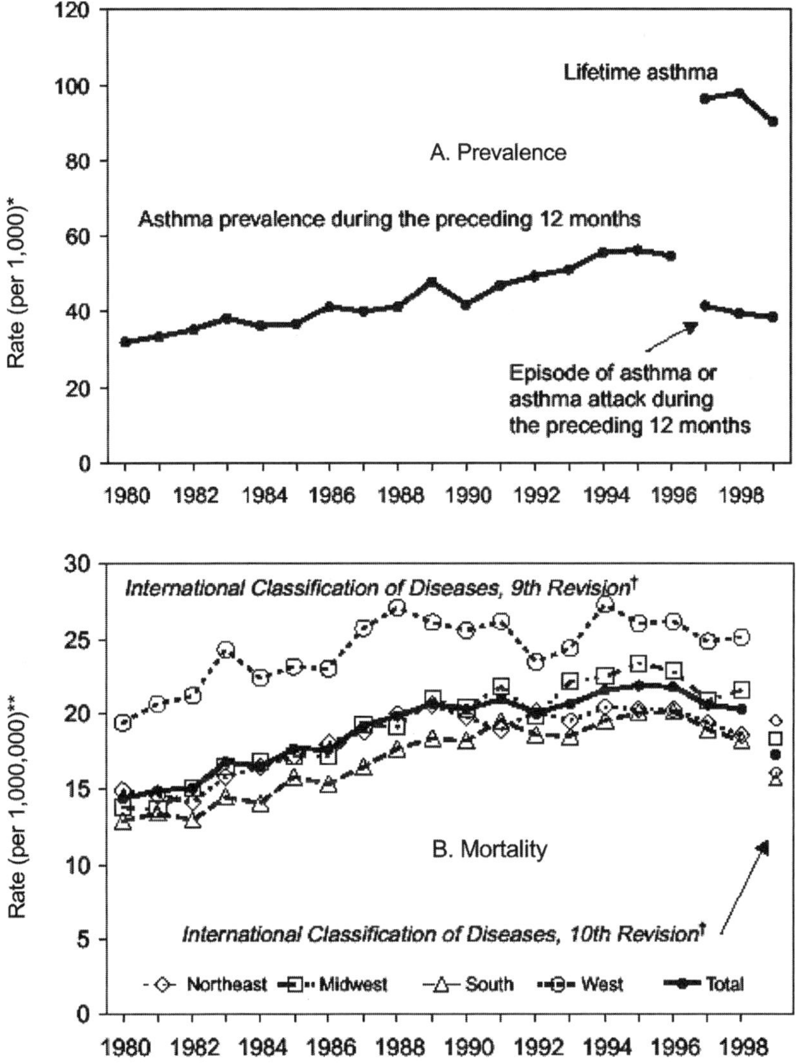

Figure 1   U.S. national statistics on asthma prevalence and mortality show that consistent increases in both these values over the last three decades may have finally reached plateaus. *Source*: Adapted from Ref. 9.

attributable signs and symptoms, there is no uniformly consistent finding present in all cases. The key components of this assessment include history, physical examination, objective measurement of airflow limitation, and quantification of early response to initial therapy. Each of these components is independently informative in the complete evaluation of the AA patient (14).

A. History

A pertinent asthma history includes assessment of onset, progression, and duration of the current exacerbation. Medication usage and compliance should be obtained. A careful asthma history also includes assessment of chronic asthma severity. While severe, labile asthmatics are at high risk, even mild asthmatics may suffer respiratory failure or die as a consequence of AA if thoughtful, attentive care is not provided. Patients at highest risk for mortality include those with recurrent hospitalizations or visits to the ED, those who have suffered life-threatening exacerbations, and patients who carry concomitant psychiatric diagnoses (15). A complete history should also assess evidence of alternative diagnoses discussed below that are commonly included in the differential diagnosis for recurrent, severe asthma.

B. Physical Examination

The general appearance of an asthmatic can reveal valuable information to the clinician. Altered mental status, the use of accessory muscles, and interrupted speech patterns have all been implicated with AA (16). In addition, inability to remain supine or diaphoresis has been shown to predict significant airflow limitation, and the combination of these findings portends lower values on objective airflow measurements (17).

Derangements in vital signs frequently accompany severe asthma exacerbations. While tachycardia and tachypnea are more frequent, a more discerning gauge of asthma severity may be the presence of an elevated pulsus paradoxus (PP) (16). An abnormal PP occurs when the measured difference in systolic pressure during the respiratory cycle is greater than 10 mmHg. Usually the PP is even higher with ranges of greater than 25 mmHg, which is highly predictive of poor airflow (18). Caution must be exercised in judging the PP, however, since PP will fall in the exhausted patient as respiratory muscle effort declines and the swings in intrathoracic pressure, which generate PP, narrow.

Central to the physical exam is auscultation of the thorax (19). This examination often reveals wheezing. In patients with severe obstruction, air movement may be so poor that there is an absence of sound. Crackles occur in asthmatics in whom airway closure or mucous plugging leads to atelectasis, but the presence of this finding should alert the clinician to the possibility of alternative diagnoses such as pneumonia or heart failure. Critical examination for alternative diagnoses should include a careful examination of the cardiovascular system for evidence of heart failure and the neck and oropharynx for stridor and tongue swelling suggestive of upper airway pathology. Clinical signs of asthma complications should also be monitored in patients with severe symptoms. Determining that the trachea is in the midline and there is no crunch on auscultation of the chest wall lowers the likelihood of barotrauma.

In total, the appearance, vital signs and direct exam of the asthmatic patient can suggest disease severity, hint at alternative diagnoses, or reveal asthma-related complications. Yet the absence of certain findings does not reduce the possibility of severe asthma morbidity. In fact, many of the above findings may disappear as a direct consequence of severe asthma progression. As mentioned above, wheezing may grow quieter as airflow is more limited, resulting in an ominously quiet chest. Similarly, increasing obtundation may allow the previously agitated, upright patient to finally assume the supine position, and fatigue may lead to lower accessory muscle use or a decrement in previously elevated PP value. It is the occurrence of these disparate findings, progressing over time as respiratory failure supervenes, that can herald a worse clinical course.

C. Pulmonary Function

Objective measurements of pulmonary function (PF) provide useful information in the assessment of severity in AA. Peak expiratory flow rate (PEFR) and FEV_1 are the commonly used measurements in EDs and acute care centers. These values can also be used to standardize inclusion criteria for studies on AA and repeated to determine response to therapy. Consensus guidelines routinely define AA with the cutoff PEFR or $FEV_1 < 50\%$ predicted with most investigations of this topic using this threshold in inclusion criteria (1). The subgroup of severe acute asthma (SAA) describes cases where measurement of PEFR or FEV_1 is below 25% or 30% of predicted.

The greatest clinical utility of PF measurements is realized when serial values are used to assess changes in airflow obstruction in response to appropriate therapy. A good response after 30 to 60 minutes of initial therapy seems to portend a favorable course (20,21). This type of response can be assessed as either the proportional response from the baseline PF value (i.e., 50 L/min increase in PEFR representing a 25% increase from baseline) or as an absolute value (i.e., FEV_1 up to 50% of predicted). It appears that patients that are able to improve to a PF measure > 45% of predicted (22) shortly after therapy have a far lower chance of hospital admission and are less likely to have a protracted clinical course.

D. Additional Data

The routine use of chest radiography as part of the initial evaluation of AA has been criticized (23). This modality should be reserved for patients with signs and symptoms of pneumonia or barotrauma. Once a patient has failed initial management and requires hospitalization, the discovery of radiographic findings that influence management is likely sufficiently high to warrant routine performance of a baseline study (24).

Routine assessment of oxygenation by pulse oximetry is recommended (1). While not entirely informative of gas exchange adequacy, pulse oximetric values over 90% are associated with very infrequent episodes of hypercarbia (25). Severity of an asthma exacerbation cannot be determined by routine pulse oximetry (26), but this monitoring modality is helpful in evaluating for pneumothorax, pneumonia, and respiratory failure.

Blood-gas analysis has a limited role in initial asthma severity scoring. Carbon dioxide retention occurs in a small proportion of cases, often when FEV_1 values are dramatically reduced (i.e., $FEV_1 < 20\%$ predicted). An ABG may be helpful is assessing detailed acid-base status when metabolic acidosis from high work of breathing or from cathecholamine therapy is suspected, or to document the degree of hypoxia if it persists despite therapy (19). Normocarbia in the patient with very significant respiratory distress may be an indicator of progression to respiratory insufficiency, but the decision to initiate mechanical ventilation is largely clinical, assisted mainly by signs, symptoms, and occasionally serial PF measurements. Blood-gas analysis should play a very minimal role in making this decision. Rather, arterial blood gases are most useful when titrating intentional hypoventilation and consequent permissive hypercapnia (PH) during mechanical ventilatory support (see below) (27).

Continuous electrocardiogram (ECG) monitoring should be employed in older patients, especially those with concomitant heart disease (1). Furthermore, screening for cocaine and heroin may help uncover cases of AA that are abrupt, severe, and sometimes life threatening. Both of these illicit substances have been shown to be associated with more severe courses in a relatively high fraction of patients presenting to urban EDs (28–30).

E. Alternative Diagnoses

While in most cases of AA, a combination of signs, symptoms, and ancillary measures correlate with a predictable clinical course, several alternative diagnoses should be entertained in the treatment of asthma in most patients, and pursued more aggressively if the setting is correct and the diagnosis of asthma is not entirely tenable. The most commonly missed diagnoses include diseases that cause airflow obstruction themselves or produce acute dyspnea that may be accompanied by wheezing, and include emphysema, chronic bronchitis, bronchiectasis, congestive heart failure, foreign body obstruction, and endobronchial lesions (31). Often, appropriate history, examination, and testing can help distinguish these processes from asthma, but sometimes patients may suffer from one or more of these diseases in addition to asthma.

The presence and activity of certain chronic conditions such as rhinitis, sinusitis, and nasal polyposis can affect the incidence of asthma exacerbations (32). The last condition, nasal polyps, may occur in a subgroup of patients that have or develop aspirin-induced asthma (AIA) via mechanisms involving the cyclooxygenase pathway (33). AIA may be present in as many as 20% of patients receiving attention for AA (34), and it should be considered during early assessment of AA as avoidance of NSAIDs and aspirin can avoid future life-threatening exacerbations (34–36). Anaphylaxis can present similarly to severe AA, although signs and symptoms in addition to those related to airflow obstruction may be present (32). Common food intolerances, insect bites, latex exposure, and medications (especially β-blockers and angiotensin-converting enzyme inhibitors) have all been implicated in asthma-like processes. The presence of stridor, rash, urticaria, or flushing can be clues to the diagnosis of anaphylaxis (32). Prompt recognition is crucial to future avoidance of the offending agent and immediate initiation of therapy for anaphylaxis.

A myriad of additional pulmonary diagnoses can mimic AA. Certain disease processes such as allergic bronchopulmonary aspergillosis (37) and the Churg–Strauss syndrome (38), occur with recurrent asthma as a prominent feature. Prevention of asthma exacerbations in these diseases depends on their proper identification to ensure adequate chronic therapy with agents such as corticosteroids (CS). Furthermore, occult, chronic thromboembolic disease may be marked by episodic dyspnea and focal wheezing (39). These processes are rarely considered in the differential of asthma and hence may be missed and inappropriately treated as simple AA.

One final disorder worth mentioning is vocal cord dysfunction (VCD) or glottic dysfunction (40). This paradoxical closure of the vocal cords during inspiration often accompanies symptoms easily confused as episodic exacerbation of asthma. Frequent ED visits and repeated corticosteroid therapy may be initiated before visualization of the vocal cords during a symptomatic episode divulges this alternative diagnosis (41). Careful auscultation of the neck may reveal stridor or abrupt cessation of sound during inspiration. Treatment for VCD involves biofeedback and speech therapy (41).

F. Near Fatal Asthma and Acute Asthma Onset

A category of asthma severity commonly investigated and reported in the literature is the "near-fatal asthma" (NFA) attack. This entity was originally proposed as part of the investigation of increases noted in asthma mortality from the 1970s on (42). Cases of NFA are more prevalent than fatalities, yet evidence suggests that these two groups may share common features, and that the former may be a useful epidemiologic marker for the latter (43). NFA is most commonly defined as asthma cases that require ventilatory assistance (42,44,45), but the term has been used to describe patients with hypercarbia, frequent hospitalization, or even severe respiratory symptoms with altered level of consciousness (46,47). Clinical characteristics that have been commonly associated with NFA include recurrent admissions, prior need for ventilatory assistance, frequent β-agonist use, and an increased incidence of psychosocial problems (48).

Variation in inclusion criteria among studies on NFA, the largely retrospective nature of their study designs, and the low frequency of asthma mortality make extrapolation of NFA data difficult. Furthermore, none of the commonly described characteristics have adequate sensitivity or specificity to be strong predictors of NFA or the need for hospitalization (31). Standardizing the definition of NFA may assist in further exploration of AA mortality risk and prevention.

Two additional asthma features that have been related to hospitalization risk or NFA include altered sense of dyspnea and a shorter onset of the asthma attack. Kikuchi et al. (49) first described that a decreased perception of dyspnea (POD) and diminished ventilatory response to hypoxia was present in a small group of patients that had suffered NFA. Subsequently Magadle et al. (50) showed that among a cohort of outpatient asthmatics, lower POD had a statistical association with more frequent ED visits, cases of NFA, and death. It can be supposed that decreased POD may be a consequence of greater asthma severity or lead to altered duration of reported symptoms in AA.

Early investigations of NFA suggested that patients with a shorter duration of asthma symptoms during an exacerbation might be at an increased risk for hospitalization or mortality. A prospective study by Rodrigo and Rodrigo (51) also supported this association. Rapid-onset asthma attacks (ROAAs) appear to be a distinctive subgroup of AA. These patients seem to have a lower rate of precipitating infection as an etiology for their exacerbation as compared to slow-onset asthma attacks (SOAA). Furthermore, ROAA patients present with more severe obstruction upon arrival to the ED but have predictably faster recovery rates after therapy is initiated. Rodrigo and Rodrigo found that this ROAA group comprised the minority of AA cases that presented to the ED (10–20%) (51,52) and were less likely to require subsequent hospitalization because of their advantageous response to therapy. It is thought that ROAAs present with more acute bronchospasm and lesser degrees of worsening airway inflammation. This is in contrast to SOAAs, where worsening airway inflammation is thought to play a more central role.

IV. Emergency Department Therapy

A. β_2-Agonists

The mainstays of initial therapy for AA are the inhaled β_2-agonists. These agents treat bronchial smooth muscle constriction and thus produce bronchodilation. This salutary effect is more pronounced with β_2-agonists than other classes of bronchodilators (53,54). Among the intermediate-acting β_2-agonists, the most commonly used agent is albuterol (or salbutamol). Other short-onset, intermediate-acting agents include pirbuterol, terbutaline, metaproteronol, and fenoterol (not used in the United States).

The most efficacious means of delivery of β_2-agonist during an acute exacerbation is the inhaled route. The peak effects of oral preparations are delayed relative to the onset (roughly five minutes) of most short-acting β_2-agonists (55). Oral agents are only advisable in situations of unavailability of other delivery methods. The role of parenteral β_2-agonists (terbutaline and epinephrine) remains controversial (56,57). The largest detriment to routine use of parenteral adrenergic agents remains concerns over a narrow therapeutic index. Tachycardia and hypertension are effects that may not be tolerated by patients with comorbid cardiac disease or in older patients. A recent meta-analysis of studies comparing the effectiveness of IV β_2-agonists to inhaled β_2-agonist or IV methylxanthines for the treatment of AA in the ED concluded that the evidence did not support the preferential use of IV β_2-agonists (58). On the other hand, Cydulka et al. (59) showed that subcutaneous epinephrine was effective and tolerated without a cardiac event in a group of 95 older adult asthmatics. Furthermore, subcutaneous epinephrine has been proven to have some benefit in AA after an initial therapeutic failure of nebulized β_2-agonists (60). Given current evidence, parenteral administration of these agents can only be recommended in cases where inhaled therapy is not feasible or where there is no therapeutic response to inhaled β_2-agonists.

Among inhaled modalities, there appears to be no measurable clinical advantage to nebulized therapy over the use of a metered-dose inhaler with a spacer (MDI/spacer) device when doses are matched (61,62). While MDI/spacer delivery requires less time at lower costs than wet nebulization, it can be argued that nebulized therapy obviates the need for close supervision of proper technique. When coupled with asthma education, a spacer, and prescription of inhaled CS at ED discharge, MDI/spacer administration of β_2-agonists has been linked to fewer short-term relapses than nebulizer use (63).

Nebulized β_2-agonist therapy is routinely given either in a continuous manner or intermittently. Based on the results of a recent meta-analysis, there appears to be no difference in hospital admission or magnitude of PF improvement between continuous or intermittent administration of nebulized albuterol (64). This review concluded that this non-difference was seen regardless of the severity of the asthma exacerbation. This meta-analysis incorporated seven studies, two of which reported an advantage to continuous administration in a more severe asthma group (65,66). While there may be no advantage with continuous nebulized therapy in most patient groups, in the most severe cases with an impending requirement for mechanical ventilation some benefit to this strategy may exist.

The optimal dose and frequency of inhaled β_2-agonist administration is not clear. Clinical effect is dose dependent and delivery of drug to distal airways is inversely related to the degree of airflow obstruction. Sequential doses given at a set frequency has been shown to have the same effect as the cumulative dose given once (67). Yet larger single doses may be associated with more side effects. Evidence supports the use of either 2.5 mg of nebulized albuterol every 20 minutes for an hour or 2.4–3.6 mg of albuterol by MDI/spacer in an hour (four to six puffs every 10 minutes) (68). With acute exacerbations of moderate to severe asthma, increasing dosage further provides little therapeutic advantage (69).

It has been repeatedly shown that roughly two of every three patients presenting to the ED with AA will have a favorable response to aggressive β_2-agonist therapy (68,70,71). This consistent finding has added to the hypothesis that two forms of AA based on predominant pathologic features may exist: one marked by acute bronchial smooth muscle contraction and the other by other progressive inflammatory features. The former type may have near-complete resolution with treatment geared to abate bronchospasm.

A relatively novel therapeutic option within this drug class is a single isomeric form of albuterol. Racemic albuterol consists of equal concentrations of R- and S-enantiomers. Preferential pulmonary retention, increased toxicity, and attenuation of bronchodilatation are all effects attributed to S-albuterol (72–75). A recent pilot study showed levalbuterol (R-albuterol) dosed at 1.25 mg produced greater bronchodilation than 2.5 and 5 mg of racemic albuterol among patients treated for AA (73,76,77). The effect of levalbuterol on clinical outcomes including ED disposition await the results of a current larger, randomized, prospective study.

Longer-acting β_2-agonists (salmeterol and formoterol) have clear roles in outpatient asthma management. These agents are not recommended for use in AA, but formoterol may have short enough onset properties that make its use in AA plausible. Further investigations are required to clarify this role.

B. Oxygen

Supplemental oxygen is routinely administered to patients with AA. It is recommended for use (1) to resolve modest hypoxemia attributed to V/Q mismatch. Significant hypoxemia ($PaO_2 \leq 55$ mmHg) appears to occur only in a minority of patients with AA (78). Recent investigation suggests that in some patients with more severe gas exchange, early administration of 100% O_2 may lead to significant worsening of hypercarbia (79,80), presumably due to resolution of hypoxic vasoconstriction and resultant increase in blood flow to low V/Q units. This is rarely, if ever, clinically significant, and severe hypoxemia, if present, should always be reversed with adequate oxygen therapy. Since hypoxemia in uncomplicated AA is due to V/Q mismatch and not intrapulmonary shunt, large concentrations of oxygen are not required clinically. In fact, if patients exhibit a requirement for large concentrations of oxygen, a complicating cause of impaired gas exchange with intrapulmonary shunt (e.g., pneumonia) should be considered.

A potential salutary consequence of oxygen therapy is protection from decreases in arterial oxygen concentration associated with inhaled β_2-agonist therapy. This modest consequence of β_2-agonist use, rarely of great clinical significance, is thought to be related to increased V/Q mismatching.

One new, small study explored the role of adding humidification to delivered oxygen in asthmatics (81). The results suggest patients with AA are prone to airway dehydration. Separately, in a group of clinically stable patients, these investigators showed that dry air led to increased bronchoconstriction in asthmatics, which was relieved by the addition of humidification.

Patients with AA should be monitored for hypoxemia noninvasively by pulse oximetry. When hypoxia is present, prudent administration of supplemental oxygen should target normoxia (i.e., $SpO_2 > 90\%$ or even higher in pregnant patients). The innocuous addition of humidification to employed oxygen delivery systems seems reasonable.

C. Corticosteroids

CS are recommended for use in moderate to severe asthma exacerbations (1). Response to initial inhaled bronchodilator therapy may be another measure in determining which patients with AA should receive systemic CS (1,68,70). Systemic CS primarily works by regulation of genes and subsequent protein synthesis. This likely explains the significant lag time of at least six hours before objective changes in PF are measurable (82–85). Management issues surrounding systemic steroid therapy include the preferred route of administration, the role of their early application in the emergency room, and their optimal dose.

There appears to be no difference in effect when steroids are given orally as opposed to intravenously for the majority of patients with asthma of moderate severity (86,87). This equivalence prompted national guidelines to favor the less invasive use of oral therapy (1). The role of early CS use upon entry into the acute setting is much more controversial. Confounders to consensus on this topic result from wide dosing differences and endpoint assessment among pertinent investigations (31). Results of a recent meta-analysis assessing early administration of steroids in the ED concluded that two groups were more likely to benefit if this therapy were given within the first hour: the more severe asthmatics and those who were steroid naïve on ED entry (88).

Whether a larger dose of systemic steroids improves outcomes or PFs is not certain (89,90). A review of the literature showed nonsignificant trends towards medium and high doses being more efficacious than low doses (82). National guidelines recommend that 120–180 mg/day of prednisolone, prednisone, or methylprednisolone be given divided over three to four doses for the first 48 hours of management. On subsequent days,

60–80 mg should be continued with the goal of therapy being a PEF at 70% of predicted (1).

Continuation of corticosteroid therapy for AA after achieving recovery is aimed at reducing relapses (91). The optimal length of therapy is unclear, but the dose of 40 mg of prednisone a day divided over two doses for 3 to 10 days is the current expert panel recommendation (1). The short end of this range can be utilized if all components of outpatient therapy and monitoring are optimally in place (92). The proper tapering technique also has no consensus recommendation, but evidence exists that it can be rapid (93,94). Limited data support the use of intramuscular steroids at the time of ED discharge (95). Although not incorporated as an option in the national guidelines (1), depot methylprednisolone led to similar rates of relapse of AA as seen in a group of patients discharged from the ED with oral methylprednisolone (96). This alternative is attractive if patient compliance is an issue.

Another modality of steroid delivery for patients with AA that has sparked recent investigation is the inhaled route. High-dose, inhaled steroids may create measurable immediate benefit by causing local vasoconstriction and thereby reducing airway edema (97). In addition, these agents may potentiate the benefit of inhaled β_2-agonists (98). Recent meta-analyses have reviewed studies on the role of ICS in the ED and upon discharge for treatment and prevention of relapse in AA. The most recent report by Edmonds et al. (99) in the Cochrane Database Review concludes that while in the ED, ICS use may reduce admissions to the hospital, but there is inconclusive evidence that it adds any benefit to concomitant use with systemic steroids. Rodrigo and Rodrigo (100) demonstrated that the addition of high-dose ICS to standard regimens of inhaled β_2-agonists and ipratroprium in the ED improved PFs and was associated with a trend towards reduction in hospitalization rates, but in this investigation no comparison of this "triple inhaler" therapy to a schedule including systemic steroid administration was made. Edmonds et al. (101) also reviewed ICS use at the time of ED discharge and cautiously reported potential benefit in a subgroup of mild asthmatics.

At the present time, there is little convincing evidence that argues for the replacement of systemic steroids in the armamentarium of AA treatment with high-dose ICS. ED investigations for ICS most often require every 10-minute administration of ICS with a spacer device. Further investigation is needed to clarify the role of ICS in AA.

D. Anticholinergics

Ipratropium bromide (IP) is the primary inhaled anticholinergic used in the treatment of AA. The bronchodilator effect is not as pronounced as that achieved by β_2-agonists (102). The majority of effect occurs within 30 minutes with duration of action around six hours (103). Importantly, routine use of this agent has been associated with virtually no side effect (103,104).

The results of a large RCT done by Rodrigo and Rodrigo showed that addition of IP to albuterol therapy in an ED was accompanied by improved PF and a lower rate of hospitalization (105). The patients that received the most advantage were those who had more severe disease. One important reason this study showed such significant benefit while others prior had not may lie in the high dosing regimen used by these investigators. Confirming these benefits, several recent meta-analyses have concluded the above advantageous effects associated with the addition of anticholinergic agents to conventional β_2-agonist therapy (106,107). Similar findings in hospitalization rate and PF among pediatric patients have been demonstrated (108,109).

Consensus guidelines recommend the addition of IP in AA patients with more severe obstruction (1,110). Administration of high doses is appropriate in these cases. Either four puffs every 10 minutes from an MDI with a spacer or 0.5 mg of nebulized ipratroprium every 20 minutes constitutes high dosage (107). Because of differences in its muscarinic receptor selectivity and duration of action, tiotropium may also find a role in the treatment of AA (111). To date, no prospective RCT has been conducted with this agent used in the treatment of AA.

E. IV Magnesium

Evidence for an adjunctive role for IV magnesium in the treatment of AA has been forthcoming from several studies. Many smaller studies in the past have shown modest bronchodilator properties of IV magnesium (112–115). Reduction of hospital admission from the ED has also been reported (115). Meta-analyses on the topic suggest PF improvement and lower hospitalization rates may be most pronounced in severe AA (116,117).

In 2002, Silverman et al. (118) published results of a large, multicenter, randomized, double-blinded study on the role of IV magnesium administration for severe AA. Two hundred and forty eight patients arriving in the ED with severe asthma ($FEV_1 < 30\%$ predicted) were enrolled. Magnesium or placebo was given after nebulized albuterol and 125 mg of IV methylprednisolone were administered. At four hours, PF improved significantly in the magnesium group with the largest differential benefit seen in the subgroup of patients with initial $FEV_1 < 20\%$. Admission rate to the hospital did not differ among treatment arms, but the authors state that the majority of patients refused admission when this was advised.

The national guidelines over the decade have changed to reflect the growing substantiation of purported advantages of magnesium sulfate in a select group of patients. While there was no mention of magnesium in the treatment algorithm in the 1997 statement (1), a more recent report suggests considering this therapy in patients with very severe asthma (110). The dose used by Silverman et al. (118) was 2 g infused over 10 to 15 minutes;

no important side effects were reported. Whether continuous dosing or repeated, interval administration would add any benefit is unknown. Furthermore, it remains unclear whether concomitant use of IP or inhaled steroids would lead to additive or muted effects on PF and outcome.

F. Leukotriene Antagonists

These agents, which are routinely used for the management of chronic asthma, may have a role in the acute setting as well. While having established benefits for mild asthma, use of these agents in the oral form has recently been linked to ED and hospital visits and greater asthma severity (1,119,120). Dockhorn et al. (121), have described interesting advantages of intravenous montelukast over its oral form. In their double-blind, single-dose comparison of mild to moderate asthmatics, IV montelukast had earlier PF improvement (as early as 15 minutes) and greater efficacy over oral montelukast. Both the early onset of action and higher efficacy suggested to the authors that IV montelukast may benefit AA patients.

To date, only one published report has demonstrated the benefit of IV montelukast in the setting of AA. Camargo et al. (122) showed that 7 mg of IV montelukast was beneficial over placebo in reducing subsequent β_2-agonist administration, corticosteroid use, improving PF and reducing the combined endpoints of hospitalization or prolonged ED therapy. The PF effect was seen as early as 10 minutes and no side effects were reported. Their methodology excluded patients who had a substantial response to initial β_2-agonist therapy (improvement by 20% predicted on FEV_1). This makes the use of this novel therapy potentially promising in those patients known to have poorer initial bronchodilator response (68,70,71). On the other hand, this exclusion makes it difficult to extrapolate general use of leukotriene antagonists for all patients with AA. Furthermore, benefit has to be determined among patients receiving steroids or oral leukotriene antagonists chronically. Given the favorable risk–benefit balance, IV montelukast should be considered in cases of AA that are not immediately responsive to bronchodilators. The only limitation to its routine use in the United States is its lack of availability in the intravenous form.

G. Methylxanthines

While longstanding mainstays in asthma therapy, theophylline and aminophylline have not consistently shown efficacy in the management of AA. β_2-agonists possess greater bronchodilator effect than aminophylline (53). While individual studies have shown some benefits from use of these agents, other studies have yielded negative results (123), and the results of two meta-analyses revealed no statistical effect on PF improvement (124,125). The more recent review suggests that side effects (palpitations, vomiting, etc.) predictably occur more frequently with methylxanthine use (124). Currently, there is no established role for routine use of these agents in the management of AA.

H. Antibiotics

The role for antibiotics in patients with AA needs to be tailored to their risk for exacerbating bacterial infection. It is accepted that most asthma-triggering infections are viral in nature. The latest National Institutes of Health (NIH) guidelines suggest that antibiotic use should be considered in patients with bacterial sinusitis, appropriate comorbid conditions, and the combination of "fever and purulent sputum" (110). In this updated consensus an effort was made to avoid associating high specificity with polymorphonuclear cell predominance in sputum with bacterial infection. The only pertinent RCT among adults suggests the routine use of antibiotics is not beneficial (126). Counter to this evidence is the observation that newer antibiotics (esp. macrolides) may have additional roles in asthma therapy through pathways curtailing inflammation or slowing metabolism of other antiasthma agents (127).

I. Heliox

Heliox is a mixture of oxygen with the inert gas helium. Commonly used concentrations of this agent utilize 60% to 80% helium (128). Its therapeutic benefit in asthma is attributed to lower turbulent flow in high-resistance airways secondary to its lower density compared with air–oxygen mixtures. More importantly, a low-density gas such as heliox decreases the pressure gradient required to achieve a given flow rate through turbulent airways. This effect could lead to partial attenuation of the increased work of breathing seen in the most severe cases of AA. In theory, initiation of MV could be obviated if patients progressing to respiratory failure could be stabilized with heliox as a result of its reduction in the overwhelming work of breathing, but this has not been shown to be true in prospective trials. Heliox can be delivered via a tight-fitting mask or through the inspiratory limb of a ventilator.

Manthous et al. (129) showed that initiation of heliox could lower measured PP and improve PEF. A number of studies have demonstrated a PF improvement after heliox use. In addition, greater inhaled bronchodilator delivery (130,131), improvement in oxygenation (132), and improvement of hypercapnic acidosis (133) have all been implicated with its use. Two reviews on the small amount of clinical trials have recently been simultaneously published. Rodrigo et al. determined that there was no overall PF benefit or hospital admission reduction among moderate to severe cases of AA (134). Ho et al. (135) suggested that there might be a modest, early benefit seen with heliox use that could be more substantial among the most severe cases.

Given its favorable safety profile, heliox should be considered in severe or extremely labile cases of AA (128). Its early administration, in these select cases, should be aimed at optimizing gas exchange and bronchodilator therapy and hence avoiding hospitalization and/or ETI (128). It may have a further role in mechanically ventilated patients (136). In these cases, care must be taken in evaluating ventilator settings. The less dense gaseous mixture will alter tidal volume measurement if flow meters are not recalibrated. Furthermore, the therapeutic effects of heliox may be lost after concentrations of helium are dropped below 70%. Further investigation in this area is needed (Table 1).

J. Non-invasive Ventilation

Marked increase in inspiratory and expiratory airflow obstruction leads to dynamic hyperinflation in severe AA (137) (Fig. 2). The cumulative cost of this is respiratory muscle fatigue that, along with the associated increase in dead space, may lead to hypercarbic respiratory failure. Noninvasive positive pressure ventilation (NIPPV) has been extensively reported to be beneficial in other forms of hypercapnic respiratory failure (138–142). While only a minority of patients with AA requires mechanical ventilation (143), such patients suffer significantly high morbidity. Unfortunately, the literature on NIPPV for AA treatment is fairly limited.

The goals of NIPPV in asthma are to reduce work of breathing and potentially decrease the degree of hyperinflation, with mechanical support conducted long enough for pharmacologic therapies to take effect. The former is accomplished in two ways. Application of continuous positive airway pressure (CPAP) or expiratory positive airway pressure (EPAP) when matched to the raised intrathoracic pressure seen as a consequence of dynamic hyperinflation [and assessed by the measurement of intrinsic positive end expiratory pressure (PEEP)] allows inspiratory flow to be initiated with lower intrathoracic pressure swings. This reduces the "inspiratory threshold load" on breathing in a dynamically inflated state. Adding inspiratory pressure support assists the exhausted asthmatic in generating adequate tidal volume and further reduces work of breathing and risk of progression to ventilatory failure. Furthermore, the addition of positive pressure may lead to decreased inspiratory time and extension of expiratory time; to the extent this occurs, gas trapping may be reduced.

Meduri et al. (144) reported findings associated with the early implementation of NIPPV in patients with severe asthma exacerbations. Tolerance of NIPPV was excellent. All but one of the 17 patients had improvements in gas exchange as measured by blood–gas analysis, and the majority had a reduction in respiratory and heart rate. While not a

Table 1 Overview of Pharmacotherapy

Standard therapies	
Albuterol	0.5 mL of 0.5% solution (2.5 mg) in 2.5 mL normal saline by nebulization every 20 minutes × 3 or 4–6 puffs by MDI with spacer every 10 minutes initially then every 20 minutes; for intubated patients, consider 10–15 mg/hr continuously and titrate to physiologic effect or side effects. The role of levalbuterol (1.25 mg by nebulization) as replacement for albuterol in patients with side effects is promising yet requires further validation.
Corticosteroids	Methylprednisolone/prednisone/prednisolone 120–180 mg/day over 3–4 doses for the first 48 hours, then 60–80mg/day until PF reaches 70% predicted or personal best.
Oxygen	1–3 L/min by nasal cannula; titrate using pulse oximeter to goal saturation > 90% and consider addition of humidification.
Anticholinergics	Ipratropium bromide 0.5 mg by nebulization every 20 minutes or 4–8 puffs by MDI with spacer as frequently as every 10 minutes initially. (Used in addition to β-agonist, not as first line therapy.)
Adjunctive therapies for consideration in severe acute asthma	
Magnesium	2 gm IV over 10–15 minutes along with standard therapy. Benefit is seen in patients with PF < 20% of predicted.
Montelukast (IV)	7 mg IV along with standard therapy. Benefit may beseen in patients who do not have substantial PF improvement with initial standard therapy.
Heliox	80:20, 70:30, or 60:40 helium:oxygen. Higher helium concentrations are needed for optimal effect.
Antibiotics	Use in patients with bacterial sinusitis or patients with appropriate comorbid conditions and fever with purulent sputum.
Theophylline	5 mg/kg intravenously over 30 minutes loading dose in patients not receiving theophylline followed by 0.4 mg/kg/hr intravenous maintenance dose. Check serum level within 6 hours of loading dose. Watch for drug interactions and disease states that alter clearance rates.
Epinephrine	0.3–0.5 mL of a 1:1,000 solution subcutaneously every 20 minutes × 3; terbutaline (0.25 mL) is favored in pregnant patients when parenteral therapy is indicated.Use with caution in patients older than 40 years of ageand in patients with coronary artery disease.

Source: Adapted from Ref. 16.

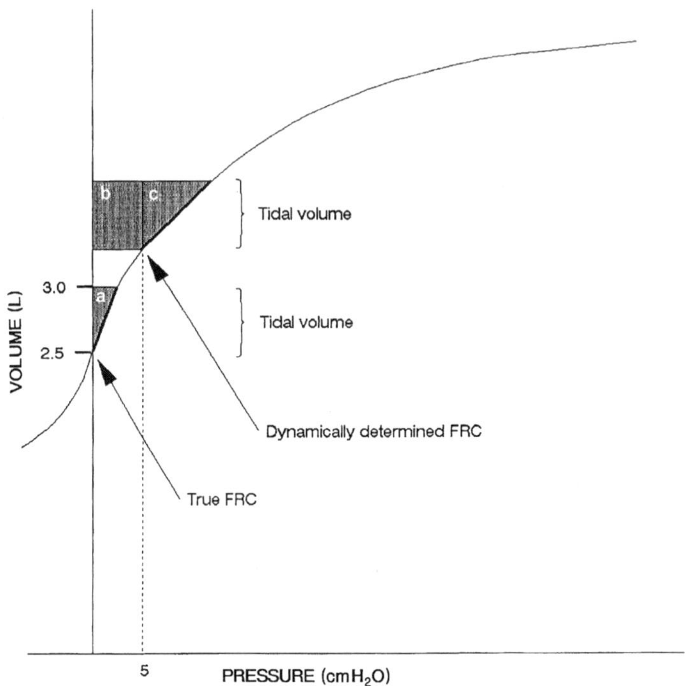

Figure 2 Dynamic hyperinflation significantly increases the work of breathing. In the absence of hyperinflation, a person taking a 0.5 L breath at the usual functional residual capacity (FRC) expends a workload equal to the shaded area (*a*). As a consequence of incomplete alveolar emptying due to limitation in airflow, asthmatic patients may begin inspiration at a less advantageous FRC. At this *dynamically determined FRC*, the work of breathing is the sum of the energy expended to bring alveolar pressures below zero (*shaded area b*) and the workload at a less compliant portion of the pressure-volume curve (*shaded area c*). *Source*: From Ref. 137.

randomized or blinded study, the patients who received NIPPV received less sedation and had a shorter length of ICU and hospital stay than a cohort of intubated, mechanically ventilated patients.

More recently, Soroksky et al. (145) showed in a prospective, randomized study that the implementation of bi-level, nasal NIPPV in the ED improved both PF in the short term and reduced hospitalization rates. Their control group included 15 patients who also wore nasally fitted masks but received sham therapy at 1 cm of IPAP and EPAP through tubing that was purposefully interrupted. Notably, inhaled therapies were administered to both intervention and control groups during brief periods of mask ventilation. This methodology allowed the investigators to evaluate the direct benefits of NIPPV use and avoid any potentially conflicting profit related to greater bronchodilator delivery with NIPPV-administered breaths.

The growing body of evidence suggests that the use of NIPPV can be attempted in AA and respiratory embarrassment. Caution should be employed in selecting appropriate patients for this ventilation modality as not all patient populations are ideal candidates for NIPPV. Patients with excessive oral secretions, recent upper airway or GI surgery, and patients who are uncooperative should not be treated with NIPPV. In addition, hemodynamic instability and inability to protect the airway are further contraindications to initiating mask ventilation (139) (Table 2). Close attention to worsening respiratory status and the need for escalation to controlled ETI is imperative if NIPPV is attempted.

Initiating NIPPV requires first fitting the mask to allow the most minimal air leak possible. Evidence exists that greater reduction in hypercapnia can be accomplished with the use of a full oronasal mask over nasal masks alone (146). Patient comfort may be higher with nasal masks or newer helmet devices over tight oronasal mask delivery of NIPPV (146,147). Patient compliance may increase if the mask is hand-placed firmly over the nose and mouth for several minutes to allow a period of accommodation before the straps are secured around the head. The appropriate snugness of the straps should be tailored to minimize air leak yet ensure comfort. Initial inspiratory and expiratory pressure ranges are 8–10 and 4–5 cm of H_2O, respectively. Since hypoxemia is uncommon in AA, the reason to titrate expiratory pressures is to offset intrinsic PEEP (PEEPi) and ease effort of breathing (148). Inspiratory pressures should be appropriately adjusted so adequate tidal volumes ($>7\,mL/kg$) are achieved and, maybe more importantly, a low respiratory rate (<20 per minute) in order to minimize air trapping (27). Total inspiratory pressures above 20 cm of H_2O are poorly tolerated, require very tight fitting masks, and can result in skin breakdown and excessive gastric insufflation.

Lacking larger prospective RCTs, current evidence suggests that among the most severe cases of AA, a trial of several hours of NIPPV may avoid ETI and prolonged hospitalization. If embarked upon, NIPPV use should be followed with early assessment of improvement or deterioration. The use of heliox in concert with NIPPV has not been thoroughly

Table 2 Contraindications to NIPPV

After respiratory arrest
Medically unstable
Unable to protect airway
Excessive secretions
Uncooperative or agitated
Recent airway or gastrointestinal surgery

Source: From Ref. 139.

investigated, but both expert opinion and anecdotal experiences seem to favor the use of this low-risk, adjunctive therapy if a brief trial is rapidly feasible.

V. ED Disposition

Clinical assessment along with serial objective PF measurement can be used to determine patient disposition from the ED to home, a medical ward, or the ICU. National guidelines utilize three categories of PF that, along with a patient's clinical picture, can be used to guide patient assignment. Good, intermediate, and poor responses are defined as PF values of >80%, 50% to 79%, and <50% of predicted values (1). In practice, observational data suggests that adherence to these strict objective criteria is poor with discharge home often occurring at a far lower value of PF. As previously noted, early response to aggressive therapy portends a greater chance for discharge. This early discriminatory tool may help delineate patients who are responsive to bronchodilatation from those that need additional protracted anti-inflammatory therapy. A final ingredient in disposition planning is assessment of confounding comorbid disease, including psychological factors and socioeconomic issues.

Patients with rapid and significant improvement of PFs and clinical symptoms should be discharged home after a sufficient observational period time from the last administered therapy ($\geq$30 minutes) ensures adequate clinical stability. Paramount ingredients to avoiding relapses include arrangement of close follow-up (within a week), ensuring patient comprehension of prescribed medication regimens, and the institution of an action plan that clearly outlines severity criteria that would prompt immediate return to medical supervision. While the majority of AA patients should be sent home on a course of steroids, a group of immediate responders may require little to no systemic CS. All patients who are discharged after an episode of AA should be transitioned to chronic anti-inflammatory therapy (i.e., inhaled CS).

VI. Hospital Ward Care

An observational period in a hospital ward is appropriate for slower, intermediate responders to ED care or after an ICU stay for the poorest responders to initial care. In addition, patients with limited access to care, concomitant psychiatric pathology, or significant cardiac comorbidity may benefit from ward admission. Pharmacologic mainstays on the wards are β-agonists, supplemental oxygen, and systemic CS. These cases of asthma likely represent a more progressive inflammatory pathogenesis pattern. Besides attention to barotrauma and nosocomial complications, ward care can be focused on untethering social barriers to medical access and reinvestigating the differential diagnosis of recurrent cases of AA. Home discharge criteria and considerations are similar to those previously discussed.

VII. ICU Care

A. ICU Admission

Admission to the ICU with SAA occurs most commonly for management of established or progressing respiratory failure. Patients with severe airflow obstruction who fail to improve significantly (final ED PF < 40% predicted) or those who continue to deteriorate despite aggressive medical therapy should be admitted to the ICU. If NIPPV has been initiated in the ED without an early dramatic reversal of clinical parameters, further monitoring in the ICU in anticipation of possible ETI is appropriate. Unfortunately, the easiest cases to triage to the ICU include patients who suffer a course of progressive obtundation or cardiorespiratory collapse.

Only a minority of all patients that present with AA require ETI. Once in the ICU, the occurrence of this therapy rises dramatically with reported incidences varying widely from 2% to 70% (31). Pooled averages from studies over the last three decades of the 20th century (31) correlate with recently published epidemiological data suggesting between 30% and 60% of ICU admissions (149,150) require ETI. While considered a life-saving therapy, ETI is associated with higher mortality rates and a number of accompanying morbidities, including barotraumas (151), hypotension, nosocomial infection, and neuromuscular disease (152).

When to proceed to ETI and invasive ventilation remains a crucial clinical judgment. The immediate requirement of ETI is clear in those patients who suffer cardiorespiratory arrest or obtundation prior to ICU or ED presentation. Elective intubation should be performed in those patients who report being or subjectively appear to be exhausted; in patients who are failing NIPPV; and in anyone who has evidence of worsening cardiorespiratory status (e.g., a fall in peak flows or PP without clinical improvement in RR, accessory muscle use or a falling arterial pH) (16,153). Normocarbia or hypercarbia can be helpful measures of respiratory system fatigue in some patients with AA, but these findings alone in the absence of clinical worsening or a falling pH rarely proceed to ETI (143).

B. Intubation

Whenever possible, time should be taken to discuss the role and consequences of ETI with the patient. ETI should be done by, or under the guidance of, an experienced airway clinician. Laryngospasm and bronchospasm are well-recognized costs of excessive airway manipulation. While there is no consensus on the route (oral vs. nasal) for intubating the AA patient, it is the opinion of these authors that oral intubation is the preferred method. This technique allows for the larger endotracheal tubes (ETTs), avoids nasal polyps, decreases the incidence of sinusitis (154), and may be performed more expediently. Larger ETTs are preferred as they add less resistance to the respiratory circuit and allow for more aggressive treatment of the asthmatic's mucous secretions (16).

In almost all cases, quick-onset sedative agents can be used for anesthetic induction prior to intubation. Rapid-sequence induction should be utilized in unstable patients that require optimal conditions for expedient airway control. The cost of this technique is the short-term use of a paralytic agent, which for reasons discussed below should be avoided whenever possible. Commonly used sedative agents prior to intubation include midazolam, thiopental, propofol, and ketamine. All of these agents have the rapid onset properties required during the peri-intubation period. Furthermore, continuous infusions of these agents (except thiopental) can be administered to assist in achieving the goals of mechanical ventilation successfully (16).

Hypotension frequently coincides with the initiation of mechanical ventilation (155). Mechanisms for this effect often include one or more of the following: hypovolemia, sedative effect, barotrauma (i.e., pneumothorax or pneumomediastinum), and decreased venous return secondary to dynamic hyperinflation (156,157). This last mechanism deserves underscoring as this often avoidable morbidity is frequently not entertained early during the acute intervention for hypotension. In fact, there is a robust literature implicating cessation of aggressive resuscitation or ventilation in obstructed patients leading to a "Lazarus syndrome" or spontaneous return of circulation (158–160). Care should be taken to avoid overaggressive Ambu-bag ventilation that may increase PEEPi. Vigorous volume challenge should be the first response to a drop in blood pressure. Concomitantly, while administering 100% oxygen, delivered minute volumes should be minimized or ventilation temporarily discontinued (60 to 90 seconds, an "apnea test") (156). Persistent hypotension should provoke a radiographic search for a tension pneumothorax.

C. Ventilator Management

The overall goals of MV are to provide adequate ventilatory support and reduce work of breathing to the tired asthmatic until time and ongoing pharmacotherapy corrects the airway obstruction. In cases of severe asthma, strategies aimed at minimizing hyperinflation have been shown to be beneficial. To this end, lowering minute volume (V_e), decreasing inspiratory time (T_i), and assuring patient–ventilator synchrony become the targets of therapy (161).

Both lowered V_e and shorter T_i aid in abating hyperinflation by lengthening expiratory time and prolonging alveolar emptying. The more powerful determinant of adequate airway emptying is minute ventilation.

Accordingly, attention should be specifically addressed to reduce administered tidal volumes and their frequency. Reasonable initial ventilator settings used to avoid lung hyperinflation are tidal volumes up to 8 cc/kg and respiratory rates between 10 and 12 breaths/min in a volume-control mode (162). In addition, inspiratory flow rate should be set between 70 and 100 L/min to further increase T_e (161). Setting flow rates to this level often occurs with the ventilator alarming as the set peak inspiratory pressure (PIP) alarm has been exceeded. Increasing the PIP alarm limit is the correct remedy in this situation. Achieving lower PIPs by decreasing V_t or flow rate has been shown to increase hyperinflation. Conversely, elevated PIPs at the ventilator setting described above are associated with theoretical risks of barotraumas that have never been clinically corroborated (163,164).

More useful measurements of hyperinflation and the consequent risk of barotrauma and hyperinflation include plateau pressure (P_{plat}) and PEEPi values (162). These measurements are made by implementing inspiratory and expiratory pauses and should be done when the ventilator circuit is uninterrupted by external sources of airflow, i.e., continuous nebulized therapy. Care should be taken in always discontinuing pauses programmed into the routine ventilator sequence after measurements are made. A persistent inspiratory pause will increase the I:E ratio and not only affect P_{plat} measurement but may also increase the degree of hyperinflation. Reasonable goals of P_{plat} are below 35 cmH$_2$O with even safer values below 30 cm H$_2$O (153). PEEPi measurements correlate with end-expiratory alveolar volumes, but due to heterogeneity of airway closure, a large proportion of alveolar units may not be in communication with the ventilator at the time of this measurement. This phenomenon likely explains the cases of underestimation of hyperinflation by PEEPi measurements (165,166).

A more accurate measurement of dynamic hyperinflation can be made by quantifying the amount of gas collected from end inspiration during a period of prolonged apnea (up to 60 seconds). This value, end-inspiratory lung volume or V_{EI}, was termed and validated by Tuxen et al. (163,167). While V_{EI} is predictably more prognostic of hypotension than PEEPi measurements, it is more difficult to routinely measure and may more frequently require paralytic use to obtain (Fig. 3).

When ventilation is completely controlled, the addition of ventilator circuit PEEP may worsen hyperinflation (168). In tenuous cases of SAA, sedation should be used to ablate patient-triggered breaths and ventilator PEEP should be set to zero (27). It has been argued that potentially beneficial effects of ventilator administered PEEP are seen as a result of dilating previously collapsed airways, hence allowing improved gas exchange (169); we have not seen this theoretical effect benefit patients and do not employ machine PEEP during the early stabilization of an asthmatic on the ventilator. As patients are aroused from induced coma and resume triggering

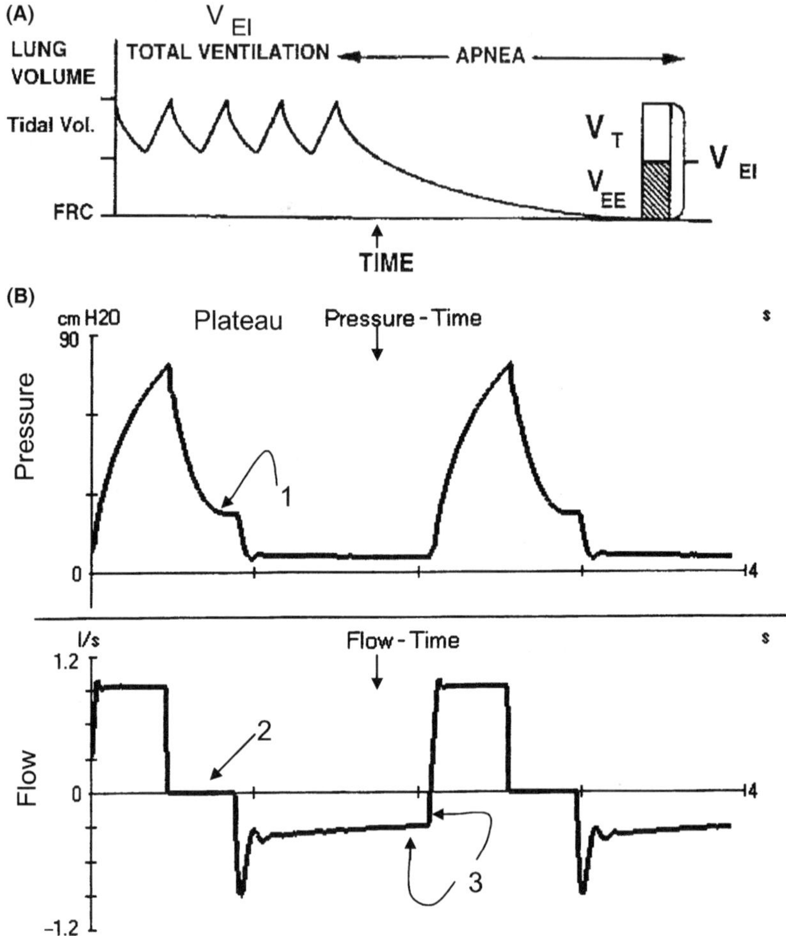

Figure 3 Measurements of dynamic hyperinflation. *Panel* (**A**): Described by Tuxen et al., end-inspiratory lung volume, VEI, can be measured during a prolonged apnea at the conclusion of a tidal volume delivery. *Panel* (**B**): An easier measurement, plateau pressure (P_{plat}) (*arrow 1*), can be determined by temporarily incorporating an end inspiratory pause into the ventilator circuit (*arrow 2*). Another clue to the presence of hyperinflation is persistent end-expiratory flow in this example (*arrow 3*). The magnitude of the auto-PEEP or PEEPi can be quantified by an end-expiratory pause maneuver (not shown). *Source*: Panel B provided by G. A. Schmidt.

breaths on the ventilator, prudent use of PEEP should be considered. At this time airflow obstruction has improved significantly, if not completely resolved, and administered PEEP may be acceptable if kept below PEEPi and its addition does not adversely affect measurements of hyperinflation (169,170).

D. Sedation

The initial mechanical ventilation settings and subsequent pressure measurements detailed above require a largely passive patient without the usual dyspnea accompanying asthma itself, intubation, and the emergence of permissive hypercapnea. To assure this level of control during a disease process that is associated with significant patient discomfort, adequate sedative administration becomes imperative. As mentioned above, short-acting benzodiazepines, and the parenterally administered anesthetics, propofol and ketamine, are the sedative agents most commonly used, given their rapid onset (27).

Among the benzodiazepines, the ultra-short onset of midazolam makes it the most common agent of this class used in the authors' ICU. Other advantageous features of midazolam and other benzodiazepines include their amnestic and anxiolytic properties. At higher doses respiratory depression can occur and may be beneficial in achieving purposeful hypoventilation (discussed below). Metabolism is slowed by poor hepatic function that delays conjugation and by renal dysfunction that leads to accumulation of the less active conjugated metabolites (171).

Propofol has become another mainstay in the sedative management of the intubated asthmatic. In addition to its rapid onset, propofol's quick offset properties allow for very adjustable titration of sedation effect. Attributable hypotension results from high doses of continuous infusion or during induction phases of anesthesia. Certain patients develop hypertriglyceridemia with prolonged propofol administration, and a high dosage of the drug given in this manner has been linked to fatalities among children. Its metabolism is not significantly delayed by hepatic or renal impairment (171).

Both midazolam and propofol can be successfully used to accomplish the goals of ventilator management detailed above (172). While both agents have comparable respiratory depressive effects with bolus administration, it appears that with ongoing, continuous use, the level of respiratory control is attenuated with propofol (173). On the other hand, comparative studies between the two agents reveal a predictably shorter time to awakening after propofol discontinuation (174–177). Duration of mechanical ventilation may not be appreciably different with either agent if a standard practice of daily sedative interruption is employed to avoid cumulative effects of midazolam infusion (178,179). Relative dosing requirements between these agents have not been described for the practice of PH detailed below.

Ketamine is a unique anesthetic that, in addition to its rapid onset and respiratory depressive effects, may have the added advantage of a direct bronchodilator effect (180,181). This airway effect has not been shown to be clinically additive to standard pharmacologic therapies employed with asthmatics (182). In addition, the catecholamine surge thought to be responsible for this result also is implicated in the hypertension and tachycardia often seen after ketamine infusion. This cardiovascular profile makes ketamine administration more advisable for pediatric populations (183).

Lower sedative requirements are achievable with concomitant analgesic use. This often forgotten adjunct to the sedative cocktail is most often implemented with the narcotics, morphine or the shorter-acting fentanyl. These agents can be exploited for their additional respiratory depressant effects, if wanted (184).

E. Paralysis

The use of neuromuscular blocking agents (NMBAs) to assure complete patient–ventilator synchrony in severe acute asthmatics has been drastically reduced given the growing certainty of their connection with myopathy (185–188). Since early reports of the link between combined corticosteroid and NMBA use and neuromuscular disease, further investigation has corroborated this association regardless of the type of NMBA used (185). The risk for myopathy appears to increase with duration of NMBA administration, with the vast majority of cases resolving over several weeks after NMBA discontinuation (185,188).

Given the significant morbidity associated with their use, NMBAs should be avoided whenever possible. Avoiding paralysis may require the use of a combination of sedatives along with an analgesic. Combinations of sedatives may be employed to avoid the implementation of paralysis. If paralytic use cannot be avoided, cisatracurium is the preferred agent, given its spontaneous serum degradation. Vecuronium and pancuronium are less commonly used. Bedside nerve stimulators should be employed to avoid over-titration of these agents (189). It is uncertain whether frequent NMBA infusion interruption or titration to lower level of blockade as measured by nerve stimulation will lower the risk for neuromuscular pathology.

F. Permissive Hypercapnia

Elevation of arterial pCO_2 can occur as a consequence of lowering minute volume. This allowed effect of controlled mechanical ventilation is not observed in all cases. Two physiologic effects may result in cumulative improvement of gas exchange. First, adequate sedation and unloading of fatigued respiratory muscles can lead to decreased CO_2 production. Second, and likely more pertinent, as dynamic hyperinflation is minimized, effective dead space is reduced. This result favors greater CO_2 elimination if the proportion decline in dead space overrides the opposing effect of decreased minute ventilation (16).

A strategy utilizing PH is well tolerated through most states of health and disease (190,191). Scenarios for which PH is commonly avoided are pregnancy, conditions leading to elevation in intracranial pressure, and severe cardiac dysfunction. Unfavorable effects on uterine (192,193) and intracranial blood flow (194) can lead to fetal distress or elevation in ICP, respectively. Furthermore, hypercapnic acidosis has several adverse cardiac effects, including myocardial depression and elevation in pulmonary arterial pressures (191). In most other cases, maintaining PH above 7.15 and pCO_2 below 90 mmHg are reasonable and safe limits to allowed acidosis and hypercapnia.

G. Inhaled Therapies

Along with ongoing corticosteroid therapy, inhaled bronchodilator treatment should be continued in the ventilated patient. Therapy frequency should be titrated down as asthma severity resolves. Routes of administration remain MDI/spacer or nebulization, both through the inspiratory limb of the ventilator. Given proper MDI administration, ventilator maneuvers, and airway circuit properties, this method of therapy can be significantly more efficient than nebulized therapy (195). Yet the required ventilator manipulations are associated with significant increases in inspiratory time fraction. The consequence of this result has not been tested in patients with severe hyperinflation. Conversely, less efficient intermittent nebulizer therapy may lead to increased direct costs and the potential for higher nosocomial infection rates related to frequent interruption of the ventilator circuit (195). Due to its ease of use, continuous delivery of nebulized medication may be a preferable way to avoid the technical issues of MDI-ventilator adaptation while overcoming the inefficiency in drug dosing of intermittent nebulization.

H. Liberation from Mechanical Ventilation

A minority of mechanically ventilated patients have rapid resolution (within 24 hours) of bronchoconstriction. The remainder of patients often require from two up to seven days for resolution of obstruction (181). Additional ventilatory requirements may be minimized by early recognition and appropriate response to dynamic hyperinflation and/or pneumothoraces and protocols to reduce sedative accumulation. Once a patient is extubated, a period of observation should precede ICU discharge.

I. Potential Adjunctive Therapies

A number of pharmacologic agents and procedures have been reported to have potential benefit among asthmatics in the ICU. The most noteworthy, unproven therapy is heliox, which has already been discussed above. The infrequent incidence of intubated asthmatics and variation in the expedient availability of helium–oxygen have made it difficult to establish evidence-based efficacy of heliox in mechanically ventilated patients. A number of anecdotal reports by experts argue for a potential role for this agent in the ICU among patients ventilated via ETI or NIPPV. Other occasionally reported therapies include inhaled anesthetics and bronchoscopy.

The common inhalational anesthetics (enflurane, isoflurane, and halothane) have all been reported to have beneficial effects via smooth muscle relaxation (196–199). Limitations on the use of these agents include lack of proper expertise among medical intensivists concerning anesthetic use and the concomitant restrictions in the applicability of anesthesia ventilators with asthmatics (200). These ventilators have flow and pressure limits that can lead to inadequate tidal volumes and longer I:E ratios in severely obstructed patients (200).

Asthma has long been considered a relative risk for morbidity when considering fiberoptic bronchoscopy (FOB) due to the possibility of worsening airway reactivity (201–203). In patients with severe asthma, irreversible airflow may in part be due to the heavy airway burden of inspissated mucus and atelectasis. Case reports and anecdotal use of FOB with lavage to help with mucus disimpaction suggests a possible therapeutic role for this procedure (204–206). Further studies need to be performed to define the therapeutic index, proper patient selection, and safety in mechanically ventilated patients before advocacy of this process is possible.

J. ICU/MV Outcomes

Predictably, outcome analyses of asthmatic patients who require ICU care reveal overall worse mortality than asthmatics who avoid ICU admission. Although rare reports of no mortality have been reported by single centers (138), recent observed ICU mortality of 7% or 8% has been reported (149,150,207,208). Consistent factors that place patients at higher risk for death include older age, female sex, higher severity of illness score, CPR or anoxic insult prior to admission, and worse gas-exchange parameters on admission to the ICU (149,150,208,209). There is some evidence that overall ICU mortality has decreased over time as a consequence of our greater understanding of pharmacologic options and proper mechanical ventilation strategies (207,210).

VIII. Conclusion

While overall mortality remains low, asthma cases are prevalent and contribute substantially to national health expenditures. The disproportionate majority of this cost occurs in a minority of asthmatics that suffer from episodes of AA requiring ED attention or hospitalization. Recent trends in mortality and hospitalization seem to have reached a plateau in the United States. Complete assessment of severity, full understanding of therapeutic options, and adequate transition to outpatient treatment are all components of AA care that may continue to contribute to currents favorable asthma trends.

References

1. National Asthma Education and Prevention Program. Expert Panel Report 2: Guidelines for the diagnosis and management of asthma. Bethesda, MD: National Institutes of Health, 1997:publication No. 55–4051.
2. Kolbe J, Vamos M, Fergusson W, Elkind G. Determinants of management errors in acute severe asthma. Thorax 1998; 53:14–20.
3. Salmeron S, Liard R, Elkharrat D, Muir J, Neukirch F, Ellrodt A. Asthma severity and adequacy of management in accident and emergency departments in France: a prospective study. Lancet 2001; 358:629–635.
4. Smith DH, Malone DC, Lawson KA, Okamoto LJ, Battista C, Saunders WB. A national estimate of the economic costs of asthma. Am J Respir Crit Care Med 1997; 156:787–793.
5. Weiss KB, Gergen PJ, Hodgson TA. An economic evaluation of asthma in the United States. N Engl J Med 1992; 326:862–866.
6. Evans R III, Mullally DI, Wilson RW, Gergen PJ, Rosenberg HM, Grauman JS, Chevarley FM, Feinleib M. National trends in the morbidity and mortality of asthma in the US. Prevalence, hospitalization and death from asthma over two decades: 1965–1984. Chest 1987; 91:65S–74S.
7. Asthma mortality and hospitalization among children and young adults—United States, 1980–1993. MMWR Morb Mortal Wkly Rep 1996; 45:350–353.
8. Mannino DM, Homa DM, Pertowski CA, Ashizawa A, Nixon LL, Johnson CA, Ball LB, Jack E, Kang DS. Surveillance for asthma—United States, 1960–1995. MMWR CDC Surveill Summ 1998; 47:1–27.
9. Mannino DM, Homa DM, Akinbami LJ, Moorman JE, Gwynn C, Redd SC. Surveillance for asthma—United States, 1980–1999. MMWR Surveill Summ 2002; 51:1–13.
10. Early Release of Selected Estimates Based on Data From the January–June 2003. National Health Interview Survey: National Health Interview Survey, 2003.
11. Smith D, Weiss K, Sullivan S. Epidemiology and costs of acute asthma. In: In: Hall JB, ed. Acute Asthma: Assessment and Management. New York: McGraw-Hill Medical Publishing Division, 2000:1–10.
12. Sly RM. Continuing decreases in asthma mortality in the United States. Ann All Asthma Immunol 2004; 92:313–318.
13. Sly RM. Decreases in asthma mortality in the United States. Ann All Asthma Immunol 2000; 85:121–127.
14. Rodrigo G, Rodrigo C. Assessment of the patient with acute asthma in the emergency department. A factor analytic study. Chest 1993; 104:1325–1328.
15. Nannini L. Morbidity and mortality from acute asthma. In: Hall JB, ed. Acute Asthma: Assessment and Management. New York: McGraw-Hill Medical Publishing Division, 2000:11–28.
16. Corbridge TC, Hall JB. The assessment and management of adults with status asthmaticus. Am J Respir Crit Care Med 1995; 151:1296–1316.
17. Brenner BE, Abraham E, Simon RR. Position and diaphoresis in acute asthma. Am J Med 1983; 74:1005–1009.

18. Pearson MG, Spence DP, Ryland I, Harrison BD. Value of pulsus paradoxus in assessing acute severe asthma. British Thoracic Society Standards of Care Committee. BMJ 1993; 307:659.

19. Rodrigo G, Rodrigo C. Emergency department assessment: severity and outcome prediction. In: Hall JB, ed. Acute Asthma: Assessment and Management. New York: McGraw-Hill Medical Publishing Division, 2000:125–138.

20. Nowak RM, Pensler MI, Sarkar DD, Anderson JA, Kvale PA, Ortiz AE, Tomlanovich MC. Comparison of peak expiratory flow and FEV1 admission criteria for acute bronchial asthma. Ann Emerg Med 1982; 11:64–69.

21. Rodrigo G, Rodrigo C. A new index for early prediction of hospitalization in patients with acute asthma. Am J Emerg Med 1997; 15:8–13.

22. Rodrigo G, Rodrigo C. Early prediction of poor response in acute asthma patients in the emergency department. Chest 1998; 114:1016–1021.

23. Sherman S, Skoney JA, Ravikrishnan KP. Routine chest radiographs in exacerbations of chronic obstructive pulmonary disease. Diagnostic value. Arch Intern Med 1989; 149:2493–2496.

24. White CS, Cole RP, Lubetsky HW, Austin JH. Acute asthma: admission chest radiography in hospitalized adult patients. Chest 1991; 100:14–16.

25. Carruthers DM, Harrison BD. Arterial blood gas analysis or oxygen saturation in the assessment of acute asthma? Thorax 1995; 50:186–188.

26. Hardern R. Oxygen saturation in adults with acute asthma. J Accid Emerg Med 1996; 13:28–30.

27. Rodrigo GJ, Rodrigo C, Hall JB. Acute asthma in adults: a review. Chest 2004; 125:1081–1102.

28. Cygan J, Trunsky M, Corbridge T. Inhaled heroin-induced status asthmaticus: five cases and a review of the literature. Chest 2000; 117:272–275.

29. Rome LA, Lippmann ML, Dalsey WC, Taggart P, Pomerantz S. Prevalence of cocaine use and its impact on asthma exacerbation in an urban population. Chest 2000; 117:1324–1329.

30. Krantz AJ, Hershow RC, Prachand N, Hayden DM, Franklin C, Hryhorczuk DO. Heroin insufflation as a trigger for patients with life-threatening asthma. Chest 2003; 123:510–517.

31. McFadden ER Jr, Acute severe asthma. Am J Respir Crit Care Med 2003; 168:740–759.

32. NHLBI/WHO workshop Report. Global Strategy for Asthma Management and Prevention. Vol. 2002. Bethesda, MD: National Institutes of Health, 2002:publication No. 02–3659.

33. Picado C. Aspirin intolerance and nasal polyposis. Curr All Asthma Rep 2002; 2:488–493.

34. Castillo JA, Picado C. Prevalence of aspirin intolerance in asthmatics treated in a hospital. Respiration 1986; 50:153–157.

35. Picado C, Castillo JA, Montserrat JM, Agusti-Vidal A. Aspirin-intolerance as a precipitating factor of life-threatening attacks of asthma requiring mechanical ventilation. Eur Respir J 1989; 2:127–129.

36. Dias MA, Biedlingmaier JF. Ketorlac-induced status asthmaticus after endoscopic sinus surgery in a patient with Samter's triad. Otolaryngol Head Neck Surg 1997; 117:S176–S178.

37. Katayama N, Fujimura M, Kasahara K, Yasui M, Kita T, Abo M, Yoshimi Y, Nishitsuji M, Nomura S, Nakao S. A case of broncho-pulmonary aspergillosis complicated by bronchial asthma attack. Nihon Kokyuki Gakkai Zasshi 2003; 41:Abstract only.
38. Noth I, Strek ME, Leff AR. Churg-Strauss syndrome. Lancet 2003; 361: 587–594.
39. Hollingsworth HM. Wheezing and stridor. Clin Chest Med 1987; 8:231–240.
40. Murray DM, Lawler PG. All that wheezes is not asthma. Paradoxical vocal cord movement presenting as severe acute asthma requiring ventilatory support. Anaesthesia 1998; 53:1006–1011.
41. Bahrainwala AH, Simon MR. Wheezing and vocal cord dysfunction mimicking asthma. Curr Opin Pulm Med 2001; 7:8–13.
42. Kallenbach JM, Frankel AH, Lapinsky SE, Thornton AS, Blott JA, Smith C, Feldman C, Zwi S. Determinants of near fatality in acute severe asthma. Am J Med 1993; 95:265–272.
43. Campbell DA, McLennan G, Coates JR, Frith PA, Latimer KM, Luke CG, Martin AJ, Roder DM, Ruffin RE. A comparison of asthma deaths and near-fatal asthma attacks in South Australia. Eur Respir J 1994; 7:490–497.
44. Mitchell I, Tough SC, Semple LK, Green FH, Hessel PA. Near-fatal asthma: a population-based study of risk factors. Chest 2002; 121:1407–1413.
45. Moore BB, Wagner R, Weiss KB. A community-based study of near-fatal asthma. Ann All Asthma Immunol 2001; 86:190–195.
46. Miller TP, Greenberger PA, Patterson R. The diagnosis of potentially fatal asthma in hospitalized adults. Patient characteristics and increased severity of asthma. Chest 1992; 102:515–518.
47. Turner MO, Noertjojo K, Vedal S, Bai T, Crump S, Fitzgerald JM. Risk factors for near-fatal asthma. A case-control study in hospitalized patients with asthma. Am J Respir Crit Care Med 1998; 157:1804–1809.
48. Molfino N. Near-fatal asthma. In: Hall JB, ed. Acute Asthma: Assessment and Management. New York: McGraw-Hill Medical Publishing Division, 2000:29–48.
49. Kikuchi Y, Okabe S, Tamura G, Hida W, Homma M, Shirato K, Takishima T. Chemosensitivity and perception of dyspnea in patients with a history of near-fatal asthma. N Engl J Med 1994; 330:1329–1334.
50. Magadle R, Berar-Yanay N, Weiner P. The risk of hospitalization and near-fatal and fatal asthma in relation to the perception of dyspnea. Chest 2002; 121:329–333.
51. Rodrigo GJ, Rodrigo C. Rapid-onset asthma attack: a prospective cohort study about characteristics and response to emergency department treatment. Chest 2000; 118:1547–1552.
52. Plaza V, Serrano J, Picado C, Sanchis J. Frequency and clinical characteristics of rapid-onset fatal and near-fatal asthma. Eur Respir J 2002; 19:846–852.
53. Rossing TH, Fanta CH, Goldstein DH, Snapper JR, McFadden ER Jr. Emergency therapy of asthma: comparison of the acute effects of parenteral and inhaled sympathomimetics and infused aminophylline. Am Rev Respir Dis 1980; 122:365–371.

54. Chaieb J, Belcher N, Rees PJ. Maximum achievable bronchodilatation in asthma. Respir Med 1989; 83:497–502.

55. Wolfe JD, Yamate M, Biedermann AA, Chu TJ. Comparison of the acute cardiopulmonary effects of oral albuterol, metaproterenol, and terbutaline in asthmatics. JAMA 1985; 253:2068–2072.

56. Williams SJ, Winner SJ, Clark TJ. Comparison of inhaled and intravenous terbutaline in acute severe asthma. Thorax 1981; 36:629–631.

57. Salmeron S, Brochard L, Mal H, Tenaillon A, Henry-Amar M, Renon D, Duroux P, Simonneau G. Nebulized versus intravenous albuterol in hypercapnic acute asthma. A multicenter, double-blind, randomized study. Am J Respir Crit Care Med 1994; 149:1466–1470.

58. Travers AH, Rowe BH, Barker S, Jones A, Camargo CA Jr. The effectiveness of IV beta-agonists in treating patients with acute asthma in the emergency department: a meta-analysis. Chest 2002; 122:1200–1207.

59. Cydulka R, Davison R, Grammer L, Parker M, Mathews JT. The use of epinephrine in the treatment of older adult asthmatics. Ann Emerg Med 1988; 17:322–326.

60. Appel D, Karpel JP, Sherman M. Epinephrine improves expiratory flow rates in patients with asthma who do not respond to inhaled metaproterenol sulfate. J All Clin Immunol 1989; 84:90–98.

61. Turner MO, Patel A, Ginsburg S, FitzGerald JM. Bronchodilator delivery in acute airflow obstruction. A meta-analysis. Arch Intern Med 1997; 157:1736–1744.

62. Raimondi AC, Schottlender J, Lombardi D, Molfino NA. Treatment of acute severe asthma with inhaled albuterol delivered via jet nebulizer, metered dose inhaler with spacer, or dry powder. Chest 1997; 112:24–28.

63. Newman KB, Milne S, Hamilton C, Hall K. A comparison of albuterol administered by metered-dose inhaler and spacer with albuterol by nebulizer in adults presenting to an urban emergency department with acute asthma. Chest 2002; 121:1036–1041.

64. Rodrigo GJ, Rodrigo C. Continuous vs intermittent beta-agonists in the treatment of acute adult asthma: a systematic review with meta-analysis. Chest 2002; 122:160–165.

65. Shrestha M, Bidadi K, Gourlay S, Hayes J. Continuous vs intermittent albuterol, at high and low doses, in the treatment of severe acute asthma in adults. Chest 1996; 110:42–47.

66. Rudnitsky GS, Eberlein RS, Schoffstall JM, Mazur JE, Spivey WH. Comparison of intermittent and continuously nebulized albuterol for treatment of asthma in an urban emergency department. Ann Emerg Med 1993; 22:1842–1846.

67. Cydulka RK, McFadden ER, Sarver JH, Emerman CL. Comparison of single 7.5-mg dose treatment vs sequential multidose 2.5-mg treatments with nebulized albuterol in the treatment of acute asthma. Chest 2002; 122:1982–1987.

68. McFadden ER Jr, Strauss L, Hejal R, Galan G, Dixon L. Comparison of two dosage regimens of albuterol in acute asthma. Am J Med 1998; 105:12–17.

69. Emerman CL, Cydulka RK, McFadden ER. Comparison of 2.5 vs 7.5 mg of inhaled albuterol in the treatment of acute asthma. Chest 1999; 115:92–96.

70. Strauss L, Hejal R, Galan G, Dixon L, McFadden ER Jr. Observations on the effects of aerosolized albuterol in acute asthma. Am J Respir Crit Care Med 1997; 155:454–458.

71. Rodrigo C, Rodrigo G. Therapeutic response patterns to high and cumulative doses of salbutamol in acute severe asthma. Chest 1998; 113:593–598.

72. Nowak R. Single-isomer levalbuterol: a review of the acute data. Curr All Asthma Rep 2003; 3:172–178.

73. Nowak RM, Emerman CL, Schaefer K, Disantostefano RL, Vaickus L, Roach JM. Levalbuterol compared with racemic albuterol in the treatment of acute asthma: results of a pilot study. Am J Emerg Med 2004; 22:29–36.

74. Page CP, Morley J. Contrasting properties of albuterol stereoisomers. J All Clin Immunol 1999; 104:S31–S41.

75. Nelson HS, Bensch G, Pleskow WW, DiSantostefano R, DeGraw S, Reasner DS, Rollins TE, Rubin PD. Improved bronchodilation with levalbuterol compared with racemic albuterol in patients with asthma. J All Clin Immunol 1998; 102:943–952.

76. Rodrigo C, Rodrigo G. High-dose MDI salbutamol treatment of asthma in the ED. Am J Emerg Med 1995; 13:21–26.

77. Rodrigo G, Rodrigo C. Metered dose inhaler salbutamol treatment of asthma in the ED: comparison of two doses with plasma levels. Am J Emerg Med 1996; 14:144–150.

78. McFadden ER Jr, Lyons HA. Arterial-blood gas tension in asthma. N Engl J Med 1968; 278:1027–1032.

79. Rodrigo GJ, Rodriquez Verde M, Peregalli V, Rodrigo C. Effects of short-term 28% and 100% oxygen on PaCO2 and peak expiratory flow rate in acute asthma: a randomized trial. Chest 2003; 124:1312–1317.

80. Chien JW, Ciufo R, Novak R, Skowronksi M, Nelson J, Coreno A, McFadden ER, Jr. Uncontrolled oxygen administration and respiratory failure in acute asthma. Chest 2000; 117:728–733.

81. Moloney E, O'Sullivan S, Hogan T, Poulter LW, Burke CM. Airway dehydration: a therapeutic target in asthma? Chest 2002; 121:1806–1811.

82. Rodrigo G, Rodrigo C. Corticosteroids in the emergency department therapy of acute adult asthma: an evidence-based evaluation. Chest 1999; 116:285–295.

83. McFadden ER Jr, Kiser R, deGroot WJ, Holmes B, Kiker R, Viser G. A controlled study of the effects of single doses of hydrocortisone on the resolution of acute attacks of asthma. Am J Med 1976; 60:52–59.

84. Fanta CH, Rossing TH, McFadden ER Jr. Glucocorticoids in acute asthma. A critical controlled trial. Am J Med 1983; 74:845–851.

85. Sue MA, Kwong FK, Klaustermeyer WB. A comparison of intravenous hydrocortisone, methylprednisolone, and dexamethasone in acute bronchial asthma. Ann All 1986; 56:406–409.

86. Jonsson S, Kjartansson G, Gislason D, Helgason H. Comparison of the oral and intravenous routes for treating asthma with methylprednisolone and theophylline. Chest 1988; 94:723–726.

87. Ratto D, Alfaro C, Sipsey J, Glovsky MM, Sharma OP. Are intravenous corticosteroids required in status asthmaticus? JAMA 1988; 260:527–529.

88. Rowe BH, Spooner CH, Ducharme FM, Bretzlaff JA, Bota GW. Early emergency department treatment of acute asthma with systemic corticosteroids. Cochrane Database Syst Rev 2001:CD002178.

89. Emerman CL, Cydulka RK. A randomized comparison of 100-mg vs 500-mg dose of methylprednisolone in the treatment of acute asthma. Chest 1995; 107:1559–1563.

90. Haskell RJ, Wong BM, Hansen JE. A double-blind, randomized clinical trial of methylprednisolone in status asthmaticus. Arch Intern Med 1983; 143: 1324–1327.

91. Rowe BH, Spooner CH, Ducharme FM, Bretzlaff JA, Bota GW. Corticosteroids for preventing relapse following acute exacerbations of asthma. Cochrane Database Syst Rev 2001:CD000195.

92. Jones AM, Munavvar M, Vail A, Aldridge RE, Hopkinson L, Rayner C, O'Driscoll BR. Prospective, placebo-controlled trial of 5 vs 10 days of oral prednisolone in acute adult asthma. Respir Med 2002; 96:950–954.

93. Lederle FA, Pluhar RE, Joseph AM, Niewoehner DE. Tapering of corticosteroid therapy following exacerbation of asthma. A randomized, double-blind, placebo-controlled trial. Arch Intern Med 1987; 147:2201–2203.

94. O'Driscoll BR, Kalra S, Wilson M, Pickering CA, Carroll KB, Woodcock AA. Double-blind trial of steroid tapering in acute asthma. Lancet 1993; 341: 324–327.

95. McNamara RM, Rubin JM. Intramuscular methylprednisolone acetate for the prevention of relapse in acute asthma. Ann Emerg Med 1993; 22:1829–1835.

96. Hoffman IB, Fiel SB. Oral vs repository corticosteroid therapy in acute asthma. Chest 1988; 93:11–13.

97. Brieva JL, Danta I, Wanner A. Effect of an inhaled glucocorticosteroid on airway mucosal blood flow in mild asthma. Am J Respir Crit Care Med 2000; 161:293–296.

98. Kumar SD, Brieva JL, Danta I, Wanner A. Transient effect of inhaled fluticasone on airway mucosal blood flow in subjects with and without asthma. Am J Respir Crit Care Med 2000; 161:918–921.

99. Edmonds ML, Camargo CA Jr, Pollack CV Jr, Rowe BH. Early use of inhaled corticosteroids in the emergency department treatment of acute asthma. Cochrane Database Syst Rev 2003:CD002308.

100. Rodrigo GJ, Rodrigo C. Triple inhaled drug protocol for the treatment of acute severe asthma. Chest 2003; 123:1908–1915.

101. Edmonds ML, Camargo CA Jr, Brenner BE, Rowe BH. Replacement of oral corticosteroids with inhaled corticosteroids in the treatment of acute asthma following emergency department discharge: a meta-analysis. Chest 2002; 121:1798–1805.

102. Gross NJ, Skorodin MS. Anticholinergic, antimuscarinic bronchodilators. Am Rev Respir Dis 1984; 129:856–870.

103. Gross NJ. Ipratropium bromide. N Engl J Med 1988; 319:486–494.

104. Cugell DW. Clinical pharmacology and toxicology of ipratropium bromide. Am J Med 1986; 81:18–22.

105. Rodrigo GJ, Rodrigo C. First-line therapy for adult patients with acute asthma receiving a multiple-dose protocol of ipratropium bromide plus albu-

terol in the emergency department. Am J Respir Crit Care Med 2000; 161:1862–1868.

106. Stoodley RG, Aaron SD, Dales RE. The role of ipratropium bromide in the emergency management of acute asthma exacerbation: a metaanalysis of randomized clinical trials. Ann Emerg Med 1999; 34:8–18.

107. Rodrigo GJ, Rodrigo C. The role of anticholinergics in acute asthma treatment: an evidence-based evaluation. Chest 2002; 121:1977–1987.

108. Osmond MH, Klassen TP. Efficacy of ipratropium bromide in acute childhood asthma: a meta-analysis. Acad Emerg Med 1995; 2:651–656.

109. Plotnick LH, Ducharme FM. Acute asthma in children and adolescents: should inhaled anticholinergics be added to beta(2)-agonists? Am J Respir Med 2003; 2:109–115.

110. National Asthma Education and Prevention Program. Expert panel report: guidelines for the diagnosis and management of asthma update on selected topics—2002. J All Clin Immunol 2002; 110:S141–S219.

111. O'Connor BJ, Towse LJ, Barnes PJ. Prolonged effect of tiotropium bromide on methacholine-induced bronchoconstriction in asthma. Am J Respir Crit Care Med 1996; 154:876–880.

112. Sharma SK, Bhargava A, Pande JN. Effect of parenteral magnesium sulfate on pulmonary functions in bronchial asthma. J Asthma 1994; 31: 109–115.

113. Okayama H, Aikawa T, Okayama M, Sasaki H, Mue S, Takishima T. Bronchodilating effect of intravenous magnesium sulfate in bronchial asthma. JAMA 1987; 257:1076–1078.

114. Noppen M, Vanmaele L, Impens N, Schandevyl W. Bronchodilating effect of intravenous magnesium sulfate in acute severe bronchial asthma. Chest 1990; 97:373–376.

115. Skobeloff EM, Spivey WH, McNamara RM, Greenspon L. Intravenous magnesium sulfate for the treatment of acute asthma in the emergency department. JAMA 1989; 262:1210–1213.

116. Alter HJ, Koepsell TD, Hilty WM. Intravenous magnesium as an adjuvant in acute bronchospasm: a meta-analysis. Ann Emerg Med 2000; 36:191–197.

117. Rowe BH, Bretzlaff JA, Bourdon C, Bota GW, Camargo CA Jr. Intravenous magnesium sulfate treatment for acute asthma in the emergency department: a systematic review of the literature. Ann Emerg Med 2000; 36:181–190.

118. Silverman RA, Osborn H, Runge J, Gallagher EJ, Chiang W, Feldman J, Gaeta T, Freeman K, Levin B, Mancherje N, Scharf S. IV magnesium sulfate in the treatment of acute severe asthma: a multicenter randomized controlled trial. Chest 2002; 122:489–497.

119. Suissa S, Dennis R, Ernst P, Sheehy O, Wood-Dauphinee S. Effectiveness of the leukotriene receptor antagonist zafirlukast for mild-to-moderate asthma. A randomized, double-blind, placebo-controlled trial. Ann Intern Med 1997; 126: 177–183.

120. Snyder L, Blanc PD, Katz PP, Yelin EH, Eisner MD. Leukotriene modifier use and asthma severity: how is a new medication being used by adults with asthma? Arch Intern Med 2004; 164:617–622.

121. Dockhorn RJ, Baumgartner RA, Leff JA, Noonan M, Vandormael K, Stricker W, Weinland DE, Reiss TF. Comparison of the effects of intravenous and oral montelukast on airway function: a double blind, placebo controlled, three period, crossover study in asthmatic patients. Thorax 2000; 55:260–265.

122. Camargo CA Jr, Smithline HA, Malice MP, Green SA, Reiss TF. A randomized controlled trial of intravenous montelukast in acute asthma. Am J Respir Crit Care Med 2003; 167:528–533.

123. Wrenn K, Slovis CM, Murphy F, Greenberg RS. Aminophylline therapy for acute bronchospastic disease in the emergency room. Ann Intern Med 1991; 115:241–247.

124. Parameswaran K, Belda J, Rowe BH. Addition of intravenous aminophylline to beta2-agonists in adults with acute asthma. Cochrane Database Syst Rev 2000:CD002742.

125. Littenberg B. Aminophylline treatment in severe, acute asthma. A meta-analysis. JAMA 1988; 259:1678–1684.

126. Graham VA, Milton AF, Knowles GK, Davies RJ. Routine antibiotics in hospital management of acute asthma. Lancet 1982; 1:418–420.

127. Beuther DA, Martin RJ. Antibiotics in asthma. Curr All Asthma Rep 2004; 4:132–138.

128. Kass JE. Heliox redux. Chest 2003; 123:673–676.

129. Manthous CA, Hall JB, Caputo MA, Walter J, Klocksieben JM, Schmidt GA, Wood LD. Heliox improves pulsus paradoxus and peak expiratory flow in nonintubated patients with severe asthma. Am J Respir Crit Care Med 1995; 151:310–314.

130. Kress JP, Noth I, Gehlbach BK, Barman N, Pohlman AS, Miller A, Morgan S, Hall JB. The utility of albuterol nebulized with heliox during acute asthma exacerbations. Am J Respir Crit Care Med 2002; 165:1317–1321.

131. Goode ML, Fink JB, Dhand R, Tobin MJ. Improvement in aerosol delivery with helium-oxygen mixtures during mechanical ventilation. Am J Respir Crit Care Med 2001; 163:109–114.

132. Schaeffer EM, Pohlman A, Morgan S, Hall JB. Oxygenation in status asthmaticus improves during ventilation with helium-oxygen. Crit Care Med 1999; 27:2666–2670.

133. Shiue ST, Gluck EH. The use of helium-oxygen mixtures in the support of patients with status asthmaticus and respiratory acidosis. J Asthma 1989; 26:177–180.

134. Rodrigo GJ, Rodrigo C, Pollack CV, Rowe B. Use of helium-oxygen mixtures in the treatment of acute asthma: a systematic review. Chest 2003; 123: 891–896.

135. Ho AM, Lee A, Karmakar MK, Dion PW, Chung DC, Contardi LH. Heliox vs air-oxygen mixtures for the treatment of patients with acute asthma: a systematic overview. Chest 2003; 123:882–890.

136. Jaber S, Fodil R, Carlucci A, Boussarsar M, Pigeot J, Lemaire F, Harf A, Lofaso F, Isabey D, Brochard L. Noninvasive ventilation with helium-oxygen in acute exacerbations of chronic obstructive pulmonary disease. Am J Respir Crit Care Med 2000; 161:1191–1200.

137. Hall JB, Schmidt GA, Wood LDH. Principles of Critical Care. New York: McGraw-Hill Health Professions Division, 1998:xxiv, 1767.

138. Brochard L, Mancebo J, Wysocki M, Lofaso F, Conti G, Rauss A, Simonneau G, Benito S, Gasparetto A, Lemaire F, Isabey A, Harf A. Noninvasive ventilation for acute exacerbations of chronic obstructive pulmonary disease. N Engl J Med 1995; 333:817–822.

139. Liesching T, Kwok H, Hill NS. Acute applications of noninvasive positive pressure ventilation. Chest 2003; 124:699–713.

140. Meyer TJ, Hill NS. Noninvasive positive pressure ventilation to treat respiratory failure. Ann Intern Med 1994; 120:760–770.

141. Meduri GU, Turner RE, Abou-Shala N, Wunderink R, Tolley E. Noninvasive positive pressure ventilation via face mask. First-line intervention in patients with acute hypercapnic and hypoxemic respiratory failure. Chest 1996; 109:179–193.

142. Meduri GU, Abou-Shala N, Fox RC, Jones CB, Leeper KV, Wunderink RG. Noninvasive face mask mechanical ventilation in patients with acute hypercapnic respiratory failure. Chest 1991; 100:445–454.

143. Mountain RD, Sahn SA. Clinical features and outcome in patients with acute asthma presenting with hypercapnia. Am Rev Respir Dis 1988; 138: 535–539.

144. Meduri GU, Cook TR, Turner RE, Cohen M, Leeper KV. Noninvasive positive pressure ventilation in status asthmaticus. Chest 1996; 110:767–774.

145. Soroksky A, Stav D, Shpirer I. A pilot prospective, randomized, placebo-controlled trial of bilevel positive airway pressure in acute asthmatic attack. Chest 2003; 123:1018–1025.

146. Navalesi P, Fanfulla F, Frigerio P, Gregoretti C, Nava S. Physiologic evaluation of noninvasive mechanical ventilation delivered with three types of masks in patients with chronic hypercapnic respiratory failure. Crit Care Med 2000; 28:1785–1790.

147. Antonelli M, Pennisi MA, Pelosi P, Gregoretti C, Squadrone V, Rocco M, Cecchini L, Chiumello D, Severgnini P, Proietti R, Navalesi P, Conti G. Noninvasive positive pressure ventilation using a helmet in patients with acute exacerbation of chronic obstructive pulmonary disease: a feasibility study. Anesthesiology 2004; 100:16–24.

148. Appendini L, Patessio A, Zanaboni S, Carone M, Gukov B, Donner CF, Rossi A. Physiologic effects of positive end-expiratory pressure and mask pressure support during exacerbations of chronic obstructive pulmonary disease. Am J Respir Crit Care Med 1994; 149:1069–1076.

149. Afessa B, Morales I, Cury JD. Clinical course and outcome of patients admitted to an ICU for status asthmaticus. Chest 2001; 120:1616–1621.

150. Gupta D, Keogh B, Chung KF, Ayres JG, Harrison DA, Goldfrad C, Brady Ar, Rowan K. Characteristics and outcome for admissions to adult, general critical care units with acute severe asthma: a secondary analysis of the ICNARC Case Mix Programme Database. Crit Care 2004; 8:R112–R121.

151. Anzueto A, Frutos-Vivar F, Esteban A, Alia I, Brochard L, Stewart T, Benito S, Tobin MJ, Elizalde J, Palizas F, David CM, Pimentel J, Gonzalez M, Soto L,

D'Empaire G, Pelosi P. Incidence, risk factors and outcome of barotrauma in mechanically ventilated patients. Intensive Care Med 2004; 30:612–619.

152. Mansel JK, Stogner SW, Petrini MF, Norman JR. Mechanical ventilation in patients with acute severe asthma. Am J Med 1990; 89:42–48.

153. Manthous CA. Management of severe exacerbations of asthma. Am J Med 1995; 99:298–308.

154. Rouby JJ, Laurent P, Gosnach M, Cambau E, Lamas G, Zouaoui A, Leguillou JL, Bodin L, Khac TD, Marsault C. Risk factors and clinical relevance of nosocomial maxillary sinusitis in the critically ill. Am J Respir Crit Care Med 1994; 150:776–783.

155. Williams TJ, Tuxen DV, Scheinkestel CD, Czarny D, Bowes G. Risk factors for morbidity in mechanically ventilated patients with acute severe asthma. Am Rev Respir Dis 1992; 146:607–615.

156. Rosengarten PL, Tuxen DV, Dziukas L, Scheinkestel C, Merrett K, Bowes G. Circulatory arrest induced by intermittent positive pressure ventilation in a patient with severe asthma. Anaesth Intensive Care 1991; 19:118–121.

157. Kollef MH. Lung hyperinflation caused by inappropriate ventilation resulting in electromechanical dissociation: a case report. Heart Lung 1992; 21: 74–77.

158. Ben-David B, Stonebraker VC, Hershman R, Frost CL, Williams HK. Survival after failed intraoperative resuscitation: a case of "Lazarus syndrome." Anesth Analg 2001; 92:690–692.

159. Lapinsky SE, Leung RS. Auto-PEEP and electromechanical dissociation. N Engl J Med 1996; 335:674.

160. Martens P, Vandekerckhove Y, Mullie A. Restoration of spontaneous circulation after cessation of cardiopulmonary resuscitation. Lancet 1993; 341:841.

161. Peigang Y, Marini JJ. Ventilation of patients with asthma and chronic obstructive pulmonary disease. Curr Opin Crit Care 2002; 8:70–76.

162. Tuxen D, Anderson M, Sheinkestel C. Mechanical ventilation for severe asthma. In: Hall JB, ed. Acute Asthma: Assessment and Management. New York: McGraw-Hill Medical Publishing Division, 2000:209–228.

163. Tuxen DV, Lane S. The effects of ventilatory pattern on hyperinflation, airway pressures, and circulation in mechanical ventilation of patients with severe air-flow obstruction. Am Rev Respir Dis 1987; 136:872–879.

164. Connors AF Jr, McCaffree DR, Gray BA. Effect of inspiratory flow rate on gas exchange during mechanical ventilation. Am Rev Respir Dis 1981; 124:537–543.

165. Leatherman JW, Ravenscraft SA. Low measured auto-positive end-expiratory pressure during mechanical ventilation of patients with severe asthma: hidden auto-positive end-expiratory pressure. Crit Care Med 1996; 24:541–546.

166. Stewart TE, Slutsky AS. Occult, occult auto-PEEP in status asthmaticus. Crit Care Med 1996; 24:379–380.

167. Tuxen DV, Williams TJ, Scheinkestel CD, Czarny D, Bowes G. Use of a measurement of pulmonary hyperinflation to control the level of mechanical ventilation in patients with acute severe asthma. Am Rev Respir Dis 1992; 146:1136–1142.

168. Tuxen DV. Detrimental effects of positive end-expiratory pressure during controlled mechanical ventilation of patients with severe airflow obstruction. Am Rev Respir Dis 1989; 140:5–9.

169. Mathieu M, Tonneau MC, Zarka D, Sartene R. Effect of positive end-expiratory pressure in severe acute asthma. Crit Care Med 1987; 15:1164.

170. Marik PE, Varon J, Fromm R Jr. The management of acute severe asthma. J Emerg Med 2002; 23:257–268.

171. Marinelli WA, Leatherman JW. Sedation, paralysis, and acute myopathy. In: Hall JB, ed. Acute Asthma: Assessment and Management. New York: McGraw-Hill Medical Publishing Division, 2000:229–256.

172. Kress JP, O'Connor MF, Pohlman AS, Olson D, Lavoie A, Toledano A, Hall JB. Sedation of critically ill patients during mechanical ventilation. A comparison of propofol and midazolam. Am J Respir Crit Care Med 1996; 153:1012–1018.

173. Weinbroum AA, Halpern P, Rudick V, Sorkine P, Freedman M, Geller E. Midazolam versus propofol for long-term sedation in the ICU: a randomized prospective comparison. Intensive Care Med 1997; 23:1258–1263.

174. Hall RI, Sandham D, Cardinal P, Tweeddale M, Moher D, Wang, Anis AH. Propofol vs midazolam for ICU sedation: a Canadian multicenter randomized trial. Chest 2001; 119:1151–1159.

175. Hann HC, Hall AP, Raphael JH, Langton JA. An investigation into the effects of midazolam and propofol on human respiratory cilia beat frequency in vitro. Intensive Care Med 1998; 24:791–794.

176. Chamorro C, de Latorre FJ, Montero A, Sanchez-Izquierdo JA, Jareno A, Moreno JA, Gonzalez E, Barrios M, Carpintero JL, Martin-Santos F, Otero B, Ginestal R. Comparative study of propofol versus midazolam in the sedation of critically ill patients: results of a prospective, randomized, multicenter trial. Crit Care Med 1996; 24:932–939.s

177. Magarey JM. Propofol or midazolam—which is best for the sedation of adult ventilated patients in intensive care units? A systematic review. Aust Crit Care 2001; 14:147–154.

178. Schweickert WD, Gehlbach BK, Pohlman AS, Hall JB, Kress JP. Daily interruption of sedative infusions and complications of critical illness in mechanically ventilated patients. Crit Care Med 2004; 32:1272–1276.

179. Kress JP, Pohlman AS, O'Connor MF, Hall JB. Daily interruption of sedative infusions in critically ill patients undergoing mechanical ventilation. N Engl J Med 2000; 342:1471–1477.

180. Hemmingsen C, Nielsen PK, Odorico J. Ketamine in the treatment of bronchospasm during mechanical ventilation. Am J Emerg Med 1994; 12:417–420.

181. Hall JB. Acute Asthma: Assessment and Management. New York: McGraw-Hill Medical Publishing Division, 2000:xvi, 378.

182. Howton JC, Rose J, Duffy S, Zoltanski T, Levitt MA. Randomized, double-blind, placebo-controlled trial of intravenous ketamine in acute asthma. Ann Emerg Med 1996; 27:170–175.

183. Lau TT, Zed PJ. Does ketamine have a role in managing severe exacerbation of asthma in adults? Pharmacotherapy 2001; 21:1100–1106.

184. Weil JV, McCullough RE, Kline JS, Sodal IE. Diminished ventilatory response to hypoxia and hypercapnia after morphine in normal man. N Engl J Med 1975; 292:1103–1106.

185. Leatherman JW, Fluegel WL, David WS, Davies SF, Iber C. Muscle weakness in mechanically ventilated patients with severe asthma. Am J Respir Crit Care Med 1996; 153:1686–1690.

186. Douglass JA, Tuxen DV, Horne M, Scheinkestel CD, Weinmann M, Czarny D, Bowes G. Myopathy in severe asthma. Am Rev Respir Dis 1992; 146:517–519.

187. Griffin D, Fairman N, Coursin D, Rawsthorne L, Grossman JE. Acute myopathy during treatment of status asthmaticus with corticosteroids and steroidal muscle relaxants. Chest 1992; 102:510–514.

188. Behbehani NA, Al-Mane F, D'Yachkova Y, Pare P, FitzGerald JM. Myopathy following mechanical ventilation for acute severe asthma: the role of muscle relaxants and corticosteroids. Chest 1999; 115:1627–1631.

189. Rudis MI, Sikora CA, Angus E, Peterson E, Popovich J, Jr., Hyzy R, Zarowitz BJ. A prospective, randomized, controlled evaluation of peripheral nerve stimulation versus standard clinical dosing of neuromuscular blocking agents in critically ill patients. Crit Care Med 1997; 25:575–583.

190. Laffey JG, Tanaka M, Engelberts D, Luo X, Yuan S, Tanswell AK, Post M, Lindsay T, Kavanagh BP. Therapeutic hypercapnia reduces pulmonary and systemic injury following in vivo lung reperfusion. Am J Respir Crit Care Med 2000; 162:2287–2294.

191. Bigatello LM, Patroniti N, Sangalli F. Permissive hypercapnia. Curr Opin Crit Care 2001; 7:34–40.

192. Walker AM, Oakes GK, Ehrenkranz R, McLaughlin M, Chez RA. Effects of hypercapnia on uterine and umbilical circulations in conscious pregnant sheep. J Appl Physiol 1976; 41:727–733.

193. Hanka R, Lawn L, Mills IH, Prior DC, Tweeddale PM. The effects of maternal hypercapnia on foetal oxygenation and uterine blood flow in the pig. J Physiol 1975; 247:447–460.

194. Rodrigo C, Rodrigo G. Subarachnoid hemorrhage following permissive hypercapnia in a patient with severe acute asthma. Am J Emerg Med 1999; 17:697–699.

195. Dhand R, Tobin MJ. Inhaled bronchodilator therapy in mechanically ventilated patients. Am J Respir Crit Care Med 1997; 156:3–10.

196. Bierman MI, Brown M, Muren O, Keenan RL, Glauser FL. Prolonged isoflurane anesthesia in status asthmaticus. Crit Care Med 1986; 14:832–833.

197. Saulnier FF, Durocher AV, Deturck RA, Lefebvre MC, Wattel FE. Respiratory and hemodynamic effects of halothane in status asthmaticus. Intensive Care Med 1990; 16:104–107.

198. Maltais F, Sovilj M, Goldberg P, Gottfried SB. Respiratory mechanics in status asthmaticus. Effects of inhalational anesthesia. Chest 1994; 106: 1401–1406.

199. Rooke GA, Choi JH, Bishop MJ. The effect of isoflurane, halothane, sevoflurane, and thiopental/nitrous oxide on respiratory system resistance after tracheal intubation. Anesthesiology 1997; 86:1294–1299.

200. Mutlu GM, Factor P, Schwartz DE, Sznajder JI. Severe status asthmaticus: management with permissive hypercapnia and inhalation anesthesia. Crit Care Med 2002; 30:477–480.

201. National Institutes of Health workshop summary. Summary and recommendations of a workshop on the investigative use of fiberoptic bronchoscopy and bronchoalveolar lavage in individuals with asthma. J Allergy Clin Immunol 1985; 76:145–147.

202. Rankin JA, Snyder PE, Schachter EN, Matthay RA. Bronchoalveolar lavage. Its safety in subjects with mild asthma. Chest 1984; 85:723–728.

203. Djukanovic R, Wilson JW, Lai CK, Holgate ST, Howarth PH. The safety aspects of fiberoptic bronchoscopy, bronchoalveolar lavage, and endobronchial biopsy in asthma. Am Rev Respir Dis 1991; 143:772–777.

204. Lang DM, Simon RA, Mathison DA, Timms RM, Stevenson DD. Safety and possible efficacy of fiberoptic bronchoscopy with lavage in the management of refractory asthma with mucous impaction. Ann Allergy 1991; 67:324–330.

205. Millman M, Goodman AH, Goldstein IM, Millman FM, Van Campen SS. Treatment of a patient with chronic bronchial asthma with many bronchoscopies and lavages using acetylcysteine: a case report. J Asthma 1985; 22:13–35.

206. Smith DL, Deshazo RD. Bronchoalveolar lavage in asthma. An update and perspective. Am Rev Respir Dis 1993; 148:523–532.

207. Braman SS, Kaemmerlen JT. Intensive care of status asthmaticus. A 10-year experience. Jama 1990; 264:366–368.

208. Marquette CH, Saulnier F, Leroy O, Wallaert B, Chopin C, Demarcq JM, Durocher A, Tonnel AB. Long-term prognosis of near-fatal asthma. A 6-year follow-up study of 145 asthmatic patients who underwent mechanical ventilation for a near-fatal attack of asthma. Am Rev Respir Dis 1992; 146:76–81.

209. Gehlbach B, Kress JP, Kahn J, DeRuiter C, Pohlman A, Hall J. Correlates of prolonged hospitalization in inner-city ICU patients receiving noninvasive and invasive positive pressure ventilation for status asthmaticus. Chest 2002; 122:1709–1714.

210. Kearney SE, Graham DR, Atherton ST. Acute severe asthma treated by mechanical ventilation: a comparison of the changing characteristics over a 17 yr period. Respir Med 1998; 92:716–721.

Index